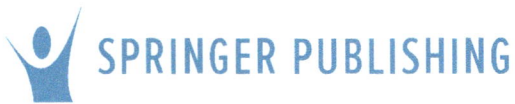 

GET THE MOST FROM YOUR BOOK

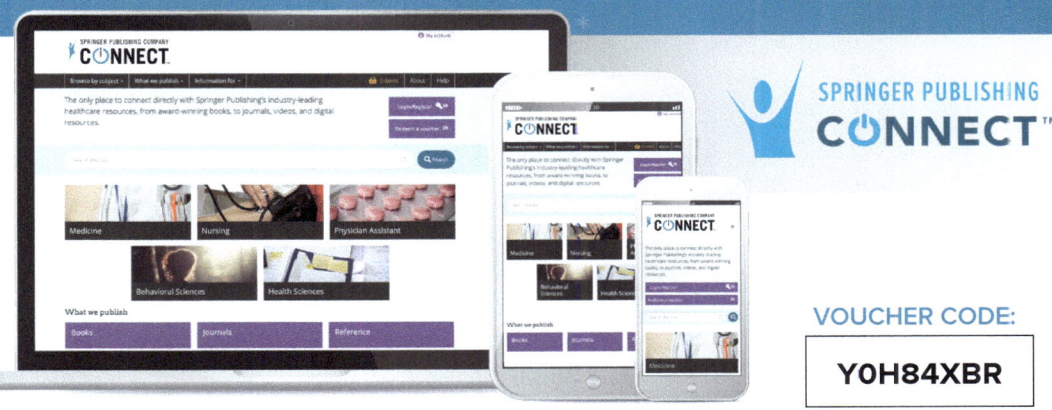

VOUCHER CODE:

Y0H84XBR

Online Access

Your print purchase of *Appraisal, Assessment, and Evaluation for Counselors: A Practical Guide* includes **online access via Springer Publishing Connect**™ to increase accessibility, portability, and searchability.

Insert the code at http://connect.springerpub.com/content/book/978-0-8261-8913-4 or scan the QR code and insert the voucher code today!

Having trouble? Contact our customer service department at *cs@springerpub.com*

Instructor Resource Access for Adopters

Let us do some of the heavy lifting to create an engaging classroom experience with a variety of instructor resources included in most textbooks SUCH AS:

      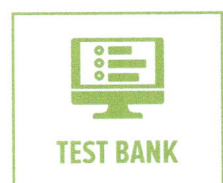

Visit **https://connect.springerpub.com/** and look for the **"Show Supplementary"** button on your **book homepage** to see what is available to instructors! First time using Springer Publishing Connect?
Email **textbook@springerpub.com** to create an account and start unlocking valuable resources.

Appraisal, Assessment, and Evaluation for Counselors

Carman S. Gill, PhD, LCMHC, NCC, ACS, is a professor and the department chair for the Department of Counselor Education at Florida Atlantic University. She obtained her PhD from the University of North Carolina at Greensboro and is licensed to practice in North Carolina. Dr. Gill is the recipient of the 2021 Association for Spiritual, Ethical, and Religious Values in Counseling (ASERVIC) Lifetime Achievement Award. Her research focus includes wellness and women's issues, as well as spirituality and religion in counseling. Carman is a past president of ASERVIC and has served that organization as conference cochair twice, as well as newsletter editor, member of the board of directors, and secretary. Dr. Gill has coauthored multiple peer-reviewed journal articles on wellness and spiritual topics. She has coedited a book on spirituality and religion in counseling, as well as the DSM-5-TR *Learning Companion for Counselors*. She has worked with client populations including individuals who are dually diagnosed, individuals with chronic mental illness, children, and those experiencing acute mental health crises.

Kelly Emelianchik-Key, PhD, LMHC, LMFT, NCC, ACS, is an associate professor of clinical mental health counseling at Florida Atlantic University. She has clinical and research experience with issues of diversity, complex traumas, intimate partner violence, couples' issues, issues of gender and sexuality, eating disorders, nonsuicidal self-injury (NSSI) behaviors, and supervision. She also has multiple book chapters, peer-reviewed journal publications, and a coauthored textbook on NSSI. Some of Dr. Emelianchik-Key's current and former leadership and service roles include serving on multiple journal editorial boards, treasurer for the Association of Counselor Education and Supervision (ACES), and treasurer for the Association of Assessment in Research and Counseling (AARC), as well as Emerging Leaders Cochair for AARC. Dr. Emelianchik-Key has previously won several prestigious national and regional awards, including the Patricia Elmore Award for outstanding article in the journal *Measurement and Evaluation in Counseling and Development*, the Outstanding Teaching and Supervisor Awards from the Southern Association of Counselor Education and Supervision, and the American Counseling Association Best Practices in Research Award.

Ayse Torres, PhD, CRC, LMHC, is an associate professor of clinical rehabilitation counseling at Florida Atlantic University. As a Florida Licensed Mental Health Counselor and a Nationally Certified Rehabilitation Counselor, she has held various leadership roles in public rehabilitation counseling settings. Notably, she has provided services to individuals, and their families, who have been impacted by a wide range of psychiatric, cognitive, and physical disabilities during her 8-year plus tenure at the agencies of Vocational Rehabilitation and Blind Services. Her research is predominantly focused on employment and vocational rehabilitation interventions, specifically tailored for individuals with disabilities. Dr. Torres has successfully secured research funding from prestigious organizations, including the National Institute on Disability, Independent Living, and Rehabilitation Research (NIDILRR); the Patient-Centered Outcomes Research Institute (PCORI); and the Rehabilitation Services Administration (RSA).

Appraisal, Assessment, and Evaluation for Counselors
A Practical Guide

Carman S. Gill, PhD, LCMHC, NCC, ACS
Kelly Emelianchik-Key, PhD, LMHC, LMFT, NCC, ACS
Ayse Torres, PhD, CRC, LMHC

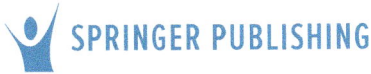

Copyright © 2025 Springer Publishing Company, LLC
All rights reserved.

No part of this publication may be reproduced, stored in a retrieval system, or transmitted in any form or by any means, electronic, mechanical, photocopying, recording, or otherwise, without the prior permission of Springer Publishing Company, LLC, or authorization through payment of the appropriate fees to the Copyright Clearance Center, Inc., 222 Rosewood Drive, Danvers, MA 01923, 978-750-8400, fax 978-646-8600, info@copyright.com or at www.copyright.com.

Springer Publishing Company, LLC
902 Carnegie Center, Princeton, NJ 08540
www.springerpub.com
connect.springerpub.com

Acquisitions Editor: Mindy Okura-Marszycki
Compositor: Amnet
Production Editor: Rachel Haines

ISBN: 978-0-8261-8912-7
e-book ISBN: 978-0-8261-8913-4
DOI: 10.1891/9780826189134

SUPPLEMENTS:

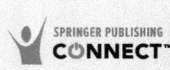 A robust set of instructor resources designed to supplement this text is located at http://connect.springerpub.com/content/book/978-0-8261-8913-4. Qualifying instructors may request access by emailing textbook@springerpub.com.

Instructor Materials:
LMS Common Cartridge–All Instructor Resources: 978-0-8261-5697-6
Instructor Test Bank: 978-0-8261-8914-1
Instructor Chapter PowerPoint Slides: 978-0-8261-8915-8

Student Materials:
Podcasts and Video: See List of Podcasts and Video at the front of this book for details.
Podcast and Video Transcripts: 978-0-8261-8458-0

24 25 26 27 / 5 4 3 2 1

The author and the publisher of this Work have made every effort to use sources believed to be reliable to provide information that is accurate and compatible with the standards generally accepted at the time of publication. Because medical science is continually advancing, our knowledge base continues to expand. Therefore, as new information becomes available, changes in procedures become necessary. We recommend that the reader always consult current research and specific institutional policies before performing any clinical procedure or delivering any medication. The author and publisher shall not be liable for any special, consequential, or exemplary damages resulting, in whole or in part, from the readers' use of, or reliance on, the information contained in this book. The publisher has no responsibility for the persistence or accuracy of URLs for external or third-party internet websites referred to in this publication and does not guarantee that any content on such websites is, or will remain, accurate or appropriate.

2024 CACREP Standards © 2023 Council for Accreditation of Counseling and Related Educational Programs (CACREP). The CACREP Standards reproduced in this textbook represent only selected parts of the 2024 CACREP Standards. Inclusion of the CACREP Standards in this textbook is in no way intended to imply CACREP endorsement or approval of the work. Use of this textbook as a teaching tool does not establish nor connote compliance with CACREP Standards for the purposes of determining CACREP accreditation of any education program.
Council for Accreditation of Counseling and Related Educational Programs. (2023). *2024 CACREP standards*. https://www.cacrep.org/for-programs/2024-cacrep-standards

Library of Congress Cataloging-in-Publication Data
Names: Gill, Carman S., author. | Emelianchik-Key, Kelly, author. | Torres, Ayse, author.
Title: Appraisal, assessment, and evaluation for counselors : a practical guide / Carman S. Gill, Kelly Emelianchik-Key, Ayse Torres.
Description: Princeton, NJ : Springer Publishing Company, LLC, [2025] | Includes bibliographical references and index.
Identifiers: LCCN 2024024474 (print) | LCCN 2024024475 (e-book) | ISBN 9780826189127 (paperback) | ISBN 9780826189134 (e-book)
Subjects: MESH: Symptom Assessment | Mental Disorders–diagnosis | Counseling–methods | Mental Disorders–rehabilitation | Counselors
Classification: LCC RC454 (print) | LCC RC454 (e-book) | NLM WM 141 | DDC 616.89–dc23/eng/20240731
LC record available at https://lccn.loc.gov/2024024474
LC e-book record available at https://lccn.loc.gov/2024024475

Contact sales@springerpub.com to receive discount rates on bulk purchases.

Publisher's Note: **New and used products purchased from third-party sellers are not guaranteed for quality, authenticity, or access to any included digital components.**

Printed in the United States of America by Gasch Printing.

Carman S. Gill
To Rob for your patience, warmth, and love.

Kelly Emelianchik-Key
*To my husband, Jared, and our wonderful children, Owen and Griffin.
Your constant encouragement, love, and patience is never taken for granted.
A special thanks to my coauthors (Carman and Ayse) for being amazing
colleagues to work with and making this process smooth.*

Ayse Torres
*To my dear husband, Juan Manuel, and our beloved son, Leo. For your support,
patience, and love, always. I am grateful for my colleagues and coauthors,
Carman and Kelly, who are a pleasure to work with.*

Contents

Contributors   xi
Preface   xiii
Acknowledgments   xv
List of Podcasts and Video   xvii
Resources   xix

SECTION I. FOUNDATIONS OF TESTING AND ASSESSMENT

1. Introduction to Assessment   3
Carman S. Gill, Kelly Emelianchik-Key, and Ayse Torres
What Is Assessment?   3
Basic Terminology   4
Assessment in Counseling   5
Guidance for Assessment in Counseling   8
Case Studies   14
Discussion Questions   16
Class Activities   16
🎙 Perspective From the Field   17
References   17

2. History and Ethics in Assessment and Appraisal   19
Kelly Emelianchik-Key, Carman S. Gill, and Ayse Torres
Historical Perspectives   19
Assessment Issues   22
Ethics and the Law   24
Legal Issues in Assessment   31
Discussion Questions   36
Class Activities   36
🎙 Perspective From the Field   36
References   37

3. Culture and Diversity Considerations in Testing and Assessment   41
Kelly Emelianchik-Key and Adriana C. Labarta
Multicultural Competence and Cultural Humility in Counseling Assessment   41
Fairness in Testing   43
High-Stakes Testing   49
Counselors as Agents of Change   51
Culturally Responsive Assessment Across Counseling Settings   58

Discussion Questions 60
Class Activities 60
🎙 Perspective From the Field 61
References 61

SECTION II. MEANINGFUL METHODS FOR COLLECTING AND APPLYING ASSESSMENT DATA

4. Methods of Assessment 69
Kelly Emelianchik-Key, Ayse Torres, and Clara Bossie
Direct and Indirect Assessment Techniques 69
Initial Interviews in Counseling 74
Guidelines for Interviews: Applying the Initial Intake Assessment 77
Other Methods of Assessment 83
Assessment Formats 86
Discussion Questions 93
Class Activities 93
References 94

5. Assessment and Diagnosis in Counseling 97
Clara Bossie and Carman S. Gill
History of Diagnosis and the Counseling Field 97
Diagnostic Assessments in Counseling: A Multifaceted Lens 101
Conducting a Diagnostic Assessment 103
Incorporating Diversity, Equity, and Inclusion Into Diagnostic Practices 112
Individualizing Care and Understanding Varying Abilities 114
Endorsing a Diagnosis 116
Discussion Questions 117
Class Activities 117
References 118

6. Test Selection, Scoring, and Statistics 123
Haley R. Ault and Kelly Emelianchik-Key
Selecting the Appropriate Tests 123
Test Administration 127
Scoring Assessments 128
Understanding Raw Scores 131
Measuring Relationships 140
Discussion Questions 146
Class Activities 146
References 147

7. Reliability, Validity, and Test Worthiness 149
Kelly Emelianchik-Key, Ayse Torres, Haley R. Ault, and Carman S. Gill
Introduction 149
Reliability 150
Estimating Reliability 154
Validity 159
Developing Quality Assessments 165

Discussion Questions   168
Class Activities   168
🎙 Perspective From the Field   169
References   169

SECTION III. ASSESSMENT TYPES

8. Assessment of Intelligence, Aptitude, Ability, and Achievement   173
Nadiya Boyce-Rosen, Ayse Torres, and Carman S. Gill
Introduction   173
Assessing Ability, Aptitude, and Intelligence   173
Common Intelligence Measures   180
Achievement, Readiness, and Aptitude Assessments in Educational Settings   183
Discussion Questions   191
Class Activities   191
🎙 Perspective From the Field   192
References   192

9. Career and Occupational Assessments and Interest Inventories   195
Ayse Torres
Career Assessments   195
Career Assessments in Online Platforms   197
Cultural Considerations in Career Assessments   198
Vocational Interest   199
Widely Used Career Assessment Tools   200
Career Assessment for Youth With Disabilities Transitioning
    From School to Adulthood   208
Career Assessment for Veterans   209
Discussion Questions   212
Class Activities   212
🎙 Perspective From the Field   213
References   213

10. Clinical Assessments and Personality Testing   217
Rebecca Nelson and Kelly Emelianchik-Key
Clinical Assessments in Counseling   217
Other Types of Clinical Assessments   228
Discussion Questions   239
Class Activities   240
🎙 Perspective From the Field   240
References   241

SECTION IV. APPLYING AND INTEGRATING ASSESSMENTS IN VARIOUS SETTINGS

11. Trauma, Harm, and Substance Abuse Assessments   247
Carman S. Gill, Ayse Torres, and Kelly Emelianchik-Key
Introduction   247

Understanding and Assessing Trauma   248
Understanding and Assessing Harm   253
Reporting Abuse and Neglect   265
Understanding and Assessing Substance Use Disorders   267
Discussion Questions   271
Class Activities   271
🎤 Perspective From the Field   272
References   272

12. The Assessment Process in Counseling   277
Ayse Torres, Carman S. Gill, and Kelly Emelianchik-Key
Intentionality in Assessment   277
An Integrated Approach to Communication   278
Integrative Case Conceptualization   283
International Classification of Functioning, Disability, and Health   288
Discussion Questions   292
Class Activities   292
🎤 Perspective From the Field   293
References   294

13. Looking Ahead: Future Direction of Assessment and Testing in Counseling   297
Clara Bossie and Carman S. Gill
From Paper Trails to Digital Footprints   298
Technological Advancements in Counseling Assessments   298
Ethics and Privacy in a Digital Age   301
Collaborative and Client-Centered Approaches   303
Evidence-Based Practices and Research   304
Counselor Education in the Era of Evolving Assessments   305
Embracing the Future of Counseling Assessments   306
Discussion Questions   308
Class Activities   308
🎤 Perspective From the Field   309
References   310

14. Resources for Assessment in Counseling   311
Carman S. Gill, Kelly Emelianchik-Key, and Ayse Torres
Diagnostic Interview   311
Case Conceptualization: Meghan   311
Percentile Conversions With Z-Scores   318
Class Activities   319
Additional Resources   320

Index   321

Contributors

Haley R. Ault, PhD, NCC Assistant Professor, Department of Leadership, Policy, and Lifelong Learning, University of South Florida, Tampa, Florida

Clara Bossie, MS, LMFT-QS Clinical Director, Wisely Wellness LLC, Boca Raton, Florida

Nadiya Boyce-Rosen Doctoral Student, Department of Counselor Education, Florida Atlantic University, Boca Raton, Florida

Adriana C. Labarta, PhD, LMHC, NCC, ACS Assistant Professor, Department of Counselor Education, Florida Atlantic University, Boca Raton, Florida

Rebecca Nelson, MA, LMHC Doctoral Student in Counseling, College of Education, Florida Atlantic University, Boca Raton, Florida

Preface

The purpose of this book is to provide a current and practical resource for counselors who are learning to integrate assessment effectively in the therapeutic process. Conducting an ethical, thorough, and accurate assessment of the client and the client system is critical in counseling. Evidence-based approaches and transparent diagnostic procedures are essential to inform counseling practice. Incorporating assessment into the therapeutic process allows counselors to gain valuable information about their clients' needs, strengths, risk and protective factors, and goals. The cultural backgrounds of our clients play a pivotal role in the assessment process and can guide the development of tailored treatment plans and interventions that address each client's unique needs. The precise and skillful integration of assessment allows counselors to monitor progress and evaluate the effectiveness of interventions over time, ensuring that clients receive the best possible care. Understanding and infusing assessment and testing skills into counseling is unlikely to occur without concrete instruction and resources. We address this need while infusing the 2024 Council for Accreditation of Counseling and Related Educational Programs (CACREP) standards. This book attempts to cover the necessary information in 14 distinct chapters, grouped into four sections, reflecting the major themes of the work:

- Section I: Foundations of Testing and Assessment
- Section II: Meaningful Methods for Collecting and Applying Assessment Data
- Section III: Assessment Types
- Section IV: Applying and Integrating Assessments in Various Settings

Within the four sections of this book, we cover the history and nature of assessment and testing as it pertains to the field of counseling and the legal and ethical implications surrounding the administration and interpretation of assessment in counseling. Cultural implications for selecting, administering, and interpreting assessment instruments and integration into diagnosis and treatment planning in counseling are discussed. Statistical concepts related to assessments in counseling, such as norm-referenced and criterion-referenced assessment, measures of central tendency, distributions, reliability, and validity related to assessment instruments, are also included. We cover the "how tos" of mental status examination, interviewing clients, risk and harm assessment, personality and psychologic assessment, career assessment, and substance abuse and addiction assessment. Understanding assessment as a process is addressed, as are future directions and technology, as well as achievement, aptitude, intelligence, and ability assessments.

At the beginning of the book, the authors present case scenarios that we will follow throughout the textbook and integrate into various chapters, providing clear examples of the content described in that chapter. These "Checking In" examples will benefit the reader by connecting content to real-life scenarios. Key terms are italicized in each chapter for easy access to definitions, and at the end of each chapter, the authors include Discussion

Questions and Class Activities to reinforce the material and extend the learning process. For chapters that include assessment information or information related to a specific specialty area, we included coauthors who are experts in that material and bring hands-on knowledge from the counseling field. Ten of the chapters have accompanying Perspective From the Field podcasts, which provide views from real-world professionals and further explore the topics discussed in the chapters. Additional resources, including an example diagnostic interview video and a sample case conceptualization, are provided in Chapter 14.

Throughout this text, the authors attempt to provide a practical resource for current and future counselors. As our world becomes more complicated, so do the needs of our clients. To fully address these needs, counselors must understand them. Appropriate, ethical, and accurate assessment of the client, client culture, and system is the first step and an ongoing part of case conceptualization, diagnosis, and ethical, appropriate, and effective treatment. Current and future counselors face an ever-changing world, which brings more complexity to practice and opportunities for new and innovative methods of approaching assessment and the counseling process. We are continually impressed by our students and future counselors who will undoubtedly improve the well-being of their clients, the client's systems, and the larger community. This work is dedicated to those students who are the future of our counseling profession. We sincerely hope that this book helps you on your journey.

Carman S. Gill
Kelly Emelianchik-Key
Ayse Torres

Acknowledgments

We wish to acknowledge all of our wonderful coauthors for working with us to make this book possible. Your knowledge, expertise, and assistance with ancillary materials are appreciated. In addition, thank you to Florida Atlantic University doctoral students Lauren Steele, Bridget Urso, and Rotem Moshe, who also assisted with videos, podcasts, and ancillary materials. We wish to thank Dr. Matthew D'Urso for his selfless assistance and Aldo Gonzalez for his technological genius. We appreciate Kirsten Elmer, Associate Content Strategist at Springer Publishing Company, for her responsiveness to all our questions and guidance through the writing and production process.

List of Podcasts and Video

Organized by chapter, podcasts are available to support readers, provide perspectives from real-world professionals, and further explore the topics discussed in the chapters. A video demonstrating a diagnostic interview is also provided with the final chapter.

Access podcasts/video via the QR code or http://connect.springerpub.com/content/book/978-0-8261-8913-4/chapter/ch00.

Chapter 1. Introduction to Assessment
Paul Peluso

Chapter 2. History and Ethics in Assessment and Appraisal
Stephanie F. Dailey

Chapter 3. Culture and Diversity Considerations in Testing and Assessment
Eleanor Su-Keene

Chapter 7. Reliability, Validity, and Test Worthiness
Tiffany Vastardis

Chapter 8. Assessment of Intelligence, Aptitude, Ability, and Achievement
Sandra Logan-McKibben

Chapter 9. Career and Occupational Assessments and Interest Inventories
Brian M. Montalvo

Chapter 10. Clinical Assessments and Personality Testing
Ali Cunningham Abbott

Chapter 11. Trauma, Harm, and Substance Abuse Assessments
Casey A. Barrio Minton

Chapter 12. The Assessment Process in Counseling
Jon Sperry

Chapter 13. Looking Ahead: Future Direction of Assessment and Testing in Counseling
Clara Bossie and Aldo Gonzalez

Chapter 14. Resources for Assessment in Counseling
Video: Diagnostic interview demonstrated by Matthew D'Urso and Lauren Steele

Resources

STUDENT RESOURCES

- **Podcasts** with content experts providing real-life perspectives are included with many chapters, plus a **video** demonstrating a diagnostic interview is included in Chapter 14. Transcripts are available for each podcast and the video.

INSTRUCTOR RESOURCES

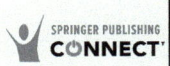 A robust set of instructor resources designed to supplement this text is located at http://connect.springerpub.com/content/book/978-0-8261-8913-4. Qualifying instructors may request access by emailing textbook@springerpub.com.

- **LMS Common Cartridge** with all instructor resources
- **Instructor Test Bank** with over 160 multiple-choice and true/false questions with answer rationales
- **Instructor Chapter PowerPoint Slides** summarizing chapter content

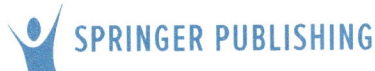

Visit https://connect.springerpub.com and look for the "**Show Supplementary**" button on the **book homepage**.

Foundations of Testing and Assessment

Introduction to Assessment

CARMAN S. GILL, KELLY EMELIANCHIK-KEY, AND AYSE TORRES

I remember when I started working as a counselor at the local mental health center. My supervisor instructed me to meet with a client and complete a biopsychosocial. Asked her what that meant, and she handed me a pen and a stack of papers with questions on them. So, I sat down with a very anxious client and asked a bunch of questions that didn't mean anything to either of us. The client didn't come back.

WHAT IS ASSESSMENT?

Sounds like a simple question that should have a simple answer, right? Wrong. Assessment may appear challenging and complex, but it doesn't have to be. In this chapter, we discuss what assessment is and isn't, we present some history, and we define types of assessments. More importantly, however, the reader will walk away with the ways in which a counselor will find assessment helpful.

Plainly speaking, *assessment* includes *appraising, evaluating,* or *gauging* information gathered to make a decision or determination about something or someone. Assessment is the overarching term that encompasses appraisal and evaluation. The *Standards for Educational and Psychological Testing* (American Educational Research Association [AERA] et al., 2014) defines assessment as the techniques used to gather data from various sources in order to make an interpretation or decision about something. AERA also defines standards for best practice when developing assessments. An additional definition of assessment, which is very similar, comes from the Council for Accreditation of Counseling and Related Educational Programs (CACREP; 2023b). They note that assessment is "the systematic gathering of information for decision making about individuals, groups, programs, or processes" (CACREP, 2023b, para 36). CACREP is the primary accrediting body for counselors recognized by the Council for Higher Education and Accreditation. We will learn more about the standards CACREP sets for counselors in training to learn about the assessment and appraisal process throughout this text. Assessment is defined using Gill and Freund's definition, "the act of determining the amount of value or importance an individual assigns to a construct," such as depression or anxiety (2018, p. 42).

In the counseling field, we measure a variety of constructs, including personality factors, career interests, and ability. Some of these constructs are easy to measure, whereas others remain challenging. For example, when we go to the doctor, they may take our blood pressure to assess how well our heart pumps blood. High blood pressure can also indicate more stress that is placed on the heart. This is a concrete number that is provided to us, and we know if our blood pressure is good or bad based on the medical profession's standard of 120/80 as an acceptable blood pressure. As counselors, when a client comes in expressing stress or conveying an emotion, like happiness or anger, how can we accurately measure this on a scale? There is no way to tell what the peak of happy, angry, or stressed is for an individual, and there is no standard number to guide us. As counselors, we rely on formal assessment tools, as well as other ways to assess, such as client self-report and informal observations that we make to fully understand and assess the extent of the situation. These factors will assist a counselor in making an inference about the client and noting the pervasiveness of a situation or problem.

BASIC TERMINOLOGY

The counseling field uses the terms *appraisal* and *assessment* synonymously. In this text, we will do the same. But keep in mind that not all fields use these terms interchangeably. We will use the terms interchangeably because they both use informal and formal techniques to gather information and decide about a construct that one is trying to measure. *Formal* or *standardized* techniques usually involve psychometrically sound assessments that are standardized and provide numerical results that counselors can compare to a norm group (Leppma & Jones, 2013). Examples include inventories, checklists, and standardized tests. *Informal* or *nonstandarized* techniques are more qualitative in nature and provide more subjective information regarding the client. These include open-ended questions, sentence completion, and even drawings. *Psychometrics* refers to the theory behind or the process of mental measurement or testing. *Psychometric properties* refer to the statistical outcomes related to operationalizing a specific construct, such as depression, using a standardized measure (Heppner et al., 2015).

A *measure* is the quantity or amount of a construct being measured. This is similar to *sampling*, which is also an example of something being measured. Many people who use assessments interchange the terms *tests*, *instrument*, and *inventory*. You are probably asking yourself, are those concepts not all the same? At the end of the day, yes, they are all tools intended to provide measurement, but they are distinctly different. A *test* will usually provide some measurement intended to evaluate and provide a number or score attached to a meaning. *Instruments* are forms of tests, such as inventories, checklists, or rating scales. As you read this textbook and start to become familiar with appraisal and assessment, you will find that many terms are similar and can sometimes be confusing to differentiate. We invite you to explore the profession's amazing resources in the area of assessment and research.

Qualitative and Quantitative Assessments

Assessments generally fall into three categorical types: qualitative, quantitative, and a combination of both. Qualitative assessments are those which measure a construct or idea using nonnumerical forms, generally focusing conversations and open-ended interactions. Some examples include genograms, ecomaps, sentence stems, open-ended questions, and lifemaps (Gill & Freund, 2018). This form of assessment can provide a holistic perspective and yield rich data regarding the client's belief systems, as well as the construct of interest. However, these are informal, often more subjective in nature, and do not provide information that is usable for general comparisons. Quantitative assessment measures differ in that they are formal, numerically focused instruments, often criterion based, and they may provide population norms, as well as reliability and validity statistics. Some examples include the Beck Depression Inventory (Beck et al., 1996), the Five Factor Wellness Evaluation of Lifestyle (Myers et al., 2004), and the Columbia-Suicide Severity Rating Scale (C-SSRS; Posner et al., 2011). With quantitative assessment comes the opportunity for comparison and for progress monitoring; however, these assessments do not provide the contextual information gathered through qualitative measures.

Norm, Criterion, and Self-Referenced Tests

Norm-referenced tests (NRT) are quantitative assessments that allow for comparison of client scores to scores of those in a "norm" group. Norm groups are established by administering these tests to a large, "typical" population to achieve a standardized sample for comparison purposes. Examples include the Graduate Record Examination (GRE; Educational Testing Service, 2016), achievement tests, and intelligence tests, such as the Wechsler Intelligence Scale for Children (WISC-V; Wechsler & Kodama, 1949). The introduction of a norm group as a standard has disadvantages, as norm groups do not always represent the person or population taking the test. Chapter 6 of this text provides a more in-depth discussion of this and other limitations, as well as an explanation of norm-referenced assessments, types of norm groups, and methods by which norm groups are typically established. *Criterion-referenced assessments* are those that are used to compare the test taker's scores to a predetermined criterion, such as a cutoff score or a body of knowledge standard, rather than a norm group. Examples of criterion-referenced assessments include any tests or quizzes that you may take as part of this class. Teachers frequently use criterion-referenced tests to determine if students have learned the course subject matter (Balkin & Juhnke, 2018). Finally, *self-referenced assessments* are used to compare results to the individual's previous performance. Counselors may use this approach as part of their assessment of the client's progress and routine outcome monitoring. As with norm-referenced tests, Chapter 6 explores criterion-referenced and self-referenced assessments in more detail.

ASSESSMENT IN COUNSELING

Do I Need to Know About Assessment as a Counselor?

The answer is simple. Yes! Counselors definitely need to know about and understand assessment. Assessments will occur from the first day you enter your counseling program. This ongoing, fluid process of giving and receiving data occurs for both the client and the counselor to varying degrees and is a fundamental part of the counseling relationship (Leppma & Jones, 2013). Further, Balkin and Juhnke argue that assessment is an unavoidable part of all human relationships (2018). Throughout this course, you may find yourself informally assessing your peers and your professors and likely taking a few formal assessments where you will explore yourself and your ideologies to get you to start thinking about why you do what you do and how it can affect your ability to be a counselor. All of this is perfectly normal and acceptable.

Assessment is one of the most vital components of successful counseling, as determining the most effective treatment is often based on choosing an appropriate measure and gathering accurate data. Effective assessment has a synergetic effect with the therapeutic alliance, as trust building is often a side effect of appropriate assessment. Bordin's model of working alliance includes bonds, goals, and tasks (1979). As trust building improves relationship bonds, the use of assessment with a strong client-centered focus can contribute to goal setting that is appropriate, is mutually agreed upon, and provides guidance for engaging in the tasks of therapy. Ongoing assessment to elicit client feedback and monitor progress works toward maintaining the tasks necessary for improving holistic wellness. As an additional benefit, assessment raises self-awareness, in some cases operating as an intervention as well. Assessment and appraisal have many functions in the counseling world, but generally speaking there are four primary purposes of assessment: (a) assessing or screening for client problems, (b) conceptualizing client cases and diagnosing, (c) treatment planning and goal setting, and (d) gauging client progress during the course of therapy.

Assess and Screen

Assessment helps counselors gather information and make decisions about treatment for clients. We start assessing clients from the moment they call to make an appointment. Interactions via phone or email form initial impressions and the information gathered is used to triage immediate and ongoing client needs. Clients may determine their personal level of commitment to the initial appointment or even long-term engagement through their own initial assessment of the interactions. While these initial assessments are often informal and based on what clients share or how they present to therapy, we use these appraisals to determine holistic client needs. Counselors must understand the problems and issues that the clients present from a holistic perspective; otherwise, we might provide treatments that are not the most effective, ultimately reducing treatment outcomes. Obtaining a complete measurement of a client's functioning and problem often requires information from multiple sources (e.g., self-reports, parent or partner reports), along with objective markers of the problem or functioning if they are available (Lambert et al., 2001). Clinicians typically utilize screenings early on in treatment because they can often save time and money by narrowing down the problem and determining further diagnostic assessment needs. Biopsychosocial assessments are typically used early on in therapy to measure biological, psychologic, and social factors that may contribute to the presenting problem. These assessments may uncover information a client might not have enough insight about to realize it impacts them as a cause of concern, adding to the problem. Biopsychosocial assessments often contain various ways to screen quickly but often leave the door open for follow-up questions that might be more open-ended when someone affirmatively answers some of the screening questions.

Conceptualize and Diagnose

A thorough assessment and screening process is necessary for counselors to conceptualize and diagnose clients (if warranted). Case conceptualization is the process of mapping and organizing client information to understand the client's problem and maladaptive patterns, informing and guiding treatment, and preparing for potential client obstacles (Gill et al., 2024). Case conceptualization is defined as "a method and clinical strategy for obtaining and organizing information about a client, understanding and explaining the client's situation and maladaptive patterns, guiding and focusing treatment, anticipating challenges and roadblocks, and preparing for successful termination" (Sperry & Sperry, 2020, p. 4). According to Sperry and Sperry (2020), case conceptualization is the heart of an evidence-based counseling process. Their definition notes that the initial step is "obtaining and organizing information about the client" (Sperry & Sperry, 2020, p. 4). Assessment is a crucial step in accurate conceptualization, as omissions or mistakes with this first step can derail the process, leading to poor treatment outcomes. Often conceptualization of the client's problem stems from our auditory understanding of the problem as reported by the client, along with our formal assessments and informal assessments, which help us to better understand the client and conceptualize the problems. Employing the most appropriate and effective measures is critical as these conceptualizations also assist in formulating an accurate diagnosis for the client.

Diagnosis refers to the process of classifying symptoms based on the counselor's conceptualization of data gathered through assessment. For mental health treatment, this formulation is typically compared to the *Diagnostic and Statistical Manual of Mental Disorders* (*DSM*). However, this system of diagnosis is sometimes contentious in the counseling field. Some counselors posit that clients are easily overdiagnosed and that a diagnosis can cause unnecessary stigma. Advocacy groups have identified specific diagnoses as problematic, such as Gender Dysphoria, which could lead to pathologizing the transgender process. While this may be true in some cases, if a diagnosis is warranted, the pros and cons should be discussed with the client, and insurance considerations need to be considered before any diagnosis is provided to the client. Accurate and ethical diagnosis will also help guide treatment for the client and allow us to use evidence-based practices that are most beneficial to produce change in the client. Whereas diagnosing certain mental illnesses, such as a traumatic brain injury, is a simple process when there is a clear physical cause that is identified through physical tests, others, such as personality disorders, require extensive assessment processes that can come from various sources and are at least partially subjective. As counselors, we must use all of the information available via formal assessments, observations, self-report, or *collateral information* (information obtained with consent through family members, physicians, or other outside sources). The more appropriate data that are collected, the greater the ability to conceptualize the client and provide a well-informed diagnosis when necessary.

Treatment Plan and Goal Set

Based on our ability to conduct case conceptualization and diagnosis, counselors create treatment plans and set goals that are unique to the client, inclusive of evidence-based practices. Effective treatment plans synthesize all factors considered during the case conceptualization process, including risk and protective factors, to achieve the desired outcomes and goals. Treatment planning also involves relying on a theoretical approach and framework as a guide. Counselors draw from the recent literature base to inform treatment plans. Treatment plans guide the therapist and client, reduce unintentional harm to clients, and provide effective billing for services. Treatment plans are referred to throughout therapy and provide clients with objectives, interventions, and a plan to monitor treatment progress. Goal setting allows for clear and well-defined direction in a treatment plan that maps the steps taken to achieve the specific goals. Counselors should set measurable goals that are cocreated with the clients. Assessment informs appropriate treatment planning and goal setting, providing the basis for routine outcome monitoring throughout the process.

Evaluation of Progress

Counselors measure treatment progress throughout the course of treatment, but formal assessments are often completed to monitor this progress. Monitoring client progress ensures that appropriate treatment interventions are used and that these interventions are helpful and not harmful. Evaluation also alerts the counselor if the client's symptoms increase due to other factors that take place outside of therapy. Routine progress monitoring assessment tools (ROMs) are becoming increasingly popular in therapy and are very effective for counselors. Medical insurance companies may require a form of progress monitoring to ensure that resources are not being wasted and the clients are improving. School administrators want to see that students are progressing and there is accountability and effectiveness with resources purchased to aid learning outcomes.

GUIDANCE FOR ASSESSMENT IN COUNSELING

As previously noted, assessment is an integral part of the counseling process. Ineffective or unethical assessment procedures can result in poor therapeutic outcomes and even be dangerous for the client. In recognition of the clear need for guidance, CACREP addresses assessment and evaluation as part of their standards. Established in 1981, CACREP's mission is to ensure quality in counselor training programs and promote counseling's professional identity (CACREP, 2023a). CACREP and other accrediting bodies use current knowledge from experts in the field to provide guidance to educational programs (i.e., colleges and universities) for the purpose of consistent, quality training. Students, graduates, and employers of these programs can expect certain outcomes as a result. CACREP's 2024 standards include the traditional six sections we expect; however, with new standards, assessment and evaluation procedures required of counseling programs move forward from the fourth section to the second section. This intentional placement seemingly gives nod to the importance CACREP places on initial and ongoing assessment, as well as quality monitoring and improvement. The Foundational Counseling Curriculum section, now moved to the third section, once again includes eight core areas, with Assessment and Diagnostic Processes remaining seventh. These 17 Assessment and Diagnostic Processes standards provide the foundation for this course and this textbook. Table 1.1 provides information as to which chapter covers each standard, along with the page numbers for easy access.

As you can see, CACREP's standards for assessment and diagnosis are infused throughout this text. However, CACREP is not the only form of guidance counselors have for these concepts. As mentioned earlier, the *Standards for Educational and Psychological Testing* are a collaborative product of AERA, the American Psychological Association (APA), and the National Council on Measurement in Education (NCME) since 1966 and considered the gold standard in testing guidance in the United States and other countries. The most recent edition was published in 2014 and includes a renewed focus on fairness and accessibility in testing by creating a new chapter and infusing appropriate language throughout. The authors acknowledged the ever-developing role of technology in testing and infused technology in testing throughout this edition. Additional structural changes included the reorganization of the *Workplace Testing and Credentialing* chapter to clarify when specific standards are related to employment and/or credentialing. This document includes 13 chapters, divided into three sections, that thoroughly cover the foundations of assessment, basic operations, and testing applications. This seventh revision of the *Standards for Educational and Psychological Testing* (AERA et al., 2014) is available in its entirety online.

The Association for Assessment and Research in Counseling (AARC) is a division of the American Counseling Association (ACA) and is specifically for counselors. They articulate their mission to advance "the counseling profession by promoting best practices in assessment, research, and evaluation in counseling" (AARC, n.d., para. 1). This organization is dedicated to the following six fundamental principles: promoting professional development in assessment, research, and evaluation; promoting appropriate use of counseling assessment, research, and evaluation; developing and distributing knowledge related to assessment, research, and

TABLE 1.1 OVERVIEW OF CHAPTER CONTENT AND CACREP STANDARDS

Section	Chapter	Chapter Name and CACREP 2024 Standards*	Page Number
Section I: Foundations of Testing and Assessment	Chapter 1	*Introduction to Assessment*	
	Chapter 2	*History and Ethics in Assessment and Appraisal*	
		3.G.1. historical perspectives concerning the nature and meaning of assessment and testing in counseling	
		3.G.6. ethical and legal considerations for selecting, administering, and interpreting assessments	
	Chapter 3	*Culture and Diversity Considerations in Testing and Assessment*	
		3.G.5. culturally sustaining and developmental considerations for selecting, administering, and interpreting assessments, including individual accommodations and environmental modifications	
Section II: Meaningful Methods for Collecting and Applying Assessment Data	Chapter 4	*Methods of Assessment*	
		3.G.9. use of environmental assessments and systematic behavioral observations	
		3.G.16. procedures to identify client characteristics, protective factors, risk factors, and warning signs of mental health and behavioral disorders	
		Clinical Mental Health Counseling	
		5.C.4. intake interview, mental status evaluation, biopsychosocial history, mental health history, and psychological assessment for treatment planning and caseload management	
		Clinical Rehabilitation Counseling	
		5.D.9. intake interview, mental status evaluation, biopsychosocial history, mental health history, and psychological assessment for treatment planning and caseload management for people with disabilities	
	Chapter 5	*Assessment and Diagnosis in Counseling*	
		3.G.7. use of culturally sustaining and developmentally appropriate assessments for diagnostic and intervention planning purposes	
		3.G.11. diagnostic processes, including differential diagnosis and the use of current diagnostic classification systems	
	Chapter 6	*Test Selection, Scoring, and Statistics*	
		3.G.2. basic concepts of standardized and non-standardized testing, norm-referenced and criterion-referenced assessments, and group and individual assessments	
		3.G.3. statistical concepts, including scales of measurement, measures of central tendency, indices of variability, shapes and types of distributions, and correlations	
	Chapter 7	*Reliability, Validity, and Test Worthiness*	
		3.G.4. reliability and validity in the use of assessments	

(continued)

TABLE 1.1 **OVERVIEW OF CHAPTER CONTENT AND CACREP STANDARDS** (*continued*)

Section	Chapter	Chapter Name and CACREP 2024 Standards*	Page Number
Section III: Assessment Types	Chapter 8	*Assessment of Intelligence, Aptitude, Ability, and Achievement* 3.G.8. use of assessments in academic/educational, career, personal, and social development	
	Chapter 9	*Career and Occupational Assessments and Interest Inventories* 3.G.8. use of assessments in academic/educational, career, personal, and social development Rehabilitation Counseling 5.G.8. career- and work-related assessments, including job analysis, worksite modification, transferable skills analysis, job readiness, and work hardening 5.G.9. evaluation and application of assistive technology with an emphasis on individualized assessment and planning	
	Chapter 10	*Clinical Assessments and Personality Testing* 3.G.10. use of structured interviewing, symptom checklists, and personality and psychological testing	
Section IV: Applying and Integrating Assessments in Various Settings	Chapter 11	*Trauma, Harm, and Substance Abuse Assessments* 3.G.12. procedures to identify substance use, addictions, and co-occurring conditions 3.G.13. procedures for assessing and responding to risk of aggression or danger to others, self-inflicted harm, and suicide 3.G.14. procedures for assessing clients' experience of trauma 3.G.15. procedures for identifying and reporting signs of abuse and neglect Addiction Counseling 5.A.3. assessment for symptoms of psychoactive substance toxicity, intoxication, and withdrawal 5.A.6. evaluating and identifying individualized strategies and treatment modalities relative to substance use disorder severity, stages of change, or recovery	
	Chapter 12	*The Assessment Process in Counseling* 3.G.17. procedures for using assessment results for referral and consultation	
	Chapter 13	*Looking Ahead: Future Direction of Assessment and Testing in Counseling* 3.E.5. application of technology related to counseling	

*CACREP 2024 Section 3 and Section 5 standards.
CACREP, Council for Accreditation of Counseling and Related Educational Programs.
Source: Standards from Council for Accreditation of Counseling and Related Educational Programs. (2023). *2024 CACREP standards.* https://www.cacrep.org/for-programs/2024-cacrep-standards

evaluation; advocacy for optimal wellness through assessment, research, and evaluation; political support for legislation to ethically advance assessment, research, and evaluation; and collaboration and enhanced communication with other counseling organizations that examine concerns related to assessment, research, and evaluation (AARC, n.d.). AARC published the Responsibilities of Users of Standardized Tests, or the "RUST" statement, to "promote the accurate, fair, and responsible use of standardized tests by the counseling and education communities" (Lenz et al., 2022, p. 227). Now in its fourth edition (RUST-4E), it offers a values-based approach to conducting responsible standardized testing, including qualification and knowledge of users, test selection and administration, scoring tests, and interpreting the results (Lenz et al., 2022). We provide a thorough discussion of this key document in Chapter 2, and it is available on AARC's website. AARC's leadership team, including counselors and counselor educators, offers additional free resources on their website including Sponsored Assessment Standards and Statements. Counselors are encouraged to follow AARC's Scientist Practitioner Model, which is available on their website and described in Chapter 2 of this book as it relates to the ethical practice of ongoing outcomes assessment. Additionally, AARC developed "Standards for Multicultural Assessment" in 2003, which has been revised with its most recent fourth edition in 2013. These standards address the impact of cultural diversity in the assessment process for counseling professionals and counselor educators. The most recent edition focuses on the role of social advocacy in assessment. These standards focus on the critical awareness that is needed to support culturally responsive assessment selection, administration, and interpretation. This is particularly significant as assessments can be used for a variety of reasons, which include "community empowerment, advocacy, collaboration, to change systems, and inform public opinion and policy" (Foster, 2017, p. 250). This information is covered in depth in Chapter 3.

Other key counseling organizations that provide guidance for assessment and evaluation in counseling include the ACA and the National Board for Certified Counselors (NBCC), both of which provide ethical guidance through the ACA (2014) and NBCC (2023) codes of ethics. The ACA is the world's largest association for counselors and has provided ethical guidance and codes for counselors since 1961. Section E of ACA's current ethical codes is dedicated to evaluation, assessment, and intervention, and includes 29 codes grouped into 13 subsections. This portion of the ACA Code of Ethics begins with guidance to counselors which specifically notes that appropriate assessment is one part of the process and that the goal of this process is to increase holistic wellness for clients and client groups (ACA, 2014). Additional codes, related to assessment and evaluation are infused through the document. Some examples are Section C.2.d, which addresses progress monitoring; codes in Section F.6. related to evaluation and remediation in counseling supervision; and Section G, which is dedicated to research and evaluation in counseling. The NBCC is the largest national credentialing body for counselors and provides a code of ethics for what they consider "minimal" ethical standards for counselors they certify (NBCC, 2023). NBCC's Code of Ethics devotes a section to Testing, Appraisal, and Research, and has 10 distinct standards specifically devoted to assessment procedures in counseling (NBCC, 2023). Additionally, guidance is given in other sections regarding evaluation for counselor supervisors, as well as evaluation and remediation by counselor educators. We will fully address these codes for ethical practice in Chapter 2.

The American School Counselor Association (ASCA) provides Ethical Standards for School Counselors (2022), with a goal of clarifying the school counseling profession's values, beliefs, and norms. These standards include guidance for school counselors regarding risk assessment (A.9.b.), as well as nine codes of ethics specific to "Evaluation, Assessment, and Interpretation" (A.14.a.–i.). Section A.14. refers to culturally sensitive and bias-free assessment; ethically selecting, administering, and interpreting assessments within their scope of practice;

confidentiality when using assessments; using age- and language-appropriate assessments; using multiple data points and providing results in an appropriate manner; conveying the purpose and impact of the assessment to both the student and caregivers; monitoring appropriate use and preventing misuse of assessment results; taking care to use the appropriate assessment and applying the correct norm group when interpreting; and continuous program assessment that increases positive impact and making the outcomes available (ASCA, 2022). Further, Code B.1.e. calls for school counselors to inform parents and guardians prior to the use of screenings, surveys, or other assessments. In similar fashion, the Commission on Rehabilitation Counselor Certification (CRCC) delineates its ethical expectations for rehabilitation counselors through their "Code of Professional Ethics for Rehabilitation Counselors" (CRCC, 2023). Section H describes 10 codes for ethical and appropriate assessment and evaluation. Further, assessment is infused throughout these codes, including assessment for employment (A.1.c.), as an ethical component of end-of-life care (A.9.), and as part of court-ordered disclosure (B.2.c.). Rehabilitation counselor educators and supervisors are charged with delivering fair, accurate, and honest assessment to students (CRCC, 2023). Chapter 2 provides a detailed description of both Codes of Ethics and implications for counselors.

The Joint Committee on Testing Practices (JCTP) was sponsored by AERA, ACA, APA, ASHA, the National Association of School Psychologists (NASP), the National Association of Test Directors (NATD), and NCME. Disbanded in 2007, the purpose of this committee was to provide an interdisciplinary approach to improving the use of testing instruments (Hood & Johnson, 2007). To this end, JCTP produced a number of noteworthy documents including the *Code of Fair Testing Practices in Education*, *Responsible Test Use*, and *Rights and Responsibilities of Test Takers*. Chapter 2 includes more details in terms of the impact of these documents. Finally, Fair Access to Testing (FACT), a multidisciplinary nonprofit, works with representatives from the Association of Test Publishers, the ACA, and the NBCC to advocate for access to psychologic testing for qualified professionals including counselors. It is important to note that there are historical and ongoing disagreements within the counseling and psychology disciplines regarding who is qualified to administer certain psychologic tests. Counseling organizations, in conjunction with FACT, play a key role in ensuring that counselors maintain the right to purchase and administer assessment instruments (Balkin & Juhnke, 2018). Chapter 2 provides a review of the history of assessment in mental health and how this history impacts current issues, such as the attempts to restrict qualifications to administer specific instruments.

Table 1.2 describes and provides links to the key assessment documents from the counseling organizations mentioned in this chapter.

TABLE 1.2 ORGANIZING AND OBTAINING KEY ASSESSMENT DOCUMENTS

Statement/ Standards	Organization	Purpose	Weblink
2024 CACREP Standards	CACREP	Standards for accrediting counseling program	www.cacrep.org/wp-content/uploads/2023/06/Combined-version-6.21.23.pdf
Standards for Educational and Psychological Testing	AERA, APA, and NCME	Testing guidance	www.testingstandards.net/uploads/7/6/6/4/76643089/standards_2014edition.pdf
Responsibilities of Users of Standardized Tests	AARC	Promote the accurate, fair, and responsible use of standardized tests	https://aarc-counseling.org/wp-content/uploads/2023/04/Responsibilities-of-Users-of-Standardized-Tests-RUST-4E.pdf

(continued)

TABLE 1.2 **ORGANIZING AND OBTAINING KEY ASSESSMENT DOCUMENTS** (*continued*)

Statement/Standards	Organization	Purpose	Weblink
Sponsored Assessment Standards and Statements	AARC	Unifying positions on testing	https://aarc-counseling.org/resources
Scientist Practitioner Model	AARC	Describe competencies for evidence-based practice	https://aarc-counseling.org/wp-content/uploads/2020/01/practitioner.pdf
Standards for Multicultural Assessment	AARC	Introduce cultural competencies for assessment and testing	https://aarc-counseling.org/wp-content/uploads/2020/04/AARC-Standards-for-Multicultural-Assessments-2018.pdf
ACA Code of Ethics	ACA	Ethical guidelines for counselors	www.counseling.org/docs/default-source/default-document-library/ethics/2014-aca-code-of-ethics.pdf
NBCC Code of Ethics	NBCC	Ethical guidelines for certified counselors	www.nbcc.org/assets/ethics/nbcccodeofethics.pdf
AMHCA Code of Ethics	AMHCA	Ethical guidelines for mental health counselors	www.amhca.org/viewdocument/2020-amhca-code-of-ethics?CommunityKey=88ff9fb7-8724-4717-8a7c-4cf1cd0305e9
AACE-AMHCA Standards for Assessment in Mental Health Counseling	AMHCA	Professional standards for assessment and evaluation in mental health counseling	https://aarc-counseling.org/wp-content/uploads/2020/04/AACE-AMHCA-Standards-for-Assessment-in-Mental-Health-Counseling.pdf
Ethical Standards for School Counselors	ASCA	Ethical guidelines for school counselors	www.schoolcounselor.org/getmedia/44f30280-ffe8-4b41-9ad8-f15909c3d164/EthicalStandards.pdf
Code of Professional Ethics for Rehabilitation Counselors	CRCC	Ethical guidelines for rehabilitation counselors	https://crccertification.com/wp-content/uploads/2023/04/2023-Code-of-Ethics.pdf
Code of Fair Testing Practices in Education	JCTP	Guidelines for professionals to provide and use fair testing appropriately	www.apa.org/science/programs/testing/fair-testing.pdf
Rights and Responsibilities of Test Takers	JCTP	Clarify expectations for test takers	www.apa.org/science/programs/testing/rights

AACE, Association for Assessment in Counseling and Education; AARC, Association for Assessment and Research in Counseling; AERA, American Educational Research Association; AMHCA, American Mental Health Counselors Association; APA, American Psychological Association; ASCA, American School Counselor Association; CACREP, Council for Accreditation of Counseling and Related Educational Programs; CRCC, Code of Professional Ethics for Rehabilitation Counselors; JCTP, Joint Committee on Testing Practices; NBCC, National Board for Certified Counselors Code of Ethics; NCME, National Council on Measurement in Education.

CASE STUDIES

The following case studies represent our efforts to provide the reader with simulated opportunities for real-world application of this text. Throughout some of the book chapters, a case study will be used to explore and process the material, with opportunities for student interaction. It is our hope that this will make difficult concepts accessible and encourage creative practice. All of the content in these case studies is entirely fictional and intended to representatively incorporate a diverse intersection of variables for readers to consider.

Case of Sarah

Sarah, a high school student, is a 17-year-old female of mixed race (White, Latin American, and African American). She comes from a middle-class family and lives with her parents and younger sister. Sarah has always been a high achiever and has excelled academically. She is involved in various extracurricular activities, is on the cheerleading team, and holds leadership positions in school clubs. However, recently, Sarah's parents noticed a significant change in her behavior and a drop in grades for certain courses. Sarah's parents have observed that she has become increasingly withdrawn and emotionally distant. She spends most of her time alone in her room, avoids family gatherings, and rarely engages in conversations. She used to be an open and communicative child, but now she has become guarded and reluctant to share her thoughts and feelings. Sarah has a few friends that she still interacts with on occasion, but she shows little interest. Sarah's parents also report that she has not had much of an appetite lately and has lost some weight, but she has also been reducing carbs because she was going to try out for captain of the cheer team and wanted to be in top shape. Her parents do not think she has a boyfriend, but she was called to the school counselor's office last week for arguing with a male classmate. The school counselor believes she is dating this classmate. The school counselor is keeping an eye on Sarah, but with her dropping grades and lack of interest in school, the counselor is concerned about her SATs that are coming up soon. Sarah received detention for this incident at school and her school counselor noticed Sarah had some marks on her arms; when Sarah saw her staring, she said, "cheer injuries." Sarah's parents are worried about her well-being and are working with the school counselor to try and understand underlying reasons for her sudden change in behavior.

Case of John

John, a 37-year-old veteran, dedicated himself to serving his country with distinction ever since he was 21 years old. As an Army combat medic, he experienced a spinal cord injury during a deployment in a war zone, which ultimately led to his early retirement from the military. Dealing with extreme back pain, as well as difficulties with balance and walking, John relies on pain medications and regular physical rehabilitation to manage his condition. In addition, he was diagnosed with posttraumatic stress disorder (PTSD) and depressive disorder. Now, over a year into his retirement, John faces the common challenge that many veterans encounter during transition to civilian life: finding a new career path. As a combat medic specialist, John skillfully provided emergency medical care in the field, both in combat and humanitarian situations. His training equipped him to act as a first responder, effectively triaging injuries and illnesses to save lives, much like a paramedic in the civilian world. Despite his desire to work, John's physical disability, a direct consequence of his service-related injury, presents further obstacles in his job search. He worries that his disability may limit his career options and hinder his chances of finding meaningful employment in the civilian sector. On a personal note, John is married and has an 8-year-old daughter who brings him joy and motivation.

Case of Arturo

Arturo is a 61-year-old cisgender male of Greek American background who identifys as heterosexual. His family devoutly observes Greek Orthodox Christianity and has been active in their local religious community for the entirety of his life. Arturo reports that his parents immigrated to the United States as teenagers, and that he remains close with them as well as his extended family, which is spread across several countries. Arturo has a bachelor's degree and worked for a long time as a general manager of a local consumer goods chain. He has consistently fallen in and out of persistent, low-level depression for as long as he can remember. He shares that this dull sadness impacted nearly every aspect of his life, including his relationships. He has recently retired from his job, and after several months of his depressive state, he began to notice his ability to feel connected to his spirituality was diminishing. Little by little, Arturo became concerned by the way his religious practices felt more like rote behaviors. Arturo reports that he currently feels like life is stale and unfulfilling. He further feels disenfranchised regarding his faith, which he had initially believed would give him both the empowerment and purpose to avoid such periods of existential boredom. He is hopeful that therapy will help him to find a renewed enjoyment of life, companionship, and lasting relationships, and alleviate his depressive symptoms.

Case of Henry

Henry is a queer 22-year-old who is the child of a White father and a Black and Apache mother. Henry had only minimal contact with his tribal culture and his African American heritage in his formative years and none at all after his mother died in a car accident when he was 8 years old. His father rarely spoke of his mother, remarried a White woman, and had two more children. As an adolescent and young adult, Henry struggled with bipolar disorder and alcohol abuse. He left home and was homeless for a few years before reestablishing shaky contact with his father. At 21 years old, Henry saw himself as a failure, did not feel he really belonged anywhere, and despaired of ever turning his life around. His first attempt at rehabilitation was marginal. He found the medication helpful but disliked group therapy and was uncomfortable with the heavy Christian slant and rigid 12-step program of Alcoholics Anonymous. He fared better when he tried individual therapy and a small dual-diagnosis group. He started to think about the many losses he had experienced in his life.

Upon entering into sobriety, Henry became aware that he was carrying certain triggers around feelings of belonging/outsidership, loss and abandonment, and cultural identity. He noticed that when in treatment groups, he would become anxious and distant during times when he was expected to show vulnerability or discuss aspects of his childhood. As a result, he would find himself shifting into anger and argumentativeness, which would often result in being spoken to by therapists and treatment center leadership. Henry additionally expressed feelings of being adrift and isolated within the larger culture and expresses bitterness that parts of himself were erased upon his mother's passing and his father's remarriage.

END-OF-CHAPTER RESOURCES

DISCUSSION QUESTIONS

1. Reflect on quantitative and qualitative assessment methods. What are the pros and cons of each? Which method might you use most frequently with clients?

2. What are the four main purposes of assessment in counseling? How would you rank these in terms of importance and why?

3. In your opinion, are there assessments that counselors should not engage in? Describe your views in terms of counseling and assessment and testing.

4. Reflect on assessment in counseling. What are your fears about engaging in this process? What part of the assessment process might you enjoy most?

CLASS ACTIVITIES

1. Using the case of Henry, engage in a classroom discussion regarding students' initial impressions of what specific elements need to be subjected to assessment and their suggestions for what kinds of strategies (quantitative and qualitative) would be best suited for this task. Upon the collection of all ideas, utilize the textbook and available digital resources to explore potential "blind spots" to assessing that may exist due to being new in learning this material.

2. Role-play a 15- to 20-minute discussion with a student who will play the role of Sarah from the first case study. Engage in an initial, general helping discussion in which the "therapist" explores Sarah's presenting problem and personality characteristics (nuances of this will change depending on the person playing the role). Following the role-play, discuss as a pair what you have learned about how this client may respond to different kinds of assessment strategies, and the relationship needs that must be fulfilled in order to foster a cohesive and productive integration of assessment and process.

3. Research the most common ethical violations in your state for mental health professionals, utilizing public records and websites, as well as any scholarly materials you may find on the subject. Reflect on the role that insufficient or unethical assessment strategies may play in some of these violations coming to fruition. What is your plan to avoid falling into these traps of therapeutic drift and malpractice?

PERSPECTIVE FROM THE FIELD

 Chapter 1 introduces assessment and evaluation in counseling. The podcast interview gives the reader more information regarding the basics and the utilization of assessment-based measures of counseling outcomes. Dr. Paul Peluso talks about the importance of measurement in counseling and research in the field. He describes his experiences of evaluation of client outcomes, as well as his experiences with the AARC. Insight is given into the findings from the ACA's task force on best practices in research. Dr. Peluso is senior associate dean in the College of Education and professor in the Department of Counselor Education at Florida Atlantic University in Boca Raton, Florida. He is the author of 10 books. He is also the series editor for a new book series in Family Counseling for Routledge Publishing. Dr. Peluso is the past-editor of the journal *Measurement and Evaluation in Counseling and Development* and author of over 25 articles and 12 chapters related to the therapeutic relationship, family therapy, couples counseling, and Adlerian theory. His areas of clinical expertise include couples therapy, infidelity, family therapy, traumatic grief and loss, and domestic violence.

Access podcasts via the QR code or http://connect.springerpub.com/content/book/978-0-8261-8913-4/chapter/ch00.

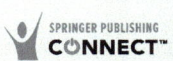 A robust set of instructor resources designed to supplement this text is located at http://connect.springerpub.com/content/book/978-0-8261-8913-4. Qualifying instructors may request access by emailing textbook@springerpub.com.

REFERENCES

American Counseling Association. (2014). *2014 ACA code of ethics*. https://www.counseling.org/docs/default-source/default-document-library/ethics/2014-aca-code-of-ethics.pdf

American Educational Research Association, American Psychological Association, & National Council on Measurement in Education. (2014). *Standards for educational and psychological testing*. https://www.testingstandards.net/uploads/7/6/6/4/76643089/standards_2014edition.pdf

American School Counselor Association. (2022). *Code of ethics*. https://www.schoolcounselor.org/getmedia/44f30280-ffe8-4b41-9ad8-f15909c3d164/EthicalStandards.pdf

Association for Assessment and Research in Counseling. (n.d.). *Our purpose*. Accessed July 26, 2024. https://aarc-counseling.org/about-us

Balkin, R. S., & Juhnke, G. A. (2018). *Assessment in counseling: Practice and applications*. Oxford University Press.

Beck, A. T., Steer, R. A., & Brown, G. K. (1996). *Beck Depression Inventory (BDI-II): Manual and questionnaire*. The Psychological Corporation.

Bordin, E. S. (1979). The generalizability of the psychodynamic concept of the working alliance. *Psychotherapy: Theory, Research, and Practice, 16,* 252–260. https://doi.org/10.1037/h0085885

Commission on Rehabilitation Counselor Certification. (2023, January 1). *Code of professional ethics for rehabilitation counselors*. https://crccertification.com/wp-content/uploads/2023/04/2023-Code-of-Ethics.pdf

Council for Accreditation of Counseling and Related Educational Programs. (2023a). *2024 CACREP standards*. https://www.cacrep.org/wp-content/uploads/2023/06/Combined-version-6.21.23.pdf

Council for Accreditation of Counseling and Related Educational Programs. (2023b). *2024 standards glossary*. https://www.cacrep.org/2024-standards-glossary-2/

Educational Testing Service. (2016). *The GRE® tests*. https://www.ets.org/gre.html

Foster, L. H. (2017). Assessment in counseling. In D. Capuzzi & D. R. Gross (Eds.), *Introduction to the counseling profession* (7th ed., pp. 233–252). Routledge.

Gill, C. S., Dailey, S. F., Karl, S., & Barrio Minton, C. (2024). DSM-5-TR *learning companion for counselors*. American Counseling Association.

Gill, C. S., & Freund, R. R. (2018). *Spirituality and religion in counseling: Competency-based strategies for ethical practice*. Routledge/Taylor & Francis.

Heppner, P. P., Wampold, B. E., Owen, J., Thompson, M. N., & Wang, K. T. (2015). *Research design in counseling*. Cengage Learning.

Hood, A. B., & Johnson, R. W. (2007). *Assessment in counseling: A guide to the use of psychological assessment procedures* (4th ed.). American Counseling Association.

Lambert, M. J., Hansen, N. B., & Finch, A. E. (2001). Patient-focused research: Using patient outcome data to enhance treatment effects. *Journal of Consulting and Clinical Psychology, 69*, 159–172. http://doi.org/10.1037/0022-006X.69.2.159

Lenz, A. S., Ault, H., Balkin, R. S., Barrio Minton, C., Erford, B. T., Hays, D. G., Kim, B. S. K., & Li, C. (2022). Responsibilities of Users of Standardized Tests (RUST-4E): Prepared for the Association for Assessment and Research in Counseling. *Measurement and Evaluation in Counseling and Development, 55*(4), 227–235. https://doi.org/10.1080/07481756.2022.2052321

Leppma, M., & Jones, K. D. (2013, January). Multiple assessment methods and sources in counseling: Ethical considerations. *VISTAS 2013*, Article 37. https://www.counseling.org/docs/default-source/vistas/multiple-assessment-methods-and-sources-in-counseling-ethical-considerations.pdf

Myers, J. E., Luecht, R. M., & Sweeney, T. J. (2004). The factor structure of wellness: Reexamining theoretical and empirical models underlying the Wellness Evaluation of Lifestyle (WEL) and the Five-Factor Wei. *Measurement and Evaluation in Counseling and Development, 36*(4), 194–208. https://doi.org/10.1080/07481756.2004.11909742

National Board for Certified Counselors. (2023). *NBCC code of ethics*. https://www.nbcc.org/assets/ethics/nbcccodeofethics.pdf

Posner, K., Brown, G. K., Stanley, B., Brent, D. A., Yershova, K. V., Oquendo, M. A., Currier, G. W., Melvin, G. A., Greenhill, L., Shen, S., & Mann, J. J. (2011). The Columbia-Suicide Severity Rating Scale: Initial validity and internal consistency findings from three multisite studies with adolescents and adults. *The American Journal of Psychiatry, 168*(12), 1266–1277. https://doi.org/10.1176/appi.ajp.2011.10111704

Sperry, L., & Sperry, J. (2020). *Case conceptualization: Mastering this competency with ease and confidence* (2nd ed.). Routledge.

Wechsler, D., & Kodama, H. (1949). *Wechsler Intelligence Scale for Children* (Vol. 1). Psychological Corporation.

History and Ethics in Assessment and Appraisal

KELLY EMELIANCHIK-KEY, CARMAN S. GILL, AND AYSE TORRES

2024 CACREP STANDARDS

3.G.1. historical perspectives concerning the nature and meaning of assessment and testing in counseling

3.G.6. ethical and legal considerations for selecting, administering, and interpreting assessments

As a counseling intern, I remember my site required me to utilize a personality assessment with all my clients. At the time, I did what I was told and gave everyone this personality assessment, even though I did not know how to score the instrument or report the results to my client. When I asked my site supervisor about the assessment tool, I was told someone else would score it, and it is just something we give all clients. Yet there was no specific information as to why this was and the purpose. Something always felt off, but as I look back, I know this practice bordered on an ethical violation. Our six ethical principles in counseling were not considered.

HISTORICAL PERSPECTIVES

Counseling and assessment have always been intricately linked. Understanding the history and development of assessing and testing in counseling will not only assist you in providing more meaningful assessment experiences for your clients but will afford a foundation for a deeper understanding of the legal and ethical issues associated with measurement today. Many of the interdisciplinary issues surrounding the administration of testing instruments have their roots buried deep in the history of the various mental health disciplines. Understanding the original intent of assessment instruments and some of the contributions and setbacks will hopefully help you with your future practice.

Human beings continually assess the data we receive through our senses in an ongoing way. We assess each other as well and this is consistent throughout our history. Some argue that the first official assessment occurred in China in 2200 B.C.E. (DuBois, 1970; Wiggins, 1973) and was likely ability testing. While this may be legend, most experts agree that written examinations began around 200–100 B.C.E. (Bowman, 1989). These examinations were used for selecting and promoting officials and eventually developed into an elaborate, formalized evaluation system. This evaluation system was associated with title granting and success led to more power. However, corruption within the system resulted in reformation attempts and eventually to its end in 1906 C.E. Noteworthy was the infusion of objectivity throughout this system, as the Chinese went to great lengths to ensure this occurred through procedures such as removing the person's name and using independent reviewers (Wainer, 1987). However, problems that impact modern testing emerged here as well, including creating expert knowledge, testing memory versus mental ability, determining implications of examinations for social mobility, examining how to measure applied problem-solving, cheating, and identifying administrator bias (Bowman, 1989). Prior to its end, this testing system spread to other countries, including France and Great Britian, and led to the Civil Service Act of 1883 passed in the United States (Wainer, 1987).

With the Age of Reason, the 1800s saw precursors to and development of modern-day psychologic assessment. As theorists became more interested in human ability, personality, and differences, noteworthy philosophers such as Charles Darwin began to develop methods of measurement focusing on their theories (Hays, 2017; Neukrug & Fawcett, 2010). Two French physicians are credited with early assessment attempts toward understanding differences in human intelligence. In 1838, Jean-Étienne Dominique Esquirol attempted to use language to identify intelligence levels. Working in Parisian mental asylums with those who had intellectual disabilities, he focused on the role of language in levels of intelligence and is credited with original attempts to establish "verbal IQ" (Neukrug & Fawcett, 2010, p. 5). Édouard Séguin built on this work, assessing a similar population, with the assumption he could identify intelligence levels through assessing characteristics such as shape concept, visual perception, and eye–hand coordination. In 1853, he developed the Seguin Form Board Test (SFBT) to measure motor control and sensory discrimination. Speed was a key factor in determining mental age and, from that, performance IQ (Koshy et al., 2017).

Darwin and his cousin, Francis Galton, both biologists, attempted to understand and measure human differences. Based off his theory of evolution, Darwin originally posited a link between human and animal development, as well as individual differences in parent/child relationship, which lead to heredity studies (Neukrug & Fawcett, 2010). Resulting from his belief that anything can be measured, Galton created standardized methods for gathering data and recording results, sometimes using a "statistical scale" (Stigler, 1989, p. 73). Galton investigated the relationship between physical characteristics, such as height, breathing capacity, arm length and weight, and mental capacity (Balkin & Juhnke, 2018; Cohen et al., 2022). Although no relationship was found, Galton routinely used statistical methods to record and evaluate his data. He confirmed that individual cognitive differences exist and invented the correlation coefficient, regression, and other mathematical concepts we use today (Stigler, 1989).

Wilhelm Wundt established the first experimental laboratory in Germany in 1879 (Balkin & Juhnke, 2018; Cohen et al., 2022). Wundt intended to identify similarities in individuals, particularly in terms of speed of thought and reaction time. He conducted experimental research, using a calibrated pendulum as a device to measure speed of thought. Wundt confirmed variation in mental processes. In addition, he focused on reducing error by controlling for extraneous variables, using techniques similar to those we use in modern day testing (Cohen et al., 2022). As a result of these controlled experiments, he is considered the founder of experimental psychology. Wundt's research, along with that of Galton, inspired James Cattell, one of Wundt's students. An American psychologist, Cattell focused on mental functions and used timed tests. He believed that physical characteristics determined intelligence levels and studied reaction time, sensation differences, memory, and other characteristics as indicators of intelligence. He is noted for coining the term *mental tests* and applying statistical concepts to people. However, his student, Clark Wissler, later determined that academic performance was unrelated to the scores on Cattell's mental tests, and response time was dismissed related to intelligence for about 70 years (Balkin & Juhnke, 2018).

Around this time, Alfred Binet, who was inspired by Esquirol and Séguin, began exploring methods for helping students who had educational deficits. Working with Theodore Simon, his goal was to identify children with intellectual disabilities (Neukrug & Fawcett, 2010). In 1905, they introduced the Binet-Simon scale, widely considered the first modern intelligence test (Hays, 2017). Lewis Terman subsequentially used this scale to gather data from children, and revised it based on this data. The ultimate outcome of the process was the Stanford-Binet scale, and the introduction of the term *intelligence quotient* or IQ (Hays, 2017). This research eventually led David Wechsler to create his Wechsler-Bellevue Intelligence Scale, later renamed the Wechsler Adult Intelligence Scale (WAIS), which is used today (Cohen et al., 2022) and is discussed in more depth in Chapter 8. Unfortunately, the Stanford-Binet scale was misused by Henry Goddard, who applied the intelligence test inappropriately to immigrants. The scale was normed using a French population, then translated to English and given to immigrants, often using translators. The result was over 80% of these immigrants identified as having low intellectual functioning (Balkin & Juhnke, 2018). Goddard's work potentially influenced policy, as he advocated for the deportation of these individuals (Hays, 2017).

The history of assessment in counseling in the United States begins with Frank Parsons. In response to the shifting paradigm of the Industrial Revolution, Frank Parsons became involved in civil service and advocated for individuals who were taken advantage of by the new industries (Wilson, 2013). Parsons was noteworthy for his role in codifying one of the first processes of counseling, which focused on vocational guidance and included use of assessment procedures and the scientific method (National Board of Forensic Evaluators [NBFE], 2022). Aimed at improving social conditions, Parsons believed that helping guide the career decisions of individuals would improve their lives substantially. As such, he relied on physical and psychologic testing to understand the individual and assist in finding the appropriate vocation based on traits (Wilson, 2013). Parsons organized the Boston Vocational Bureau in 1908. He based his work around trait and factor assessments and the theory of career counseling. So integral to counseling was the use of assessment that these first spaces dedicated to counseling were named "counseling and testing centers" (NBFE, 2022). In 1913, the National Vocational Guidance Association (NVGA) evolved from the Vocational Bureau's conferences (Wilson, 2013). This association became one of the four independent associations forming the American Personnel and Guidance Association (APGA), which later became the American Counseling Association (ACA; n.d.).

In addition to Parson's trait and factor assessments, other researchers began to investigate the connection between interest and career choice. In 1912, American psychologist Edward Thorndike published a study on elementary school students' interest. In 1922, J. B. Miner developed one of the first group interest inventories for high school students while working at the Carnegie Institute of Technology (DuBois, 1970; Neukrug & Fawcett, 2010). Another person working at this institution with a team of researchers, Edward Strong, created the Strong Vocational Interest Blank, published in 1927. Later renamed the Strong Interest Inventory, this assessment is widely used in career counseling today.

As the roots of our profession began to take hold, intelligence, achievement, and psychologic testing continued to develop as well. During World War I (WWI), intelligence testing was identified as a way to improve the military, but individual testing was impractical. As a result, group intelligence testing was developed. Robert Yerkes headed a committee that constructed two such tests, Army Alpha and Army Beta, for identifying cognitive ability. Army Beta, which relied on form boards and mazes, was used when the test taker could not read (Neukrug & Fawcett, 2010). These tests were eventually released to the public, as group testing became more prevalent, particularly in the school setting. Educational settings began to rely heavily on assessments for determining student future success. The Scholastic Aptitude

Test (SAT) was developed through the College Entrance Examination Board (CEEB) and based in James Conant's belief that these types of tests would reduce inequality. CEEB later became Educational Testing Service (ETS); the organization published the Graduate Record Examination (GRE) and continues to do so (Hays, 2017). Thorndike was credited with introducing achievement testing, leading to the development of the Stanford Achievement Test.

The rise in personality and psychologic testing grew out of both the need during and following WWI and public interest in testing. The Woodworth Personal Data Sheet was developed to detect and understand emotional instability in military members (DuBois, 1970). Woodworth later developed the Woodworth Psychoneurotic Inventory, the first commonly used self-report measure of personality (Cohen et al., 2022). Woodworth's Personal Data Sheet was followed by Hathaway and McKinley's Minnesota Multiphasic Personality Inventory (MMPI; Ben-Porath & Tellegen, 2020) in 1940 (DuBois, 1970). Created using groups of psychiatric patients to detect mental illness and diagnose, the MMPI preceded the development of multiple personality tests, including the NEO Personality Inventory (NEO-PI). Differing from symptom-based assessments, the NEO focuses on the "Big Five" theory of personality, a five-factor model based on neuroticism, extraversion, openness, agreeableness, and conscientiousness (Balkin & Juhnke, 2018). Projective tests, which rely on the assumption that individuals place their unconscious beliefs upon ambiguous stimuli, became popular during this time. In 1921, Hermann Rorschach (1921) introduced a project psychologic test based on his use of inkblots to understand and diagnose mental issues. The Rorschach Inkblot Test is perhaps the most well-known of these assessments.

The following decades saw an increased interest in both personality and clinically focused assessment measures, many of which are commonly used today. Whereas there are copious instruments available, we cover specific assessments of personality and clinical issues in Chapter 10. These instruments include those assessments based upon diagnosis, such as the Generalized Anxiety Disorder 7 (GAD-7; Spitzer et al., 2006), Eating Disorders Inventory 3 (EDI-3; Garner, 2004), and Conners' Adult ADHD Rating Scales (Conners et al., 1998), as well as personality inventories such as the Minnesota Multiphasic Personality Inventory-3 and the Myers-Briggs Type Indicator (MBTI; I. B. Myers et al., 1998). As counseling moved to a wellness-based paradigm, assessments to measure this concept were developed as well. J. E. Myers and Sweeney posited the Indivisible Self strengths-based model of wellness, grounded in Adlerian theory, specifically for counselors. This model was originally presented in a circular design and called the "Wheel of Wellness." However, analysis revealed a factor structure with one overarching factor, five discrete second-order factors, and 17 third-order factors (J. E. Myers et al., 2004). Because of the inseparable nature of the high order factor, this model is called "The Indivisible Self: An Evidence-Based Model of Wellness (ISWEL)." Further, the Five Factor Wellness Inventory (5F-WEL: J. E. Myers & Sweeney, 2005) was designed to measure overall wellness, as well as levels of wellness for secondary and tertiary factors. While multiple measures of wellness are available, this instrument is noteworthy due to the evidence-based nature of the instrument and the underlying model's focus on the counseling profession.

ASSESSMENT ISSUES

The history of assessment illuminates testing issues and ethical concerns that affect present day counselors. For example, lack of control of extraneous or external influences impacted measurement and testing outcomes, leading to inaccurate conclusions. The mistaken assumption that intelligence is related to specific physical characteristics is similar to the inaccurate and biased notions that later emerged relating race to intelligence (discussed more in depth in Chapter 3). Goddard's misuse of testing underscores the deleterious impact of administrator bias in testing and of applying instruments inappropriately on populations for which they were created. Questions regarding who is qualified to administer tests and issues of control over testing rights is under debate today. These and other issues highlight the need for ethical guidelines around the use of testing instruments, which are explored later in this chapter.

Diversity and Disability

Most assessment tools used in healthcare and counseling have been developed for English-speaking respondents with relatively high levels of education. These measures may raise concerns regarding their applicability to culturally and linguistically diverse groups, as well as individuals with disabilities (Nápoles-Springer & Stewart, 2006). To compare different groups, it is necessary for the measures to be conceptually and psychometrically equivalent among the groups being studied. Conceptual equivalence refers to an instrument having the same meaning and content across comparison groups (Weech-Maldonado et al., 2001). Assuming cultural universality often leads to bias and errors in constructing instruments and interpreting assessment results (González-Calvo et al., 1997).

The lack of representation of diverse groups during test construction and norming has historically limited the usefulness of many assessment tools in counseling. This limitation is particularly relevant for counselors working with clients who have cognitive and psychiatric disabilities, as well as those from diverse cultural backgrounds. It is crucial for counselors to be aware of the challenges and limitations associated with the use of traditional assessments with these unique client groups to avoid misinterpretations. For instance, assessing English language learners with learning disabilities presents significant issues, such as inaccuracy, lack of validity, absence of test and item fairness, and the disproportionate referral of English language learners to special education. The scores obtained using these traditional assessment tools are often not appropriate, meaningful, or useful (Huang et al., 2011).

Traditional assessment methods pose challenges when applied to individuals with significant physical, cognitive, and emotional disabilities. However, for individuals with mild to moderate disabilities, assessment information can be valuable in enhancing their self-understanding, encouraging exploration, and identifying potential educational, social, interpersonal, and employment opportunities that may have gone unnoticed before (Strauser, 2021). A more in-depth analysis of these issues and other ethical issues is provided in the subsequent chapter.

Our Role in Assessment

The intersection of counseling and assessment has not always been a clear one. Other mental health professionals, such as psychologists, have questioned counselors' training and abilities regarding certain assessments to limit access (Balkin & Juhnke, 2018). Controlling the scope of practice regarding certain types of tests, including psychologic assessments, resulted in contention between the two mental health disciplines. For example, as all 50 states established licensure laws, scope of practice or privilege to practice became an issue, particularly where psychologic testing is concerned. Following the implementation of counseling licensure in all 50 states, attempts were made to use licensure standards as a method for restricting access to testing, typically through limiting the scope of practice or exploiting ambiguous licensure requirements. State licensure boards provide some guidance through their "scope" of practice for licensed counselors. However, certain areas of testing remain controversial. Projective test administration is controversial in particular, with some states restricting administration to psychologists (Balkin & Juhnke, 2018). ACA (Watson & Sheperis, 2010) and the NBFE (2022) all provided strong support and guidance for testing and assessment remaining within the counselor's purview. However, access to fair testing is an issue for which counselors must continue to advocate.

ETHICS AND THE LAW

In counseling, we are governed professionally by a *code of ethics*. Ethics refers to a system of principles and rules of conduct recognized and accepted by a specific group or culture, dealing with right and wrong. A code of ethics gives us guidelines to follow to ensure that we practice professionally, follow a set of standards for all, and provide quality care for all clients. Professional organizations each have their code of ethics. In the counseling field, ACA (2014) has a code of ethics that is our profession's predominant set of standards to ensure ethical practice and responsibilities for counselors and counselors in training; it also provides services to assist in taking courses of action during ethical dilemmas, helps support the mission of ACA, and serves as the basis of inquiries for ethical complaints. Additionally, the following organizations and divisions also have specific codes of ethics that contain ethical guidelines related to assessment practices (see Chapter 1, Table 1.2): the American Mental Health Counselors Association (AMHCA; 2020), the American School Counselor Association (ASCA; 2022), the National Board for Certified Counselors (NBCC; 2023), and the Commission on Rehabilitation Counselor Certification (CRCC; 2023).

The relationship between ethics and law is complex, and while there is an overlap, ethics is not simply a subset of the legal system. The law differs from our ethical codes, but they can often work hand in hand. The *law* is a set of rules that govern the people's matters within a country or state (Corey et al., 2014). These are minimum standards allowed, whereas ethics represents idea standards. As such, laws are more prescriptive in nature than ethical codes (Remley & Herlihy, 2019). Laws provide a set of rules and regulations of what can be done within each profession, and they also offer consequences if they are discovered to be broken. Law enforcement lies in the legal system's hands, and ethical violations typically defer to professional associations and licensing boards to ensure compliance and ethical practice. As a counselor in practice, you should always read and understand your state laws that pertain to your counseling practice. This includes all assessment practices and record keeping. State laws will always supersede an ethical code. If you find that laws do conflict with your code of ethics, it is strongly encouraged that you seek legal counsel, in addition to using the various ethical codes and decision-making strategies that we detail in the text that follows. While both share the goal of creating and maintaining social good, they are distinct concepts. Counselors carefully consider the interaction of state law and ethical codes. For example, a counselor is ethically required to keep information confidential, but it may not be legal to do so. Following the adoption of Florida's HB 1557, school personnel are required to notify parents of any "change in the student's services or monitoring related to the student's mental, emotional, or physical health or well-being" (CS/CS/HB 1557, 2022, p. 3), including change in use of pronouns. School counselors are not exempt from this law, which also targets any reference to sexual orientation or gender identity; these rules were originally applicable before third grade, and have now been expanded to 12th grade with specific exceptions. This disclosure may not be in the best interest of building trust, helping the client to improve, and fostering an open therapeutic relationship, which are all core ethical values for counselors.

The counseling profession has many ethical codes and standards, particularly within divisions and associations. Each organization and division can have its own set of ethical codes that are unique and specific to the mission and purpose of the organization or division. However, most have the same or very similar underlying principles that are connected to ACA's ethical codes and morals of the counseling profession. Please look back at Chapter 1, Table 1.2, for a list of key organizations in the profession and their ethical guidelines pertaining to assessment. In this chapter, we will focus our attention on the ACA Code of Ethics, code E. (2014), pertaining to the ethical principles of evaluation, assessment, and interpretation. There are 13 areas within this section of the Code of Ethics that specifically cover assessment practices for counselors.

Ethical Decisions and Codes

The ACA Code of Ethics (2014) contains six ethical principles that were built on the work of Kitchner (1984) and are now considered foundational for ethical behavior and decision-making (Meara et al., 1996). These fundamental principles should be considered in all roles of the counseling profession, especially testing and assessment. These ethical principles are as follows:

- autonomy, or fostering the right to control the direction of one's life;

- nonmaleficence, or avoiding actions that cause harm;

- beneficence, or working for the good of the individual and society by promoting mental health and well-being;

- justice, or treating individuals equitably and fostering fairness and equality;

- fidelity, or honoring commitments and keeping promises, including fulfilling one's responsibilities of trust in professional relationships; and

- veracity, or dealing truthfully with individuals with whom counselors come into professional contact (ACA, 2014, p. 2).

In conjunction with the use of an appropriate ethical decision-making model (i.e., *The Practitioner's Guide to Ethical Decision Making* by Forester-Miller and Davis [2016]; "A Social Constructivism Model for Ethical Decision Making in Counseling" by Cottone [2001]; ASCA's ethical decision-making model in the "ASCA Ethical Standards for School Counselors" [ASCA, 2022]), these six ethical principles are essential to consider when resolving any ethical dilemma, including those related to testing and assessment practices. These ethical principles should be at the core of ethical decision-making with all clients. When it comes to assessments, clients need to be informed of the purpose, potential risks, and consequences of taking the assessment tool, and then they should have the *autonomy* to decide the best course of action. Further, the assessments should be individually selected for the needs of each unique and diverse client and promote their mental health. Ensuring *nonmaleficence* requires that the assessment does not cause further harm or psychologic distress. Part of this includes the counselors' knowledge about the assessment's content and ensuring we score the assessment and interpret the results with our clients. Counselors mindfully weigh the benefits of assessment to the client's well-being, focusing on promoting *beneficence* as a central part of the process. *Justice* applied to assessment means that we are treating all clients fairly and equally. Counselors should be offering the same services and assessments to all clients who meet a need to take that assessment or test. They should not only be provided if the client has insurance or can pay out of pocket for the assessment. As counselors, we need to advocate for fair and equitable treatment interventions for all clients and account for the influence of various factors, such as measurement bias and differential representation of items in assessment tools. Counselors honor the principle of *fidelity* in our relationships by providing clients with a trusted professional helping relationship, where we honor our commitments and expectations as a professional counselor. If we give an assessment and tell the client we will score the results and interpret it with them, we must follow through, even if we do not find anything meaningful in the scores. Last, we should be *truthful* in our relationship with clients, including why we select specific tests or assessments and what we suspect we might find. As counselors, we should not be deceptive or hide anything that we suspect might be going on with a client. These six ethical principles must be considered in the entire assessment process of selection, administration, scoring, and interpretation of results.

Client Rights

Codes E.1.a. and E.1.b. of the ACA Code of Ethics (2014) provide the general introduction to this section; they explain the purpose of quantitative and qualitative assessment in counseling and include guidance on client decision-making, treatment planning, and forensic proceedings. For example, if we suspect a client has depression, we could use the Beck Depression Inventory, Second Edition (BDI-II; Beck et al., 1996), to assess if the client has elevated levels of depression. If they do, this will inform our treatment plan and the interventions we will use with this client. This section also discusses the misuse of assessment results and interpretations and respect for the client's right to know the results and interpretation. When providing our client with the BDI-II (Beck et al., 1996), we must discuss why we are using this assessment, the purpose, and the results of the assessment. The client should be informed each step of the way and be made aware of how this assessment will benefit treatment. Clients have a right to their results, but we must always consider what is in their best interest. If knowing the results of an assessment score would increase anxiety significantly, we could decide to wait to tell a client during the most appropriate time when the client could be better equipped to discuss the results.

Along with the benefits of treatment, the client is also notified if using the assessment could negatively impact them in any way. For example, if a client attends therapy and uses insurance, a diagnosis is often required by third-party payers along with a treatment plan. This is something that the client would need to be aware of as it does affect confidentiality.

Competence

Codes E.2.a., E.2.b., and E.2.c. of the ACA Code of Ethics address competence to use and administer assessment tools to clients. Counselors should be competent to administer and interpret assessments, including selecting the appropriate assessment, scoring, interpretation, and use of assessment instruments based on the client's needs. Counselors are responsible for scoring on their own or through technology-assisted services. All decisions based on the assessment measures should be constructed from the results, as the counselor should understand the psychometric properties of the selected instrument.

Being a responsible and ethical counselor requires practicing within their scope of competence. This requires personal and professional monitoring. As a counselor coming from a CACREP accredited program, you will have taken a course in assessment practice. However, that does not mean you will feel competent in administering, scoring, and interpreting all tests. Counselors should know the instruments they provide and ensure they have the proper training and skill level to use the instruments with clients. Some test publishers will require the users to show that they are qualified to administer assessments before they are sold, but many do not. It is incumbent upon the test user to determine if they meet qualifications. Additionally, we are responsible for managing the use of assessments in our profession. Suppose we become aware of others using assessments they are not qualified to administer. In that case, we should address an ethical decision-making model and develop the most appropriate course of action.

The Association of Assessment in Research and Counseling has redefined its Responsibilities of Users of Standardized Tests (RUST-4E; Lenz et al., 2022). Within these standards, they outline the responsible use of standardized tests for counselors to implement (see Table 1.2 in Chapter 1 for the link to these standards). The American Psychological Association (APA; 1954) developed a three-tiered system that established the qualifications of those administering tests; Turner et al. (2001) define APA's Guidelines for Test User Qualifications. This three-tiered system has evolved and is quite extensive. However, the former three-tiered system is still used widely due to its simplicity. In the three-tiered system, tests in Level A can be administered, scored, and interpreted by any nonpsychologist who diligently reads the testing materials and is familiar with the test, as well as its purpose, use, and scoring. This level would apply to all master's level counselors and includes educational achievement tests. Level B requires comprehension of test development procedures and psychometrics, as well as advanced coursework in psychology or counseling. For counselors, an assessment course in a master's program would meet this standard. Level C calls for a license as a psychologist or an advanced degree in psychology (APA, 1954). Counselors from master's level programs would not meet this qualification.

Informed Consent and Privacy

Codes E.3. and E.4. of the ACA Code of Ethics (2014) address informed consent in assessment. Informed consent requires a detailed and clear explanation to the client on the purpose of testing, the release of the results to appropriate recipients, and the release of data to those qualified to interpret the results. Informed consent is a process that starts from day one with your clients. Clients should have all parts of the counseling process thoroughly explained to them, including assessments utilized. The nature and purpose for using the assessment results should be provided to clients and permission must be obtained. There are some instances where clients do not need to provide explicit consent, such as achievement testing in schools or with a court-ordered client, but this does not exempt counselors from fully informing clients of the process before testing (even though consent is not required). Along with informed consent, privacy is a concern. The assessment process can invade a client's privacy, especially if the client does not know how the counselor will use assessment information and who will be privy to the test results. Clients should understand the relevance of the selected assessments. They must have the ability to agree or decline the assessment through the informed consent process. If we think back to the example at the beginning of the chapter, every client at my internship site was assessed, no matter what. This underscores the relevancy and need for informed consent. If the client was not fully informed as to the purpose of the assessment and the assessment is not relevant to their goals for therapy, then they should have the opportunity to decline taking that assessment. Additionally, depending on when the results are conveyed, the client could feel as if their privacy were invaded. Clients often take assessments as part of the counseling intake process to be cooperative, but they may not have appropriate informed consent.

Diagnosis of Mental Health Disorders

Codes E.5.a., E.5.b., E.5.c., and E.5.d. in the ACA Code of Ethics (2014) address diagnosing mental disorders. When attempting to diagnose and determine the course of treatment, assessment techniques should be done with care and attention to detail in selection. These ACA codes stress the importance of selecting the appropriate and culturally sensitive test, in addition to understanding the complex ways that culture is expressed, which is not part of the diagnostic criteria for mental health disorders. This includes bias and prejudice in diagnosing mental health disorders and pathologizing certain groups due to the stigma inherent in the diagnostic process. Counselors should also refrain from making or reporting a diagnosis if they believe it could cause a client more harm than good. Additionally, once a client is provided a formal diagnosis based on an assessment tool, this becomes part of the medical record and the law requires that the client must self-report this diagnosis on various applications (for example, when applying for a medical or counseling license in their home state). Clients should be informed of their rights before a counselor uses assessments to diagnose mental health disorders.

Stigmatization and Client Rights

The American Educational Research Association's (AERA's) *Standards for Educational and Psychological Testing*, standard 8.8, notes that "when score reporting includes assigning individuals into categories, the categories should be chosen carefully and described precisely. The least stigmatizing labels, consistent with accurate representation, should always be assigned" (AERA et al., 2014, p. 88). Diagnostic labels can significantly impact a client and should be carefully considered because they can influence if a client can receive treatment for a diagnosis. For many health insurance companies, a diagnosis determines if treatment options will be paid for by the insurance company, or if the client is responsible for some or all of these charges. Insurance payment or reimbursement is important for some clients, yet the presence of a diagnosis can carry stigma and other barriers for clients, resulting in challenges such as the loss of peer and family relationships, creation of barriers to employment, and creation of internalized stigma, which impacts self-esteem and self-worth (Huggett et al., 2018; Moses, 2010; Overton & Medina, 2008).

Selecting Appropriate Instruments

Codes E.6.a. and E.6.b. of the ACA Code of Ethics (2014) pertain to selecting appropriate instruments and making referrals. Counselors must choose assessments with the appropriate psychometric properties and consider all known instrument limitations. This includes the assessment's efficacy with diverse cultural populations, if there are multiple forms of the assessment, the validity and reliability of the instrument, confidence intervals and score norms, and if scoring information and guidance is readily available. Additionally, suppose we are not competent, or properly trained, to provide the assessment ourselves. If this is the case, counselors must provide appropriate referral information to the third party, such as specific referral questions and objective data, to ensure that proper tests are utilized. According to RUST-4E Standards (Lenz et al., 2022), responsible test selection requires "establishing a clear and defensible connection between (a) the nature and purpose of a testing request, (b) user qualifications, (c) expected characteristics of the testing environment, (d) test content, processes, and intended use of test scores, and (e) test taker characteristics" (p. 231). When selecting an instrument, counselors must do their due diligence to search all available assessments that meet the unique client's needs. The fit of the instrument should be based on the client, the construct you are trying to capture further, and the assessment that would most benefit the client.

Administering Assessments

Codes E.7.a., E.7.b., E.7.c., and E.7.d. outline the considerations for assessment administration (ACA, 2014). The prior section of these ethical codes addressed instrument selection, but how we administer and provide client assessments is equally critical. Counselors should conduct assessments as they were designed to be administered during the development process. When unable to do so, counselors document this in the interpretation, and they consider that the results might have questionable validity. An example of this situation is if a test was adjusted or adapted to help a client who is disabled. The results could be invalid based on the adjustment made to assist the client, because the test was not standardized in this manner.

Counselors should also ensure the environment and setting for test administration is appropriate for the client and free of distraction, which could result in invalid or skewed results. If the test is administered electronically, all equipment should be working correctly to produce accurate results. Last, as previously noted, the test should be administered as designed, including a supervised or unsupervised administration per the testing instructions. Specific supervision instructions are often the case with many achievement and aptitude tests.

Multicultural and Diversity Issues in Assessment

Code E.8. of the ACA Code of Ethics requires that counselors select and use assessments with normed populations. Counselors recognize that administration of the instrument to diverse groups for which an instrument was not normed could result in differences in test administration and interpretation (ACA, 2014). Age, race, gender, disability, language, culture, and religion should all be considered before selecting and administering the instrument. If a clinician still decides to administer the instrument, the interpretation needs to reflect how these various contexts could impact results.

Consider the history of the Stanford-Binet scale and Goddard's misuse of this intelligence assessment. The result of this misuse underscores the importance of considering your clients' identities and the population the instrument was normed with. The authors of the assessment tools often describe this in the development and validation publication for their assessment tool. They should specifically note if the test scores and interpretations should be adjusted to account for diversity in clients. Diversity of clients and the ways in which these identities need to be considered in selection, administration, and interpretation will be detailed in Chapter 3.

Scoring and Interpretation of Assessments

When selecting and administering assessments, counselors are required to score and interpret the results in meaningful ways that facilitate client care. Code E.9.a. of the ACA Code of Ethics (2014) provides the reporting requirements for counselors when sharing the results of an assessment. The client's culture, understanding, and impact of the results should all be considered. Counselors should make the scores understandable and report inconsistencies with the tests, in addition to helping the client understand the norm and norm groups for scores. Many of us recall receiving test results either electronically or on a piece of paper, without context. This "plop phenomenon" does not lead to meaningful interpretations and can have the opposite effect, even resulting in damage to the therapeutic relationship. Counselors always engage with the client in meaningful ways when conveying the results of an assessment. Further, code E.9.b. requires counselors to exhibit caution in interpreting results and sharing the instrument's purpose and any concerns around reliability and validity with the client. Counselors who provide assessment, scoring, and interpretation are required to verify such interpretations' validity, including the assessment purpose, norms, validity, reliability, and applications of the procedures, as well as any special qualifications applicable to their use (code E.9.c.). Mistakes or errors outside of our control will happen when scoring and interpreting test results. It is critical that you document any errors that arise and note any considerations or accommodations made to account for them when interpreting results. If the error is pervasive, it might be in the client's best interest to communicate the reservations to the client and potentially invalidate the test score. The test may need to be repeated.

Test Security and Integrity

The ACA Code of Ethics, code E.10., informs counselors that they are responsible to maintain test security consistent with contractual obligations when the test was purchased, or permission was granted for use (2014). Tests should not be modified, changed, or reproduced without permission from the publisher, even when assessment measures are lengthy. When a counselor believes that the client would benefit from one portion of an assessment, the counselor is responsible for determining if part of the test has the proper psychometrics to use alone, as this is not the case for many standardized instruments. Along with test integrity is code E.11., which prohibits counselors from using outdated data or test results. Obsolete measures should not be used with clients. When newer versions are available, clinicians must learn about the latest version and administer the updated version (ACA, 2014). Counselors should not continue to administer the old version and must do their due diligence to become familiar with the new version. We must also consider that errors and newly established norms come with new versions. As discerning counselors, we may want to wait for the publisher of the new version to report an established research base and psychometric integrity. Last, code E.12. also speaks to the integrity of tests and reminds counselors to use assessments that have gone through the rigors of scientific testing in their development and publication process. To preserve the integrity and security of tests and protocols, we must follow the highest professional standards. All tests and protocols should be stored in a secure environment, such as a locked filing cabinet or on a password-protected computer in a locked office.

CHECKING IN WITH ARTURO

Arturo has been to therapy in the past. He states that one of his former counselors was through his church. As Arturo begins to describe the counselor, you wonder if this person was a trained professional counselor or a lay helper. Arturo tells you that the counselor found assessments online and would make him take them electronically or at times print them and change the wording around to add things related to his Christian worldview. Arturo does not like using computers and isn't as savvy as he would like around technology. Arturo reports never getting a score or hearing how he performed. Some of the assessments he took were more than 20 years old or described things that did not seem relevant to the reasons he attended counseling. Arturo reports he does not want to do any more testing since he did not find this to be a useful way to spend his time and the thought of more makes him anxious.

1. What are some of the ethical violations of this "counselor"? Explain why you believe each of these items are ethical violations.

2. How would you describe the testing and assessment process to Arturo to make him feel more comfortable and be open to testing and assessment in the future?

Forensic Evaluation

The last subsection of the assessment standards in the ACA Code of Ethics (2014) is code E.13., which addresses the process for forensic evaluations. Counselors are obligated to produce objective findings supported by information and techniques suitable to the evaluation (code E.13.a.). Counselors should form professional opinions based on their professional knowledge and expertise, evidenced by the data gathered in evaluations. They must explain the limits of their reports. Code E.13.b. addresses the consent for the evaluation and notes that written informed consent should be provided to and obtained from the client (parent or guardian if under age 18 or the client is not capable of giving consent). Consent must include an explanation that the relationship is for evaluation purposes and is not therapeutic in nature, while detailing those who will receive the report. The only time informed consent is not needed is if the assessment is court mandated.

Ethical codes E.13.c. and E.13.d. explicitly state that counselors should not evaluate current or former clients, the romantic partners of clients, or a client's family members or friends. Additionally, if you are in a counseling relationship, the other person needs to find their own counselor to evaluate. Potentially harmful relationships of any kind should be avoided with anyone you have provided a forensic evaluation for currently or in the past. These standards sound easy, but they can be challenging. Often clients who need an evaluation come to therapy with the sole purpose of obtaining that evaluation but do not initially disclose the need for a forensic evaluation. In your initial informed consent for therapy, forensic evaluation should be discussed, and the parameters for receiving an evaluation should be addressed in terms of being a current client and posttermination so that there is no surprise to the client. The client can then make an informed decision regarding a therapeutic or evaluative relationship.

LEGAL ISSUES IN ASSESSMENT

Client confidentiality is critical in the counseling process. *Confidentiality* is the right to privacy clients have regarding any information discussed in counseling sessions. Keeping assessment outcomes confidential should be no different than any information we verbally obtain from clients. The release of information to a third party can only occur with the client's consent or if the client is a minor. Counselors do have an obligation to inform parents and guardians of any assessments we provide, and we should discuss the measures in general with them. The only time we must break confidentiality and share information from an assessment would be if we were required to due to state laws. Some conditions under which confidentiality could be broken include harm to self or others, if the client is a minor and that state requires information to be shared with parents or guardians, and if the client asks the counselor to break confidentiality and signs written permission for that counselor to do so. Further, if the counselor is required to defend themselves in court against a legal proceeding from that client, or if the counselor is court ordered and privileged communication does not exist in that state, then the counselor can break confidentiality.

Privileged communications is a legal term referring to the client's privilege to confidentiality regarding any conversation that federal or state law considers protected from court disclosure (i.e., counselor and client, lawyer and client, married partners; Remley & Herlihy, 2019). Each state has its own laws regarding confidentiality and privileged communications. It is incumbent upon the counselor to know what their state laws say, and when confidentiality may not apply for reporting a client's assessment results. Privileged communication laws stemmed from the case of *Jaffee v. Redmond*, WL 315 841 (U.S. 1996). In this case, the Supreme Court, in a unanimous decision, recognized the existence of a psychotherapist–patient privilege under federal common law for all licensed therapists. The Court held that confidential communications between the social worker (in this case) and her client for assessment, diagnosis, or treatment are generally protected from compelled disclosure in a court of law, but also acknowledged that the privilege is not absolute and can be overcome in certain circumstances. The case affirmed the importance of confidentiality in the therapeutic relationship and recognized the potential benefits of protecting private communications between patients and their psychotherapists (Corey et al., 2023; Remley & Herlihy, 2024).

The Health Insurance Portability and Accountability Act

The Health Insurance Portability and Accountability Act (HIPAA) of 1996 is a federal law that protects the privacy and security of individuals' health information and sets standards for healthcare providers and organizations to ensure the confidentiality of patient data. HIPAA does not directly address assessments and tests specifically. However, it does have provisions that relate to the privacy and security of individuals' health information, including any data collected during assessments and tests. Under HIPAA, healthcare providers and organizations must ensure the confidentiality of patient data, including any records or results from assessments and tests. HIPAA is an essential guideline for counselors to follow as all client records would be included under it (U.S. Department of Health and Human Services, 2023).

Family Educational Rights and Privacy Act

The Family Educational Rights and Privacy Act (FERPA), which is a federal law in the United States, gives students and their families certain rights and privacy safeguards when it comes to their educational records. It was passed in 1974 and applies to schools and universities that receive federal funding. FERPA sets rules for how student information can be collected, used, and shared by these institutions. This law plays an important role in safeguarding the privacy and confidentiality of student academic records. With FERPA in place, students have control over who has access to their information while also ensuring transparency and easy access to their own academic records. Critical points of FERPA include (a) rights of access to review and inspect educational records; (b) control over the disclosure of records, with parents and students having control of the release to third parties; (c) directory information, which allows schools to designate certain information in school directories, such as name, email, and phone numbers; (d) written consent requirements from parents and the child to disclose identifiable information from educational records; and (e) enforcement and compliance by the U.S. Department of Education (U.S. Department of Education, 2023). In addition to these federal laws, counselors are guided by a variety of laws and court cases when engaging in assessment. Table 2.1 lists these by name, purpose, and weblinks for obtaining additional information.

TABLE 2.1 KEY LAWS AND COURT CASES FOR ASSESSMENT PRACTICES

Name	Purpose	For More Information
Laws and Education in Assessment		
The Protection of Pupil Rights Amendment of 1978 (PPRA)	The PPRA aims to ensure that parents have the right to inspect instructional materials, surveys, and other information-gathering instruments used in schools. It also seeks to protect students' privacy rights when it comes to the collection, disclosure, and use of personal information.	U.S. Department of Education https://studentprivacy.ed.gov/faq/what-protection-pupil-rights-amendment-ppra
The No Child Left Behind Act of 2001	This act was designed to improve educational outcomes and hold schools accountable for student achievement. It includes school performance ratings, hiring qualified teachers, school of choice, annual yearly progress targets, high-stakes testing, and federal funding laws and requirements.	U.S. Department of Education https://www2.ed.gov/nclb/landing.jhtml
Every Student Succeeds Act (ESSA) in 2015	This replaced the No Child Left Behind Act and focused on state control of educational policy and academic standards, accountability and assessments being high quality, school improvement plans, support for English learners, early childhood education, and educator preparation and support.	U.S. Department of Education www.ed.gov/essa?src%3Drn
Laws and Culture in Assessment		
The Freedom of Information Act Amendments (1996)	This provides individuals with the right to access information held by government agencies and public institutions, such as schools and universities. It gives access to testing and assessment information, scope of information for written documents, exemptions to withholding information, requests to process records, and appeals processes.	U.S. Department of State https://foia.state.gov/learn/foia.aspx
Civil Rights Acts of 1991	This series of federal laws addresses and protects civil rights and equal treatment for all individuals, regardless of protected characteristics such as gender and race. Employers can administer and use test results if they do not discriminate against individuals based on protected characteristics. It encompasses the Civil Rights Act of 1964, the Voting Rights Act of 1965, the Fair Housing Act of 1968, the Civil Rights Act of 1991, and the Americans with Disabilities Act (ADA) of 1990.	U.S. Department of Labor www.archives.gov/milestone-documents/civil-rights-act

(continued)

TABLE 2.1 **KEY LAWS AND COURT CASE FOR ASSESSMENT PRACTICES** (*continued*)

Name	Purpose	For More Information
Vocational Education Act of 1984	Known as the Carl D. Perkins Act of 1984, this federal law funds vocational and technical education programs in the United States. Within the act, each state is required to establish performance measures to evaluate the effectiveness of career and technical education programs.	U.S. Department of Education www.congress.gov/bill/98th-congress/house-bill/4164
Laws and Disability Assessment		
Americans with Disabilities Act of 1990 (ADA)	This federal law in the United States prohibits discrimination against those with disabilities. It ensures that people with disabilities can fairly pursue opportunities such as requiring testing facilities to offer exams with accommodations for those in need.	U.S. Department of Labor www.ada.gov
Guidelines of Equal Employment Opportunity Commission (EEOC)	These federal laws prohibit employment discrimination based on various protected characteristics, such as race and gender. They provide guidelines for a uniform set of principles employers can use for tests.	Equal Employment Opportunity Commission www.eeoc.gov/laws-guidance
Individuals with Disabilities Education Improvement Act of 2004 (IDEIA)	This law makes free public education available to eligible children with disabilities and ensures special education and related services are available to children, such as testing and assessment. It requires schools to come up with Individualized Education Programs (IEPs) for any student with a disability.	U.S. Department of Education www.congress.gov/bill/108th-congress/house-bill/1350
Important Court Decisions		
	Result	
Testing Bias and Placement	*Larry P. v. Riles* (1979): This case challenged the use of IQ tests that placed African American students in special education. The court deemed the tests as culturally biased and that the use led to the disproportionate representation of African American students in special education. As a result, the court ordered IQ tests to be discontinued for the placement of African American students.	*Multicultural Education* https://files.eric.ed.gov/fulltext/EJ1065426.pdf
Cultural Fairness	*Castañeda v. Pickard* (1981): A three-pronged test, known as the Castañeda test, was established by the court to determine whether an assessment is fair for students from culturally and linguistically diverse backgrounds. The test considers if the assessment has a valid purpose, if it is administered fairly, and whether appropriate accommodations are offered for students.	*Language Policy* https://link.springer.com/article/10.1007/s10993-021-09604-1
Diversity in Education	**Parents Involved in Community Schools v. Seattle School District No. 1 (2007):** This Supreme Court case addressed the use of race in school assignment plans. However, the Court also ruled that race could be considered a factor in college admissions to achieve diversity. This established the "diversity rationale" as a constitutional basis for affirmative action.	American Civil Liberties Union www.aclu.org/cases/parents-involved-community-schools-v-seattle-school-district-no-1-and-meredith-v-jefferson

(*continued*)

TABLE 2.1 KEY LAWS AND COURT CASE FOR ASSESSMENT PRACTICES (continued)

Name	Purpose	For More Information
Affirmative Action Practices	***Regents of the University of California v. Bakke* (1978):** This case dealt with affirmative action and racial quotas in college admissions. The court determined that affirmative action was lawful, a ruling that it upheld multiple times, including in the 2003 case *Grutter v. Bollinger,* which allowed schools to use affirmative action in admission processes to promote diversity, and in the 2013 and 2016 cases *Fisher v. University of Texas.*	Library of Congress https://tile.loc.gov/storage-services/service/ll/usrep/usrep438/usrep438265/usrep438265.pdf
Affirmative Action Practices	***Students for Fair Admissions, Inc. v. President and Fellows of Harvard College and Students for Fair Admissions, Inc. v. University of North Carolina* (UNC; 2023):** On June 29, 2023, the Supreme Court ruled that race-based admissions adopted by both Harvard University and UNC were deemed unconstitutional under the Equal Protection Clause of the Fourteenth Amendment.	Supreme Court of the United States www.supremecourt.gov/opinions/22pdf/20-1199_hgdj.pdf
Minimum Competency	***Deborah P v. Turlington* (1981):** This case, also known as the "Florida Student Assessment Test (F-SAT) Case," challenged the constitutionality of Florida's student assessment test as a graduation requirement for high school students. The court ruled the F-SAT violated the Equal Protection Clause and was discriminatory. It was then appealed and then reversed, noting the F-SAT did not violate the equal protection rights of the students. This case highlighted the challenges and concerns associated with high-stakes testing and the potential for disproportionate impacts on certain student populations.	Florida Department of Education www.fldoe.org/accountability/assessments/k-12-student-assessment/archive/history-fl-statewide-assessment/hsap1983.stm
Right to Privacy	***Soroka v. Dayton Hudson* (1991)—aka "Target Case":** Target stores identified problematic emotional characteristics in security guards and intended to use the Minnesota Multiphasic Personality Inventory (MMPI) and the California Psychological Inventory with job applicants. This was deemed by the court to violate privacy rights and was settled out of court.	*Psychological Reports* https://journals.sagepub.com/doi/epdf/10.2466/pr0.1995.77.2.595
Fairness in Testing	***Griggs et al. v. Duke Power Co.* (1960s):** This case involved Duke Power implementing a policy mandating employees to possess a high school diploma or pass specific IQ tests for certain positions with the company. This landmark ruling established "disparate impact," which pertains to discriminatory practices that affect protected groups, irrespective of intent. The decision emphasized the use of valid and job-related criteria when making hiring and promotion decisions to prevent inadvertent discrimination.	Library of Congress https://tile.loc.gov/storage-services/service/ll/usrep/usrep401/usrep401424/usrep401424.pdf

END-OF-CHAPTER RESOURCES

DISCUSSION QUESTIONS

Counselors use a variety of formalized tests in a variety of settings. For example, counselors may administer the BDI-II (Beck et al., 1996) or the Substance Abuse Subtle Screening Inventory-4 (SASSI-4; Lazowski & Geary, 2016).

1. Have you used any of the instruments mentioned in this chapter? Reflect on your experience.
2. What are the assessment instruments that you might utilize in your practice?
3. Are there any that you might not use?
4. How will you engage in testing in a way that avoids repeating the mistake from history?
5. What are critical ethical considerations that counselors must take into account when using psychologic testing and assessment tools with their clients? How can counselors ensure that they are using these tools in a culturally sensitive and appropriate manner?"

CLASS ACTIVITIES

1. In groups of three or four, consider the history of assessment described in this chapter. Choose a recorder and respond to the following questions: What surprises you about these historical facts? What would you like to know more about? How do you see history impacting current testing and assessment issues?
2. Remain in the same groups. Compare and contrast FERPA and HIPAA. Which of these is more difficult to maintain? How is FERPA broken? How is HIPAA broken? What are the consequences of violating these laws?

PERSPECTIVE FROM THE FIELD

 In Chapter 2, we discuss a brief history of assessment and how that history lays the groundwork for ethical issues in assessment today. We provide an overview of ethical issues associated with assessment and testing, including codes of ethics from key associations. In this podcast, we reflect on assessment as a broad range of activities that counselors can conduct in an ethical manner with a preventative approach. Dr. Stephanie F. Dailey reflects on common ethical mistakes when engaging in assessment and offers concrete resources for beginning counselors. Dr. Dailey is a licensed professional counselor and assistant professor of counseling at George Mason University. Dr. Dailey is a former cochair of the American Counseling Association Ethics Committee; a past-president of the Association

for Spiritual, Ethical, and Religious Values in Counseling; and former chair of the American Counseling Association Foundation. Dr. Dailey's research and clinical work is directed at better understanding trauma-informed response protocols for mass casualty events, increasing resilience in first responders, and working with individuals diagnosed with severe mental illness and complex trauma. Her work at the federal level has included trauma-informed mitigation protocols for public schools during active shooter events, officer wellness programs aimed at improving use-of-force decision-making, and stress inoculation training to increase resilience in military medical providers. Dr. Dailey also coleads a national school-based program to address current K–12 school shooter vulnerabilities. She has published and presented extensively on the *Diagnostic and Statistical Manual of Mental Disorders* (*DSM*), counseling assessment, and case conceptualization.

Access podcasts via the QR code or http://connect.springerpub.com/content/book/978-0-8261-8913-4/chapter/ch00.

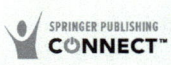

A robust set of instructor resources designed to supplement this text is located at http://connect.springerpub.com/content/book/978-0-8261-8913-4. Qualifying instructors may request access by emailing textbook@springerpub.com.

REFERENCES

American Counseling Association. (n.d.). *Our history*. https://archive.counseling.org/about-us/about-aca/our-history

American Counseling Association. (2014). *2014 ACA code of ethics*. https://www.counseling.org/docs/default-source/default-document-library/ethics/2014-aca-code-of-ethics.pdf

American Educational Research Association, American Psychological Association, & National Council of Measurement in Education. (2014). *Standards for educational and psychological testing*. /https://www.testingstandards.net/uploads/7/6/6/4/76643089/standards_2014edition.pdf

American Mental Health Counselors Association. (2020). *AMHCA code of ethics*. https://www.amhca.org/events/publications/ethics

American Psychological Association. (1954). Technical recommendations for psychological tests and diagnostic techniques. *Psychological Bulletin, 51*(2, Pt.2), 1–38. https://doi.org/10.1037/h0053479

American School Counselor Association. (2022). *ASCA ethical standards for school counselors* (Rev. ed.). https://www.schoolcounselor.org/getmedia/44f30280-ffe8-4b41-9ad8-f15909c3d164/EthicalStandards.pdf

Balkin, R. S., & Juhnke, G. A. (2018). *Assessment in counseling: Practice and application*. Oxford University Press.

Beck, A. T., Steer, R. A., & Brown, G. K. (1996). *Beck Depression Inventory (BDI-II): Manual and questionnaire*. The Psychological Corporation.

Ben-Porath, Y. S., & Tellegen, A. (2020). *Minnesota Multiphasic Personality Inventory-3 (MMPI-3): Manual for administration, scoring, and interpretation*. University of Minnesota Press.

Bowman, M. L. (1989). Testing individual differences in ancient China. *American Psychologist, 44*(3), 576–578. https://doi.org/10.1037/0003-066X.44.3.576.b

Cohen, R. J., Schneider, W. J., & Tobin, R. M. (2022). *Psychological testing and assessment: An introduction to tests and measurement* (10th ed.). McGraw Hill.

Commission on Rehabilitation Counselor Certification. (2023). *Code of professional ethics for rehabilitation counselors*. https://crccertification.com/wp-content/uploads/2023/04/2023-Code-of-Ethics.pdf

Conners, C. K., Erhardt, D., & Sparrow, E. (1998). *Conners' adult ADHD rating scales*. Multi-Health Systems.

Corey, G., Corey, M. S., & Corey, C. (2023). *Issues and ethics in the helping professions* (9th ed.). Cengage Learning.

Corey, G., Corey, M. S., Corey, C., & Callanan, P. (2014). *Issues and ethics in the helping professions* (11th ed.). Cengage Learning.

Cottone, R. R. (2001). A social constructivism model of ethical decision making in counseling. *Journal of Counseling & Development, 79*(1), 39–45. https://doi.org/10.1002/j.1556-6676.2001.tb01941.x

Council for Accrediting Counseling and Related Educational Programs. (2023). *2024 CACREP standards*. https://www.cacrep.org/wp-content/uploads/2023/06/Combined-version-6.21.23.pdf

CS/CS/HB 1557: Parental Rights in Education, 2022 Florida House of Representatives. (Fl. 2022). https://www.flsenate.gov/Session/Bill/2022/1557/BillText/er/PDF

Dubois, P. (1970). *A history of psychological testing*. Allyn and Bacon.

Forester-Miller, H., & Davis, T. E. (2016). *Practitioner's guide to ethical decision making* (Rev. ed.). American Counseling Association. https://www.counseling.org/docs/default-source/ethics/practioner-39-s-guide-to-ethical-decision-making.pdf

Garner, D. M. (2004). *Eating Disorder Inventory™ 3: Professional manual*. Psychological Assessment Resources, Inc. https://www.parinc.com/products/EDI-3

González-Calvo, J., Gonzalez, V. M., & Lorig, K. (1997). Cultural diversity issues in the development of valid and reliable measures of health status. *Arthritis & Rheumatism: Official Journal of the American College of Rheumatology, 10*(6), 448–456. https://doi.org/10.1002/art.1790100613

Hays, D. G. (2017). *Assessment in counseling* (6th ed.). Wiley.

Huang, J., Clarke, K., Milczarski, E., & Raby, C. (2011). The assessment of English language learners with learning disabilities: Issues, concerns, and implications. *Education, 131*(4), 732–739.

Huggett, C., Birtel, M. D., Awenat, Y. F., Fleming, P., Wilkes, S., Williams, S., & Haddock, G. (2018). A qualitative study: Experiences of stigma by people with mental health problems. *Psychology and Psychotherapy: Theory, Research and Practice, 91*(3), 380–397. https://doi.org/10.1111/papt.12167

Jaffee v. Redmond, 518 U.S. 1 (1996). https://supreme.justia.com/cases/federal/us/518/1/

Kitchener, K. S. (1984). Intuition, critical evaluation and ethical principles: The foundation for ethical decisions in counseling psychology. *The Counseling Psychologist, 12*(3-4), 43–55. https://doi.org/10.1177/0011000084123005

Koshy, B., Thomas, H. M., Prasanna, S., Sarkar, R., Kendall, S., & Kang, G. (2017). Seguin form board as an intelligence tool for young children in an Indian urban slum. *Family Medicine and Community Health, 5(4)*, 275–281. https://doi.org/10.15212/FMCH.2017.0118

Lazowski, L. E., & Geary, B. B. (2016). Validation of the Adult Substance Abuse Subtle Screening Inventory-4 (SASSI-4). *European Journal of Psychological Assessment, 35*(1), 86–97. http://doi.org/10.1027/1015-5759/a000359

Lenz, A. S., Ault, H., Balkin, R. S., Barrio Minton, C., Erford, B. T., Hays, D. G., Kim, B. S. K., & Li, C. (2022). Responsibilities of Users of Standardized Tests (RUST-4E): Prepared for the Association for Assessment and Research in Counseling. *Measurement and Evaluation in Counseling and Development, 55*(4), 227–235. https://doi.org/10.1080/07481756.2022.2052321

Meara, N. M., Schmidt, L. D., & Day, J. D. (1996). Principles and virtues: A foundation for ethical decisions, policies, and character. *The Counseling Psychologist, 24*(1), 4–77. https://doi.org/10.1177/0011000096241002

Moses, T. (2010). Being treated differently: Stigma experiences with family, peers, and school staff among adolescents with mental health disorders. *Social Science & Medicine, 70*(7), 985–993. https://doi.org/10.1016/j.socscimed.2009.12.022

Myers, I. B., McCaulley, M. H., Quenk, N. L., & Hammer, A. L. (1998). *MBTI manual: A guide to the development and use of the Myers-Briggs Type Indicator* (3rd ed.). Consulting Psychologists Press.

Myers, J. E., Luecht, R. M., & Sweeney, T. J. (2004). The factor structure of wellness: Reexamining theoretical and empirical models underlying the Wellness Evaluation of Lifestyle (WEL) and the Five-Factor Model. *Measurement and Evaluation in Counseling and Development, 36*, 194–208. https://doi.org/10.1080/07481756.2004.11909742

Myers, J. E., & Sweeney, T. J. (2005). *The Five Factor Wellness Inventory*. Mindgarden, Inc.

Nápoles-Springer, A. M., & Stewart, A. L. (2006). Overview of qualitative methods in research with diverse populations: Making research reflect the population. *Medical Care, 44*(11), 5–9. https://doi.org/10.1097/01.mlr.0000245252.14302.f4

National Board for Certified Counselors. (2023). *NBCC code of ethics*. https://www.nbcc.org/assets/ethics/nbcccodeofethics.pdf

National Board of Forensic Evaluators. (2022). *Can licensed mental health counselors administer and interpret psychological tests?* https://www.nbfe.net/resources/Documents/Can%20Counselors%20Test.pdf

Neukrug, E. S., & Fawcett, R. C. (2010). *Essentials of testing & assessment: A practical guide for counselors, social workers, and psychologists* (2nd ed.). Brooks/Cole Cengage Learning.

Overton, S. L., & Medina, S. L. (2008). The stigma of mental illness. *Journal of Counseling & Development, 86*(2), 143–151. https://doi.org/10.1002/j.1556-6678.2008.tb00491.x

Remley, T. P., & Herlihy, B. (2019). *Ethical, legal, and professional issues in counseling* (6th ed.). Pearson.

Remley, T. P., & Herlihy, B. (2024). *Ethical, legal, and professional issues in counseling* (7th ed.). Pearson.

Rorschach, H. (1921). *Psychodiagnostik* (H. Huber, Trans.). Bircher. (Original work published 1942).

Spitzer, R. L., Kroenke, K., Williams, J. B., & Löwe, B. (2006). A brief measure for assessing generalized anxiety disorder: The GAD-7. *Archives of Internal Medicine, 166*(10), 1092–1097. https://doi.org/10.1001/archinte.166.10.1092

Stigler, S. M. (1989). Francis Galton's account of the invention of correlation. *Statistical Science, 4*(2), 73–86. https://doi.org/10.1214/ss/1177012580

Strauser, D. R. (2021). *Career development, employment, and disability in rehabilitation: From theory to practice*. Springer Publishing Company.

U.S. Department of Education. (2023). *Family Educational Rights and Privacy Act (FERPA)*. https://www2.ed.gov/policy/gen/guid/fpco/ferpa/index.html

U.S. Department of Health and Human Services. (2023). *Health Insurance Portability and Accountability Act*. https://www.hhs.gov/hipaa/index.html

Wainer, H. (1987). *The first four millennia of mental testing: From ancient China to the computer age*. Educational Testing Services. https://www.ets.org/research/policy_research_reports/publications/report/1987/hwps.html

Watson, J. C., & Sheperis, C. J. (2010). *Counselors and the right to test: Working toward professional parity* (ACAPCD-31). American Counseling Association.

Weech-Maldonado, R., Morales, L. S., Spritzer, K., Elliott, M., & Hays, R. D. (2001). Racial and ethnic differences in parents' assessments of pediatric care in Medicaid managed care. *Health Services Research, 36*(3), 575–594. https://www.ncbi.nlm.nih.gov/pmc/articles/PMC1089243

Wiggins, J. S. (1973). *Personality and prediction: Principles of personality assessment*. Addison-Wesley.

Wilson, F. (2013). *The creation of the National Vocational Guidance Association*. National Vocational Guidance Association. https://www.ncda.org/aws/NCDA/page_template/show_detail/74076?model_name=news_article

Culture and Diversity Considerations in Testing and Assessment

KELLY EMELIANCHIK-KEY AND ADRIANA C. LABARTA

2024 CACREP STANDARD

3.G.5. culturally sustaining and developmental considerations for selecting, administering, and interpreting assessments, including individual accommodations and environmental modifications

As a counselor, cultural competence is something that I need to practice mindfully to ensure that I am not missing a critical piece of the puzzle in assessment, diagnosis, and treatment. I strive to engage in assessment questions that are sensitive to the client's cultural identity, values, and beliefs. Open-ended questions are an easy strategy that allows clients to share their cultural perspective and experiences in a way that is consistent with the assessment process. Culturally competent assessment practices help the counselor create a safe and inclusive environment for the client, which fosters trust and rapport. This is critical as counselors often provide assessments early on in therapy, setting the tone for the client. If assessment practices are not culturally responsive, it could lead to early termination and a failure to build rapport.

MULTICULTURAL COMPETENCE AND CULTURAL HUMILITY IN COUNSELING ASSESSMENT

In Western cultures, there is an overarching assumption that those who perform better on tests are also better or more capable regarding the subject matter. For example, two applicants for a job take an aptitude test. They both perform well, but one scores much better than the other. The one that scored better was a White male in his 30s. The other applicant was a Hispanic male in his 30s, but English is not his first language. Would it be safe to say that the White, middle-aged male will perform better and should receive the job? Not exactly.

The previous example illustrates why multicultural competence (MCC) and cultural humility (CH) in assessment practices is of utmost importance. By assuming that the White male applicant is the better candidate, we have not considered the various other factors that could have played a role in the assessment process. The assumption that people who perform better on tests will perform better in specific roles is not uncommon; however, it does not account for background and culture. The diverse identities of the client will always impact test outcomes, and these factors must be considered before giving any tests. In this example, the person providing the assessment should know about the test and determine if it has been normed on diverse populations, or if it has been translated into other languages.

Lenz and colleagues (2022) define *standardized testing procedures* in the Responsibilities of Users of Standardized Tests, Fourth Edition (RUST-4E), standards as the "processes for administering, scoring, and interpreting standardized tests according to a manual that is consistently reflective of the guidelines and strategies depicted by the developers of standardized tests for use across instances. These procedures commonly include reference to the testing setting, environment, protocol delivery, recording activities, interpretation, and representation of scores" (p. 2). Standardized tests and testing procedures are commonly used to assist counselors in making decisions or inferences for clients. Testing has been at the center of attention over the years due to the inherent biases in testing and the lack of consideration for diverse test takers. This has led to many legal cases over the past several decades, which have set a precedent for fair testing practices and resulted in laws and amendments that give people rights regarding testing in various domains (see Chapter 2, Table 2.1). According to the American Counseling Association (ACA) Values and Statements, a core professional value of the counseling profession is "honoring diversity and embracing a multicultural approach in support of the worth, dignity, potential, and uniqueness of people with their social and cultural contexts and promoting social justice" (ACA, 2022, para. 1). Further, the profession's values include engaging in culturally responsive assessment practices that consider clients' intersecting identities (i.e., race, ethnicity, disability, gender identity, sexual orientation, etc.) and how these factors contribute or play a role in assessment outcomes.

As professional counselors, developing *multicultural competence* (*MCC*) is critical. MCC is defined as the awareness, knowledge, skills, and action to perform counseling services with skill and effectiveness to culturally diverse clients (Drinane et al., 2016; Ratts et al., 2016). MCC does not exist in a vacuum, and one does not become culturally competent through a single course or counseling experience. This practice requires going beyond competence and engaging in *cultural humility* (*CH*). CH is a counselor's self-reflective practice of nonjudgmental compassion and sensitivity, helping them remain open to cultural encounters and experiences in multiple contexts (Davis et al., 2018; Zhu et al., 2023). Paired together, MCC and CH are powerful skills that help counselors implement more inclusive and equitable approaches. MCC and CH must be infused into every facet of professional counseling practice, including testing and assessment. To build your knowledge and work toward MCC assessment practices, you will take courses throughout the CACREP curriculum and engage in continuing education. However, CH in assessment will take more personal growth work. As you begin to learn about MCC in assessment and what that will look like for you as a professional counselor, consider the following questions to promote your practice of CH:

1. What are my own cultural values, beliefs, and biases, and how did these develop? Reflect on your cultural background, upbringing, and experiences. Consider how these factors shape your worldview and influence your interactions with others.

2. What assumptions, preconceived notions, biases, or stereotypes do I hold about different cultures or communities? Challenge these and gain a deeper understanding of how to avoid passing these onto others.

3. In what ways do I interact with individuals from different cultures? What is my communication style, including verbal and nonverbal cues? Consider if your communication patterns and style may inadvertently communicate authority, superiority, or insensitivity.

4. Do I actively listen? Assess your listening skills and your ability to hear and understand the experiences, perspectives, and wants of others. Practice active listening by suspending judgment, being authentic, asking clarifying (not curious) questions, and showing genuine interest.

5. What are some of the ways I have worked through cultural differences and conflicts? Reflect on how you respond to these situations. Do you handle these situations with a beginner's mind, openness, and a willingness to learn, or do you default to defensiveness?

6. How do I seek ongoing ways to educate and learn about different cultures? Reflect on whether you connect in continuing learning through reading, attending cultural events, personal engagement, or seeking diverse perspectives.

7. What are some of the ways that I actively seek diverse perspectives and engage with people from different backgrounds? Assess the diversity of your personal and professional networks.

8. In what ways do I respond to feedback or critique regarding cultural competence? Assess your receptiveness and openness to feedback related to cultural competence. Reflect on whether you respond with defensiveness or if you use it as an opportunity for growth and learning. Be bold and ask someone for feedback or ask a supervisor for feedback on your receptiveness to feedback related to cultural competence.

9. Do I advocate for equity, social justice, and inclusion? Consider whether you take action to address systemic barriers, biases, and inequities that exist within marginalized populations. Reflect on whether you use your privilege to strengthen marginalized voices and promote inclusivity.

FAIRNESS IN TESTING

I remember when I was a teenager sitting in the cafeteria with all the other students taking the Standardized Achievement Test (SAT). The proctor read all the directions and explained the nature of it being a timed test. Then she stated, "Those with accommodations can continue taking the test past the timer." I thought to myself, "Wait a minute, that doesn't seem fair." Being a teenager, what was fair and unfair was skewed by the lens of my adolescent perspective, which lacked knowledge of fair testing practices. Little did I know that this was an opportunity to promote fairness in testing for those with disabilities.

In the United States, fairness in testing and assessment has been a significant consideration in educational testing and evaluation for at least the last 50 years (Dorans, 2017). In the context of testing among racial groups, assessment refers to the utilization of test scores to make judgments, diagnoses, selections, or other decisions that impact the life circumstances of individual African American, Latinx American, Asian American, or Native American (ALANA) test takers (Helms, 2006). For instance, imagine working with an African American male who has been brought in due to disorderly behavior at home and in school. An assessment is conducted, and the diagnosis and treatment plan are subsequently based on the results of that assessment, which indicate that he has attention deficit hyperactivity disorder (ADHD). However, his score is compared to the mean or standardized scores, and the test mean was normed with a White sample population. Mean scores to which a person or persons are being compared are influenced by racial or cultural factors that were not intended to be assessed by the test (referred to as construct-irrelevant variance). Therefore, the test may produce unfair scores for that individual or group. This client may not actually have ADHD, yet the test might be assessing race or cultural factors. Even when tests are normed specifically for certain populations, it's important to recognize that people are unique, and each person's experiences, while sharing similarities, can be internalized differently. This can lead to variations in scores and can make it challenging to compare test results using normative standards.

The American Educational Research Association (AERA; 2014) defines fairness as the elimination of bias and the fair treatment of all test takers in the assessment process, including equity in the opportunity to learn the material (AERA et al., 2014). Various perspectives on defining fairness can be found in the literature on psychometrics, yet there is a large amount of ambiguity that exists in social sciences when it comes to racial-ethnicity group performance testing. This confusion arises from the intertwined nature of fairness and validity as conceptualized constructs, with only validity being quantifiable (Helms, 2006). Testing fairness broadly encompasses many components beyond the test taker simply taking an exam. It can encompass test content, test construction and design, psychometric properties of the test (reliability and validity), administration, and scoring, as well as appropriate coverage of relevant material and equal opportunities for learning and access to testing (Roever & McNamara, 2006; Irwing & Hughes, 2018). At the core of fairness are validity issues that necessitate consideration in all test development and use stages. There are several models to evaluate fairness in tests, such as the Helms Individual Differences (HID) fairness model (Helms, 2003). More recently, Balkin et al. (2014) developed a model for evaluating test bias and fairness specifically in counseling practice and assessment. The steps in this model include evaluating the theoretical evidence (i.e., content validity), evaluation of psychometric properties, evaluation of the normative sample, and evaluation of factor invariance. The model for evaluating test bias and test fairness encourages counselors to be aware of the theory involved in creating instruments and awareness of the essential psychometric qualities to validate the instrument. These include (a) conceptual linkages of fairness and validity, (b) fairness models, and (c) impressionistic definitions. We encourage you to review Table 3.1, which explores key terms and considerations to evaluate test fairness.

Fairness in Treatment During the Testing Process

Historically, test standardization, administration conditions, and scoring procedures are a few common ways to safeguard that test takers have equal contexts to perform on a test. All of these safeguards should be set in place by the test developers and be clearly laid out for administrators. Think back to any formal standardized test that you have taken in school. What were some of the things that were done to ensure consistency for all? These might include clear directions, time limits placed on the test, rules about taking breaks, specific requirements for proctors, and so on. Test standardization is essential, so test takers have the same opportunities. All clients taking an assessment should be treated with ACA's (2014) six core values of autonomy, justice, fairness, beneficence, nonmaleficence, and veracity. Counselors are responsible for being ethical and following all guidelines for testing and assessment with clients. Intervention is needed if inappropriate behavior or bias from a standardized test proctor or staff member occurs. The same is true if test irregularities or disruptions occur during the testing process. This must be addressed promptly; for example, if a student is taking a national counseling exam and the fire alarm sounds during the administration, the proctor must decide the best course of action following the incident. As an example, the student may be offered an opportunity to retake the test at a later date before scores were calculated. At times, test standardization procedures need to be flexible and appropriate measures should be taken to minimize any adverse impact on test takers.

TABLE 3.1 **EVALUATING TEST FAIRNESS**

Key Considerations in Evaluating Test Fairness
1. *Validity:* Does the test effectively measure what it was intended to assess, and does it align with the desired outcomes? For a test to be considered valid, it must accurately evaluate the knowledge, skills, or competencies that it aims to measure.
2. *Reliability:* Is the assessment consistent (or reliable)? It is important for a test to produce stable results over time and among different individuals or evaluators. Reliable assessments minimize the impact of measurement errors.
3. *Bias and Stereotypes:* Is the assessment subject to any form of bias, including biased language and content? It is crucial to recognize and mitigate any biases or stereotypes that may influence the evaluation process. Those responsible for administering the test should thoroughly scrutinize questions, prompts, and scoring criteria to identify any potential biases that could unfairly disadvantage specific individuals or groups.
4. *Accessibility:* Ensuring equal access to assessments is crucial, particularly for individuals with disabilities or special needs. To promote fairness and equity, appropriate accommodation should be made available, such as extended time or assistive technologies, in order to address specific requirements of test takers. This helps ensure that everyone has an equitable opportunity to participate in the assessment process.
5. *Cultural Sensitivity:* Does the test consider the cultural backgrounds and experiences of test takers as a means to avoid cultural bias? This can be achieved by reading up on the assessment, thoroughly reviewing the test content, and ensuring that normed samples are representative of diverse cultural perspectives. Taking these steps will help promote inclusivity in testing practices.
6. *Transparency:* Are the test instructions and purpose clear, brief, and unambiguous? This ensures that test takers comprehend the expectations and can function to the best of their abilities.
7. *Standardization:* Uniform administration, scoring, and analysis of assessments are vital for fairness. Standardized procedures must be followed to guarantee that all test takers are treated equally and that results can be evaluated fairly.
8. *Test-Taker Preparation:* Are the test takers prepared with access to appropriate resources and preparation materials to familiarize themselves with the assessment content? This step allows for measuring their abilities rather than testing format familiarity and ease.
9. *Scoring:* Do you know how to accurately score the assessment, convert scores (if needed), and make meaning out of the scores? This step is important as it reflects the proficiency and expertise of those responsible for scoring the test. Reliable and valid tests should provide a scoring key that outlines this information. It is crucial for individuals who are scoring the assessment to possess knowledge and skills in translating scores into meaningful information that can be effectively used in counseling sessions and shared with clients.
10. *Feedback and Appeals:* Can you provide clear and constructive feedback to test takers to help them understand their performance and what it means comparatively? It is essential to provide transparent and constructive feedback to test takers in order to help them comprehend their performance and its relative significance. Additionally, it is crucial for test takers to have the opportunity to appeal assessment outcomes if they believe there were inaccuracies or instances of unfairness during the evaluation process.
11. *Ongoing Evaluation:* Do you consistently evaluate if assessments have been updated or retested? It is essential to periodically review and assess assessments for their fairness, validity, and impact. When new versions of assessments are released, test administrators should familiarize themselves with the latest version, scoring system, and interpretation procedures. Feedback from various stakeholders such as test takers, educators, and experts should be considered to make revisions that enhance fairness and maintain high quality standards.

Additionally, flexibility is required to provide equivalent opportunities for other test takers. A standardized test might need some adaptation due to the client's disability status, culture, language, race, ethnicity, or socioeconomic status. Scoring procedures might also need to be adjusted if standardized procedures require it to address the needs of test takers without impact on the validity or reliability of the results. For example, a test might need to be read aloud to a test taker who cannot read, or it may need to be translated into a first language for a test taker who speaks English as a second language. Fairness in the individual test-taking process requires that test takers are treated comparably, which implies *equity*. Equity, however, is not synonymous with equal. For example, some students may need accommodations because English is not their first language, whereas others may need accommodations because they have a diagnosis of ADHD. For scores to be comparable, the accommodations will be different for each, to lessen disadvantages while not creating advantages. Equity is unique to each test taker's specific circumstances (Camilli, 2013). Test taking has expanded in various ways, with technology being a constantly evolving process in test administration. We must ensure each client's understanding of the technology before engaging in the test-taking process on computerized or web-based test versions that they are familiar with. For example, our test results could be biased if we asked our 75-year-old client, who has never used a computer before, to take a web-based assessment.

Fairness as Deficit of Instrument, Measurement, or Cultural Bias

Measurement bias, also known as bias in testing, is defined as "construct underrepresentation or construct irrelevant components of tests that differentially affect the performance of different groups of test takers and consequently the reliability/precision and validity of interpretations and uses of their test scores" (AERA et al., 2014, p. 216). Plainly speaking, any error or distortion during the assessment process causes an incorrect result on the assessment for the client. The two areas of measurement bias are *accessibility bias* and *universal design bias*. Accessibility bias is each client's or test taker's equal chance to demonstrate their ability to perform on the test construct. The universal design is the design of the test and its ability to consider the things that might inhibit a test taker from performing to the best of their ability. These factors can influence a test taker's score and cause a measurement bias.

When a test consistently produces different results for groups or individuals based on aspects such as demographics or culture, the test measures that aspect of the person's demographic or culture, not the construct it was designed to measure. This instrument would be labeled as having *content bias*, as the constructs are not being measured appropriately within the item content on the test. Ways to check for content bias include statistical procedures called *differential item functioning* (DIF). DIF are various statistical methods that test developers can use to analyze the difficulty of the items for various groups of people (e.g., men and women or different racial groups; Penfield & Camilli, 2006). The statistic seeks to determine if people of equal abilities contrast in their probabilities of responding to a test item correctly as a product of group membership. When an item is complicated or discriminatory for one group compared to another, regardless of their underlying abilities, it implies that item or content bias may exist. *Item bias* can arise due to cultural or linguistic differences, prior experiences, or other factors. Items that have DIF do not always indicate bias; there needs to be a reasonable explanation that accounts for the differences. An example of DIF might be on an IQ test. Maybe a question asks the test taker, "What is a football?" For someone from the United States, that might be an oval-shaped ball used to play a sport. For someone from Spain, it might be a round ball that those in the United States call a soccer ball. If a test contains too many items with DIF for different groups, it will result in *differential test functioning* (*DTF*) where groups of items function differently for defined groups. When DTF occurs, those from different groups (racial or cultural) with the same standing do not have the same projected test score.

The occurrence of groups performing inversely when examining patterns in test scores is differential prediction or *predictive bias*. There may be concerns about bias in the inferences drawn from test scores when there is evidence of differences in the associations between test scores and other variables for different groups. For example, imagine that a company administers a pre-employment assessment to applicants to forecast their future job performance. The assessment consists of multiple-choice questions examining cognitive abilities. Over time, the company observed that applicants under 30 years of age score better than applicants over the age of 40. The company then decides to evaluate performance on the job after a year of employment. They find that the assessment scores correlate with job performance for younger and older employees. Still, when examining equally qualified older and younger employees with identical assessment scores, they discover that older employees consistently perform better than predicted, while younger employees perform worse than predicted. The predictive bias occurs because the assessment overestimates the future job performance of younger applicants and underestimates the performance of older applicants, even though both groups have identical assessment scores.

Other forms of bias include social desirability bias, examiner's language bias, inequitable social consequences, and insufficient standardization practices (Reynolds & Suzuki, 2012). *Social desirability bias* is when test takers try to respond in a certain way to fit in with desirable responses. For example, clients from cultures that perceive mental health issues as shameful may downplay their symptoms or give socially desirable answers that are acceptable in their culture and would not flag a mental health condition, rather than reporting their true experiences. *Examiner's language bias* is the use of unfamiliar or confusing language, stemming from linguistic or cultural differences, that can lead to inaccurate test results that do not reflect the individual's abilities or knowledge, but rather their language proficiency or cultural familiarity with the examiner's communication style. *Inequitable social consequences* arise when test results and interpretations result in unfair advantages or disadvantages for groups because they were based on stereotypes, past experiences, or factors such as race, ethnicity, socioeconomic status, gender, or cultural background. *Insufficient standardization practices* refers to inadequate or inconsistent methods used in the development, administration, scoring, and interpretation of tests (or test norming). These insufficient practices can lead to unreliable test results, compromised validity, and potential unfairness to test takers.

Fairness in the Constructs Measured

Fairness in the constructs measured refers to the objective that all test takers have the potential to be assessed accurately and represent the construct being measured in the assessment. Promoting fairness in the measured constructs demands careful reflection of the assessment's purpose, relevance, diversity, and cultural sensitivity. There are a few different issues in test construction and fairness concerns that could result in skewed results. *Construct underrepresentation* is when the test measures part of the intended construct and omits important knowledge or skills, thus not capturing the full extent of the construct. *Construct-irrelevant variance*, another type of error in test construction, describes when a test measures other constructs irrelevant to the intention of the assessment (Sireci & Randall, 2021). Therefore, construct underrepresentation would be when a test is unfair due to a lack of content or depth, whereas construct-irrelevant variance is when the test might measure something that is culture-specific, which will not produce a true score based on content.

Testing construct and fairness are all outlined by the AERA, the American Psychological Association (APA), and the National Council on Measurement in Education (NCME), all of whom jointly publish the *Standards for Educational and Psychological Testing*, in addition to other organizations listed in Chapter 1, such as the Joint Training and Certification Program (JCTP). Some key recommendations to promote fairness in the constructs measured include: (a) alignment of items with the purpose of the assessment; (b) relevance and meaning in the context of the use of the assessment (e.g., testing an applicant for a cashier position on math skills); (c) representation of diversity in those assessed; (d) cultural sensitivity; (e) avoiding stereotypes and remaining mindful of any implicit or explicit biases; (f) validity evidence that supports the constructs being measured; (g) stakeholder involvement in the development process; and (h) ongoing evaluation and improvement of the constructs being measured based on feedback, research, and evolving needs.

Fairness in Validity of Interpretations

Interpretation of test scores is an essential part of the testing process. Counselors can do everything correctly, but if they do not interpret the scores of a test in an accurate and unbiased manner, all efforts are for nothing. Fairness in validity and interpretations refers to ensuring that the interpretation and use of assessment results are fair, accurate, and free from bias or discrimination. Test administrator bias can be eliminated by being vigilant in avoiding discrimination or bias in the interpretation of assessment results. For example, it is important to ensure that interpretations are free from stereotypes, assumptions, or prejudices based on race, ethnicity, gender, or other protected characteristics. Interpretations should be based solely on relevant assessment evidence and not influenced by irrelevant factors. As professional counselors and test administrators, we are responsible for minimizing bias and prioritizing the client's best interest. When we generalize and interpret across groups (e.g., English-speaking students), it is done for convenience and not to imply homogeneity in all group members or that all group members should be treated similarly when making interpretations. This also applies to the scoring of tests that are completed through electronic means. Electronic means can reduce bias in the test administrator, but technology also has its faults and does not allow for flexibility of standardization if necessary. The test administrator or counselor should review the scores to ensure errors in technology have not occurred.

Other Methods to Promote Fairness and Minimize Bias

Minimizing bias within testing and assessment practices is critical to ensure fair and accurate assessments. We will continue to discuss fairness in testing in several chapters. While some of these may seem redundant, it is crucial to consider all strategies to reduce and minimize bias. The following list contains recommendations to minimize bias in testing practices:

- When developing tests, writers and test editors should be from diverse cultural and ethnic groups. Additionally, different disciplines should be included to minimize bias in test materials and help identify and address potential biases that they may notice from their own cultural perspectives.

- When developing assessments, test developers will seek outside expert reviewers. We will talk about test development more in Chapter 7 but remember to seek out a diverse panel of subject matter expert reviewers.

- Limit language discrepancies between test administrators and test takers. Reducing language barriers that are within your control will help reduce language-related biases and ensure that assessments are fair.

- Avoid assuming that everyone has general knowledge and define terms that cannot be assumed.

- Seek multiple ethnic groups for norming data from the start.

- Identify tests with strong psychometric properties to help eliminate construct biases.

- Train those administering and scoring tests on the intended use of scores to help ensure that assessments are interpreted and used in a fair and unbiased manner.

HIGH-STAKES TESTING

Now that we have discussed the importance of recognizing bias and fairness in assessment, let's explore a relevant topic that has significantly impacted clients, families, educators, and counselors alike: high-stakes testing. *High-stakes testing* describes assessments that evaluate the performance of students and educators. *Mandated* refers to tests that "are required by local, state, and/or federal authority," whereas *high-stakes* indicates "that the assessments have direct and significant consequences for the person or institution being tested or addressed" (Duffy et al., 2009, p. 54). For example, high-stakes tests might include college entrance exams (e.g., SAT) or exit examinations for high school graduation, impacting both the test taker and the school or institution.

High-stakes testing is commonly associated with the *No Child Left Behind* (NCLB) *Act of 2001*, which increased the use of high-stakes assessments to measure academic achievement across schools (see Chapter 2, Table 2.1). The purpose of the NCLB Act was to close the achievement gap and ensure that all children had access to quality education; however, scholars, educators, and policy makers raised concerns regarding fairness and equity in high-stakes testing practices. Reflecting on high-stakes testing and the NCLB Act, the American School Counselor Association (ASCA; 2017) indicated that "When high-stakes assessments are used in this manner, they have a direct and significant effect on the academic future of the student being assessed and, increasingly, on the teacher's career and reputation and the school's status in the community, as well as access to local, state and federal school funding" (para. 3). In 2015, the *Every Student Succeeds Act* (*ESSA*) replaced the NCLB Act in an effort to address equity-related issues by using multiple measures to assess student success, improving accountability for schools and ensuring protections for underserved students (U.S. Department of Education, n.d.), signifying a step forward to enhancing fairness in high-stakes testing.

Understanding the history of high-stakes testing is essential, as standardized assessments impact various facets of our work as counselors as well as the lives of our clients. Although standardized tests can provide helpful information, counselors should recognize that they are solely one facet of a student's learning. As such, ASCA (2017) strongly encourages the use of multiple assessments, such as classroom performance, recommendation letters, personal statements, teacher feedback, and portfolios, to provide a more comprehensive picture of a student's performance. Regardless of their work setting, it is vital that counselors are familiar with the implications of high-stakes assessments and their systemic impacts if not utilized appropriately. As counselors, our ethical duty to advocate for marginalized clients plays a crucial role in understanding how to implement and utilize standardized assessments to empower and facilitate students' and clients' growth. Table 3.2 outlines some of the common pros and cons for the use of high-stakes assessments.

TABLE 3.2 **PROS AND CONS OF HIGH-STAKES TESTING**

Pros	Cons
Accountability: High-stakes tests hold schools, teachers, and students accountable by focusing on improving instruction and student learning outcomes.	**Narrow Curriculum:** High-stakes testing can lead to "teaching to the test," whereby educators focus solely on the material that will be assessed. This practice neglects other essential aspects of education, such as critical thinking, creativity, and problem-solving, and limits teachers' flexibility and creativity in the classroom.
Advancement: For schools, doing well on standardized tests can increase funding. For students, scores on high-stakes tests can mean advancing to the next grade level. For teachers, high-stakes testing can influence salary and promotional opportunities.	**Cutbacks:** For schools, poor performance on standardized tests may restrict public funding. For students, poor performance on high-stakes tests can mean being held back. For teachers, high-stakes testing can have implications for their salary and promotional opportunities.
Data-Driven Decisions: High-stakes testing generates data to assess the effectiveness of educational programs and policies, guiding improvements in curriculum, teaching methods, and resource allocation.	**Stress and Anxiety:** The pressure of high-stakes testing can cause stress and anxiety among students, hindering genuine learning and engagement and potentially leading to negative mental health outcomes.
Improved Performance: Results can aid teachers in creating learning plans based on students' needs.	**Unintended Consequences:** The emphasis on high-stakes testing may incentivize unethical behavior, such as cheating or manipulating test scores, to avoid negative consequences.
Standardization: High-stakes tests can establish a common standard for learning across different schools and districts, ensuring that all students are exposed to a certain level of knowledge and skills.	**Labeling and Misinformed Information:** Low-performing schools and students can face negative labeling and stigmatization, which may not accurately reflect their overall abilities and misinform the public.
Incentives for Improvement: Improved school rankings or increased funding can motivate schools and teachers to strive for better educational outcomes.	**Bias and Inequity:** High-stakes tests may be culturally biased or favor certain socioeconomic groups, leading to inequitable outcomes and perpetuating existing disparities.
Identifying Disparities: High-stakes testing can highlight achievement gaps among different demographic groups and inform specific interventions to meaningfully address these disparities.	**Narrow Assessment:** High-stakes tests often focus on a limited range of skills and knowledge, neglecting important life skills, character development, and other forms of intelligence that are not easily measured by standardized tests.

COUNSELORS AS AGENTS OF CHANGE

As we discussed in Chapter 2, ethical and culturally responsive assessment requires sensitivity to diverse factors, such as racial and ethnic identity, acculturation, age, ability status, gender identity and expression, language, body size, and sexual orientation. If these factors are neglected, assessments can potentially harm and disempower diverse clients and communities. Conversely, when counselors strive to understand clients' diverse cultures, identities, and lived experiences, assessment can serve as a form of advocacy and empowerment. In the following sections, we discuss different factors to consider when assessing diverse client populations. Corresponding recommendations, including informal and formal assessments, and relevant resources for each factor are provided in Table 3.3.

TABLE 3.3 RECOMMENDATIONS AND RESOURCES FOR CULTURALLY RESPONSIVE ASSESSMENT

Diversity Factors	Recommended Assessment Strategies	Helpful Resources
Acculturation and Language	Informal: • Discuss the client's view of the presenting problem from their own cultural framework. • Consider client's acculturation patterns, including how they might vary across contexts and over time. • Explore how various aspects of the client's identity interact with the acculturation process. • Consider sociocultural issues that may influence the client's acculturation process (e.g., discrimination; legislation impacting cultural communities). Formal: • Cultural Formulation Interview (CFI; *Diagnostic and Statistical Manual of Mental Disorders* [5th ed., text revision]; *DSM-5-TR*; American Psychiatric Association, 2022) • Multicultural Acculturation Scale (Wong-Rieger & Quintana, 1987) • Abbreviated Multidimensional Acculturation Scale (Zea et al., 2003) Translator Guidelines (Paniagua, 2014): • Use a translator that shares the client's racial/ethnic background and has training in mental health concerns. • Allow the client and translator to establish rapport. • Establish a structure for the interview, provide sentence-by-sentence translations, and avoid the use of technical terms. • Plan ahead for additional time as needed. • Avoid utilizing a client's friend or relative as a translator, which could lead to misinterpretations.	• *Multicultural and Social Justice Counseling Competencies* (MSJCC; Ratts et al., 2016): www.counseling.org/docs/default-source/competencies/multicultural-and-social-justice-counseling-competencies.pdf?sfvrsn=20 • *Translation and Cross-Cultural Adaptation of Assessments for Use in Counseling Research* (Lenz et al., 2017)

(continued)

TABLE 3.3 **RECOMMENDATIONS AND RESOURCES FOR CULTURALLY RESPONSIVE ASSESSMENT** (*continued*)

Diversity Factors	Recommended Assessment Strategies	Helpful Resources
Sexual Orientation and Gender Identity	Informal: • Understand the presence of heterosexism and transphobia in society, including their potential influence on counseling assessment and diagnosis. • Explore the intersection of gender identity, sexual orientation, and other cultural and social identities that clients hold. • Avoid assuming that all LGBTQ+ clients present to treatment with concerns regarding sexuality or gender. • Review intake paperwork and measures to ensure inclusive language throughout. Formal: • Gender Minority Stress and Resilience Measure (Testa et al., 2015) • The Daily Heterosexist Experiences Questionnaire (Balsam et al., 2013) • Minority Strengths Model (Perrin et al., 2020)	• *Transgender & LGBQQIA Competencies* (Burnes et al., 2010; Harper et al., 2013): https://saigecounseling.org/competencies-2 • *Standards of Care in Assessment of Lesbian, Gay, Bisexual, Transgender, Gender Expansive, and Queer/Questioning (LGBTGEQ+) Persons* (Goodrich et al., 2017)
Disability	Informal: • Infuse a strengths-based approach into the assessment process. • Acknowledge and avoid ableist assessment practices (e.g., viewing disability as a deficit). • Understand the provision of accommodations for testing within your specific setting. • Consider accommodations when interpreting test results. Formal: • Supports Intensity Scale-Children's Version (SIS-C; Thompson et al., 2016) • Supports Intensity Scale-Adult Version, Second Edition (SIS-A; Thompson et al., 2023)	• *Disability-Related Counseling Competencies* (Chapin et al., 2018): www.counseling.org/docs/default-source/competencies/arca-disability-related-counseling-competencies-v51519.pdf
Body Size	Informal: • Engage in self-assessment of anti-fat attitudes that can interfere with the counseling process. • Understand the role of sociocultural factors (e.g., fatphobia in the media, pathologization of larger bodies) and internalized weight bias as risk factors for mental health concerns. • Challenge the use of body mass index (BMI) as a primary indicator of health and avoid the pathologization of larger bodies. • Assess client wellness from a more size-inclusive, holistic lens, inclusive of mental health, physical health, spiritual health, relational health, and so on. Formal: • Anti-Fat Attitudes Test (Lewis et al., 1997) • Weight Bias Internalization Scale (Durso & Latner, 2008)	• *Association for Size Diversity and Health:* https://asdah.org • *National Association to Advance Fat Acceptance:* https://naafa.org

(*continued*)

TABLE 3.3 **RECOMMENDATIONS AND RESOURCES FOR CULTURALLY RESPONSIVE ASSESSMENT** (*continued*)

Diversity Factors	Recommended Assessment Strategies	Helpful Resources
Aging Populations	Informal: • Understand the impact of ageism on counseling by expanding medical models of aging and incorporating wellness into assessment. • Assess the client's current level of wellness using a multidimensional framework. • Utilize a holistic wellness lens to collaborate on treatment goals and identify areas of focus. • Implement strengths-based assessment strategies (as an alternative to deficit-based ones) to explore client's resources. Formal: • Clinical Assessment Scales for the Elderly (CASE; Reynolds & Bigler, 2000) • Mini-Mental State Examination (MMSE; Folstein et al., 2001)	• *Growing Older: Providing Integrated Care for an Aging Population* (Substance Abuse and Mental Health Services Administration & Health Resources and Services Administration, 2016): https://store.samhsa.gov/sites/default/files/d7/priv/sma16-4982.pdf

Acculturation

Culturally responsive counselors acknowledge that assessment constructs may hold different meanings to diverse individuals across various contexts (Hays et al., 2014; O'Hara et al., 2016). If we solely rely on Westernized definitions of mental health and distress, we will likely miss important information on the client's understanding of their presenting concerns. One related construct crucial to multicultural assessment, case conceptualization, and treatment is *acculturation*. Definitions of acculturation have evolved over time, with scholars recognizing its multifaceted and complex nature. For instance, Berry (2017) defined acculturation as "the dual process of cultural and psychological change that takes place as a result of contact between two or more cultural groups and their individual members. At the cultural group level, it involves social structures and institutions and in cultural norms. At the individual psychological level, it involves changes in people's behavioral repertoires (including their food, dress, language, values, and identities) and their eventual adaptation to these intercultural encounters" (p. 15). Berry (1980) also described four corresponding acculturation patterns, which are defined in the list that follows.

- *Integration*: Client integrates values/beliefs from both their original culture and the dominant culture.

- *Assimilation*: Client identifies with the values/beliefs of the dominant culture and rejects those of their original culture.

- *Separation*: Client identifies with the values/beliefs of their original culture and rejects those of the dominant culture.

- *Marginalization*: Client rejects both their original culture and the dominant culture.

Although these acculturation patterns can be useful for client conceptualization, it is also important to remember that people are highly diverse, hold various intersecting identities, and experience cultural and contextual factors that influence their acculturation process. Acknowledging the multidimensional and complex nature of acculturation, Garcia et al. (2020) proposed the Integrated Acculturation Model (IAM), which encompasses psychologic (affective and cognitive components of identity development), instrumental (norms and values of each cultural identity, including language), contextual (contextualizing factors that influence a person's acculturation process, such as social climate), and developmental levels (consideration of ever-changing life-span issues) of interaction. Specifically, Garcia et al. sought to address the gaps in acculturation models by combining existing frameworks, expanding the construct to include other cultural identities (in addition to race and ethnicity), and accounting for larger contextual and systemic factors. For example, a South Asian adolescent who immigrated to the United States with his family feels a greater sense of belonging (*psychologic level*) at home than at school (*contextual level*). As such, he might feel pressured to speak English across contexts to assimilate into the dominant American culture (*instrumental level*). During this initial transition, he struggles with *acculturative stress*, or stress that is linked to factors associated with the acculturation process, such as learning a new language, negotiating differences across cultures, experiences of discrimination, and the conflict with integrating one's original culture with the dominant culture (Katsiaficas et al., 2013). As he moves into young adulthood, however, he begins to develop meaningful connections with people of diverse racial/ethnic identities, influencing his acculturation process and leading to the integration of his South Asian and American cultural identities (*developmental level*). As we can see from this example, there are various factors at play that can influence an individual's acculturation process, potentially influencing their lived experience of mental health and wellness throughout the life span.

Language

Language plays a crucial role in our everyday lives, influencing how we communicate, connect with others, and make meaning of our experiences. In counseling, language helps us understand our clients' struggles, goals, and needs within the therapeutic setting. Therefore, ensuring that assessments are cross-culturally valid is imperative. Consider the example earlier in this chapter regarding the two male job applicants. On the surface, one might assume that the White male is the stronger applicant. However, a culturally responsive approach encourages us to look beyond scores and consider contextual factors influencing an individual's performance. Since the Hispanic male applicant's first language is not English, equity and fairness in testing should be addressed. By not providing the opportunity for the applicant to complete the test in his first language, we receive an incomplete picture of his skills or strengths, potentially leading to a biased assessment of his future job performance.

Counseling professionals are responsible for ensuring that all test takers are provided with the same opportunities. Thus, one must determine if English is the test taker's first language. We would not want to interpret the test score based on the person's ability to read, write, or interpret the English language, unless the test's purpose was to interpret English proficiency. An example when this is really important to consider is when deciphering a learning disability or neurodivergence. We would not want the score to be based on understanding of the language or culture.

There are a few options that a counselor might consider when working with clients with limited English proficiency, including the use of a translator, test adaptation, or test translation. However, there can be limitations to using a translator in counseling (e.g., misinterpretation, inability to capture the client's thoughts, client discomfort). Interpreting written tests ourselves before or after a client takes them could also become problematic due to difficulty in interpreting directions, a lack of translating back to the original language, and the translations of some terms that are not universal across cultures. An example of this is the term *bully*, which has no direct equivalent in Portuguese. To combat some of these challenges, Paniagua (2014) provides helpful recommendations to consider, some of which are included in Table 3.3. Furthermore, many counseling assessments have now been adapted to incorporate the needs of underrepresented groups (who may have not been included in the original norming samples) or translated into different languages, promoting greater accessibility for use across cultures.

Sexual/Affectional Orientation

Sexual or affectional orientation is another relevant diversity factor to consider regarding counseling assessment. Imagine the following scenario: A lesbian couple begins couples counseling at a local community agency. As they complete the couples counseling intake forms, they notice heterosexist language, such as "wife" and "husband," throughout the items on a relationship satisfaction scale. Even if the agency had adopted a widely used measure, heteronormative bias remains a crucial limitation. As a result, the couple may feel frustrated and unseen before they enter their session. This example not only sheds light on the importance of inclusive language and terminology, but also the need for instruments that are validated on sexual or affectional minority populations.

Heteronormativity describes the assumption that heterosexual identities or relationships are the standard in society, thus silencing and marginalizing LGBQ+ identities. This prevailing assumption can be harmful to sexual minority individuals, potentially leading to internalized stigma or an internalized negative view of one's sexuality (e.g., internalized homophobia; Puckett & Levitt, 2015). For example, research shows that sexual minority individuals may experience *minority stress*, or the distress related to experiences of oppression, which are associated with adverse mental health (Meyer, 2003). Minority stress distinguishes between two different stressors that an individual might experience: distal and proximal. *Distal stressors* are processes that are external to the individual, including discrimination, harassment, and rejection. *Proximal stressors*, on the other hand, are those that are internal, including internalized homophobia, concealment of sexual orientation identity, and hypervigilance due to safety concerns. Meyer's (2003) minority stress theory provides a helpful framework to understand significant health disparities within LGBQ+ communities and to explore potential stressors that might be impacting a client's mental health. Assessment of coping strategies and social support are also inherent in the minority stress theory, such as LGBQ+ community connectedness. For example, Alessi's (2014) proposed framework for incorporating the minority stress into treatment includes a two-part assessment process. First, counselors examine four components of minority stress (i.e., exposure to prejudice, internalized homophobia, sexual orientation concealment, and stigma), followed by the client's coping, emotion regulation, and social and cognitive processes.

Gender Identity

Gender identity is how one fundamentally understands and describes their own gender. It is the gender that a person intrinsically views themselves as, whether that be male, female, a combination of both, or neither. A person's gender identity may align with the sex they were assigned at birth, or it may differ (Human Rights Campaign, n.d.). The intersection of gender and assessment has been widely studied in the mental health professions. Gender roles and norms can impact the way that individuals perceive mental health concerns. For example, femininity is often associated with qualities like sensitivity, emotionality, and passivity, whereas masculinity is associated with aggressiveness, emotional toughness, and dominance. If biases are left unchecked, socially constructed gender norms can impact the assessment and diagnosis process in serious ways.

Gender is a common factor that can lead to misdiagnosis in assessment of clients (Bruchmüller et al., 2012; Fruzzetti, 2017). A recent study examining competence in treating teen dating violence (TDV) discovered *gender bias* in counseling students' responses to prompts on male and female client case vignettes (Emelianchik-Key et al., 2023). Although the case vignettes were identical (with only the client/survivor's pronouns changed), students were more likely to identify the female client as a survivor of TDV. Overall, the researchers found major differences in diagnosis, conceptualization, and treatment of the fictitious client. This is just one example of gender biasing on informal assessment of a client. Counselor biases and misdiagnosis can have harmful consequences on the treatment process, perpetuating stigma associated with specific diagnoses and potentially leading to client disempowerment.

Additionally, stereotype threat can cause test takers to perform worse on assessments. The test takers will perform worse on tests due to anxiety surrounding the stereotypes that are associated with their gender. Socialization and cultural norms around gender-related differences can also influence test results as well as differences in gender-related self esteem and self efficacy. Tests can also be biased and favor one gender over another as mentioned earlier in the discussion about measurement bias and DIF.

Similar to heteronormativity and homophobia, transphobia is another construct that is relevant to assessment with transgender and gender diverse clients. *Transphobia* describes prejudice toward transgender individuals, or those who do not identify with traditional cisgender identities. Transgender and gender nonconforming individuals may experience internalized transphobia, or an internalized negative view of their gender identities. Indeed, Meyer's (2003) minority stress theory was expanded to encompass minority stress experiences in transgender communities, resulting in the development of the Gender Minority Stress and Resilience scale (Testa et al., 2015). Such formal assessments can be helpful for counselors to understand the potential role of gender minority stress on clients' mental health and well-being, as well as resilience strategies that serve as protective factors (e.g., community connectedness and pride). Efforts to minimize gender-based disparities in assessment scores should focus on creating equitable learning environments, addressing biases, and promoting a growth mindset to help all students reach their full potential regardless of their gender.

Disability

In the United States, persons with disabilities (PWD) comprise one of the largest minority groups, including more than one in four adults (28.7%; Centers for Disease Control and Prevention, 2024) and about one in five children (19.4%; U.S. Census Bureau, 2022). There are various types of disabilities, including vision, hearing, cognitive, ambulatory, self-care, and independent living difficulties (U.S. Census Bureau, 2021). Section 504 of the Rehabilitation Act of 1973 provides protections for individuals with disabilities and forbids organizations and employers from engaging in discriminatory practices that inhibit PWDs from receiving equal access and opportunities. For instance, within a school setting, a student with a diagnosis of ADHD may qualify for accommodations for testing, such as extended time or a separate testing area. Such accommodations are developed collaboratively by school staff, caregivers, and the student, and documented in a 504 plan. The student's school counselor would also serve an instrumental role in this process by consulting with school staff, participating on multidisciplinary teams to assess student needs, and advocating for students with disabilities in the school community (ASCA, 2022b).

Despite the prevalence of disability, PWDs are often overlooked across counseling specialty areas (Emir Öksüz & Brubaker, 2020). Ensuring accessibility during the assessment process is of utmost importance across counseling settings. If counselors proceed with standardized administration without consideration of a client's disability, assessment results may be invalid (Chapin et al., 2018). It is recommended that counselors consult with their client, in addition to other professionals with relevant expertise, to determine appropriate accommodations as needed. Chapin et al. (2018) also encourage counselors to approach counseling assessment from a strengths-based perspective when working with PWDs, which is in contrast to the medical model focusing on "fixing the individual" (Emir Öksüz & Brubaker, 2020, p. 165). As such, an empowerment-based and collaborative approach is imperative to effective counseling assessment with clients with disabilities.

Body Size

Body size is a dimension of identity that is often disregarded in multicultural counseling scholarship. Nonetheless, it is a critical construct that counselors should be familiar with to promote culturally responsive assessment. To illustrate the importance of body size, let us consider the following scenario: A young adult client with a larger body presents to her university's counseling center for an intake appointment. Upon meeting with the counselor, she primarily reports feelings of sadness, isolation, and disconnection from others. The client also indicates that she has struggled with her weight throughout her life and feels dissatisfied with her body. The counselor proceeds to further assess the client's "wellness practices," specifically inquiring about her current diet and exercise. At the end of the session, the counselor recommends short-term therapy for depressive symptoms and provides a referral to the on-campus dietician for weight management.

Although the counselor may have been well-intentioned with their recommendations, this example illustrates the presence of weight bias in counseling. *Weight bias* describes negative beliefs, attitudes, or assumptions toward people in larger bodies. Weight bias is pervasive in Western culture due to sociocultural standards of beauty and the idealization of thinner bodies. In the previous scenario, the counselor neglected to further assess the client's relationship with her body, which may have potentially led to a conversation about internalized weight bias, experiences of discrimination, and subsequent feelings of disconnection from others. Instead, the counselor's assumption may have been that the client can achieve happiness or wellness if she better manages her weight. Indeed, research has shown that counselors are not immune to weight bias in counseling, with clients of size sharing experiences of microaggressions from counselors (Akoury et al., 2019). Although assessment-related sizeism scholarship is lacking in the counseling field, researchers are increasingly recognizing the importance of addressing weight bias in counseling (e.g., Kerl-McClain et al., 2022; McHugh & Chisler, 2019).

Aging Populations

According to the U.S. Census Bureau (2020), about 16.8% of the U.S. population are 65 and older, marking an increase of 50.9 million since 1920. As the need for mental health services grows alongside the rise in aging populations, the assumption that older adults' needs are mainly physiologic impacts care in myriad ways, such as overemphasizing physical well-being rather than holistic well-being (Ng et al., 2015). Scholars posit that such perceptions may lead to *ageism*, or discrimination toward older adults, in counseling (Fullen, 2018). Imagine, for instance, that a 68-year-old man begins counseling at a private practice agency. He reported struggling with his recent transition to retirement as he grew accustomed to a very active and busy life. The client also indicated experiencing fatigue and restlessness over the past few months. Adopting a medical conceptualization of the aging process may help with understanding physical health concerns. Yet, it may overlook the connection between the client's physical and emotional concerns in the context of his recent transition to retirement.

In response to this gap, Fullen (2019) developed a framework for aging well, including the following eight dimensions: (1) developmental, (2) physical, (3) emotional, (4) relational, (5) contextual, (6) vocational, (7) spiritual, and (8) cognitive. This multidimensional framework can be introduced to clients during the initial assessment process to explore various facets of wellness and identify needs and goals. For instance, counselors can pose the following question to generate discussion: "Previous research shows that having a positive perception of aging is related to longevity. How would you describe your perceptions of growing older?" (Fullen, 2019, p. 70). Although more research and validated wellness assessments for older adults are needed, scholars have provided helpful assessment recommendations for counseling older adults, which are included in Table 3.3.

CULTURALLY RESPONSIVE ASSESSMENT ACROSS COUNSELING SETTINGS

Regardless of the setting within which you work, culturally responsive assessment is an ethical imperative. In addition to the ACA (2014), the codes of ethics across counseling specialty areas, including the ASCA (2022a), the Commission on Rehabilitation Counselor Certification (CRCC; 2023), the American Mental Health Counselors Association (AMHCA; 2020), and the International Association of Marriage and Family Counselors (IAMFC; 2017), underscore the role of multicultural assessment. Even so, biases remain in the field of counseling assessment. Counselors will encounter clients of diverse, intersecting cultural identities across settings, highlighting the need to ensure appropriate and ethical utilization of counseling assessments. We also acknowledge that there are other identity factors that were not discussed in this chapter, such as socioeconomic status, religious/spiritual identity, and education level. These are also important considerations to better understand our clients and related risk and protective factors.

Counselors can work toward adopting more culturally sensitive assessment practices, including formal and informal strategies, that meet the needs of diverse populations. Although we discussed various recommendations for multicultural counseling, several themes can be highlighted:

1. Counselors should understand that not all assessments have been normed on diverse client groups; as such, assessments should be selected with this in mind.

2. Various forms of bias can exist within formal counseling assessment. Counselors serve an important role in using assessment as a form of advocacy rather than a form of disempowerment.

3. Assessments on marginalized populations have historically focused on deficits or risk factors. While these are important to consider, counselors should also assess clients' strengths by adopting strengths-based assessment approaches.

4. No single assessment can fully capture all clients' experiences. Therefore, counselors should consider using multiple assessment methods to ensure a comprehensive picture of the client's presenting concerns and resources and explore these collaboratively with the client.

As you continue reading this text, we encourage you to continue reflecting on ways that you can use counseling assessment to connect with and empower your clients. Although assessment is an ongoing process, counseling often begins with an intake or biopsychosocial evaluation. Counselors can initiate the assessment process with CH, curiosity, and openness, creating an inclusive environment for clients with diverse identities across the life span.

CHECKING IN WITH HENRY

When Henry was 10 years old, his father sent him to a psychiatrist to "fix" what was wrong with him, stating that he "was acting up and not the same kid that he was before his mother died." Upon the initial phone call, the psychiatrist said he knew what was happening and would evaluate further during Henry's appointment. The psychiatrist spent 20 minutes with Henry's father and about 20 minutes with Henry. He gave Henry two assessments, but Henry struggled to answer the questions on the first and refused to take the second one. The psychiatrist then noted, "It was exactly as I initially thought," and diagnosed Henry with a conduct-related disorder. Black youth are diagnosed with conduct and behavioral-related disorders more often than their White counterparts (Ballentine, 2019; Liang et al., 2016).

Henry's father sent him to counseling for a brief period of time before he left home at 18 years of age. During this time, the counselor connected with Henry and strongly felt that he did not have a conduct disorder. She recognized that Henry's "acting up" behaviors were manifestations of his grief, identity concerns, and lack of support. Henry connected with his female counselor, feeling supported and less angry when he was with her. Ultimately, he was able to open up about his mother. However, Henry did not receive the support he needed at home and was continually compared to his stepsiblings, who often teased Henry for being different. This is when Henry dropped out of therapy and began to engage in alcohol use.

1. What types of bias did Henry experience in the assessment process with his psychiatrist?

2. What types of questions should the psychiatrist have asked Henry during the assessment process and before diagnosing him?

3. What therapeutic qualities or approaches helped facilitate a positive relationship between Henry and his counselor?

4. How does acculturation play a role in Henry's presenting problem?

END-OF-CHAPTER RESOURCES

DISCUSSION QUESTIONS

1. Name three ways that counselors can facilitate an inclusive, affirming, and collaborative intake interview with their clients. How can counselors continue to integrate these strategies to promote ongoing assessment with clients?

2. Identify potential risks of using assessments that have not been normed or validated on culturally diverse populations. How might these risks impact the counseling and treatment process?

3. Reflect on potential opportunities and challenges with integrating culturally responsive assessment practice across counseling settings, including schools, inpatient facilities, community agencies, or private practices. How can you use assessment as a form of advocacy within your specific setting?

CLASS ACTIVITIES

1. **Reflection and Discussion:** Assign the *Multicultural and Social Justice Counseling Competencies* (MSJCC; Ratts et al., 2016) as a pre-class reading. Together, discuss how these competencies can be integrated into the assessment process with diverse clients. Consider and review the developmental domains (i.e., counselor self-awareness, client worldview, counseling relationship, and counseling and advocacy interventions) and aspirational competencies (i.e., attitudes and beliefs, knowledge, skills, and action) of the MJSCC model, particularly in the context of counseling assessment.

2. **In-Class Role-Play:** Ask students to work in pairs and practice broaching culture in the assessment process using the case of Henry. Each student will take turns playing the role of Henry and the counselor. Then, process the overall experience as a class. Consider the following questions in your overall discussion:

   a. As the counselor, what were your strengths as the counselor? What challenges did you encounter?

   b. As the client, what strategies did your counselor use that were helpful and affirming?

   c. How will this activity inform the way you will approach counseling assessment in the future?

3. **Group Project:** Divide students into small groups and assign a specific cultural identity to research in more depth (e.g., race/ethnicity, LGBTQ+, body size, etc.). Each student will identify a different peer-reviewed article related to their population and collaborate on a brief presentation, including the following: (a) key aspects from the literature, (b) discussion questions to facilitate reflection, and (c) strategies for building cultural competence. Students will deliver their presentations to the class to facilitate deeper insight into various cultural identities.

PERSPECTIVE FROM THE FIELD

The primary goal of this chapter was to examine the importance of culture and diversity in the assessment process, with an emphasis on ensuring fair and equitable testing practices. As discussed, high-stakes testing is critical in schools, posing several benefits, limitations, and consequences for students, educators, and other stakeholders. In this podcast, chapter coauthor Dr. Adriana C. Labarta interviews Dr. Eleanor Su-Keene to better understand these issues. Dr. Su-Keene is a former public school teacher and an interdisciplinary researcher interested in school improvement from a health and social justice perspective. She utilizes her former training in the biological sciences and educational leadership to examine the impacts of job-related stress on personal health and self-efficacy in the principalship and the enactment of socially just leadership to improve schools for marginalized students. Dr. Su-Keene is currently an assistant professor at Texas A&M University in the Department of Teaching, Learning, and Culture. In this podcast, Dr. Su-Keene shares her practitioner experiences with high-stakes testing and explores existing challenges.

Access podcasts via the QR code or http://connect.springerpub.com/content/book/978-0-8261-8913-4/chapter/ch00.

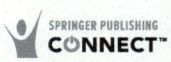 A robust set of instructor resources designed to supplement this text is located at http://connect.springerpub.com/content/book/978-0-8261-8913-4. Qualifying instructors may request access by emailing textbook@springerpub.com.

REFERENCES

Akoury, L. M., Schafer, K. J., & Warren, C. S. (2019). Fat women's experiences in therapy: "You can't see beyond . . . unless I share it with you." *Women & Therapy, 42*(1–2), 93–115. https://doi.org/10.1080/02703149.2018.1524063

Alessi, E. (2014). A framework for incorporating minority stress theory into treatment with sexual minority clients. *Journal of Gay & Lesbian Mental Health, 18*(1), 47–66. https://doi.org/10.1080/19359705.2013.789811

American Counseling Association. (2014). *2014 ACA code of ethics*. Author. https://www.counseling.org/docs/default-source/default-document-library/ethics/2014-aca-code-of-ethics.pdf?sfvrsn=55ab73d0_1

American Counseling Association. (2022). *Values and statements*. Author. https://www.counseling.org/about-us/about-aca/values-and-statements

American Educational Research Association, American Psychological Association, & National Council on Measurement in Education. (2014). *Standards for educational and psychological testing*. https://www.testingstandards.net/uploads/7/6/6/4/76643089/standards_2014edition.pdf

American Mental Health Counselors Association. (2020). *AMHCA code of ethics*. https://www.amhca.org/events/publications/ethics

American Psychiatric Association. (2022). *Diagnostic and statistical manual of mental disorders* (5th ed., text rev.). https://doi.org/10.1176/appi.books.9780890425787

American School Counselor Association. (2017). *The school counselor and high-stakes testing*. https://www.schoolcounselor.org/Standards-Positions/Position-Statements/ASCA-Position-Statements/The-School-Counselor-and-High-Stakes-Testing

American School Counselor Association. (2022a). *ASCA ethical standards for school counselors*. https://www.schoolcounselor.org/About-School-Counseling/Ethical-Responsibilities/ASCA-Ethical-Standards-for-School-Counselors-(1)

American School Counselor Association. (2022b). *The school counselor and students with disabilities*. https://www.schoolcounselor.org/Standards-Positions/Position-Statements/ASCA-Position-Statements/The-School-Counselor-and-Students-with-Disabilitie

Balkin, R. S., Heard, C. C., Lee, S., & Wines, L. A. (2014). A primer for evaluating test bias and test fairness: Implications for multicultural assessment. *Journal of Professional Counseling: Practice, Theory & Research, 41*(1), 42–52. https://doi.org/10.1080/15566382.2014.12033932

Ballentine, K. L. (2019). Understanding racial differences in diagnosing ODD versus ADHD using critical race theory. *Families in Society, 100*(3), 282–292. https://doi.org/10.1177/1044389419842765

Balsam, K. F., Beadnell, B., & Molina, Y. (2013). The Daily Heterosexist Experiences Questionnaire: Measuring minority stress among lesbian, gay, bisexual, and transgender adults. *Measurement and Evaluation in Counseling and Development, 46*(1), 3–25. https://doi.org/10.1177/0748175612449743

Berry, J. W. (1980). Acculturation as varieties of adaptation. In A. M. Padilla (Ed.), *Acculturation: Theory, models and some new findings* (pp. 9–25). Westview Press.

Berry, J. W. (2017). Theories and models of acculturation. In S. J. Schwartz & J. Unger (Eds.), *The Oxford handbook of acculturation and health* (1st ed.). Oxford University Press.

Bruchmüller, K., Margraf, J., & Schneider, S. (2012). Is ADHD diagnosed in accord with diagnostic criteria? Overdiagnosis and influence of client gender on diagnosis. *Journal of consulting and clinical psychology, 80*(1), 128–138. https://doi.org/10.1037/a0026582

Burnes, T. R., Singh, A. A., Harper, A. J., Harper, B., Maxon-Kann, W., Pickering, D. L., Moundas, S., Scofield, T. R., Roan, A., & Hosea, J. (2010). American Counseling Association competencies for counseling with transgender clients. *Journal of LGBTQ Issues in Counseling, 4*(3), 135–159. http://doi.org/10.1080/15538605.2010.524839

Camilli, G. (2013). Ongoing issues in test fairness. *Educational Research and Evaluation, 19*(2-3), 104–120. https://doi.org/10.1080/13803611.2013.767602

Centers for Disease Control and Prevention. (2024). *Disability impacts all of us*. https://www.cdc.gov/ncbddd/disabilityandhealth/infographic-disability-impacts-all.html

Chapin, M., McCarthy, H., Shaw, L., Bradham-Cousar, M., Chapman, R., Nosek, M., Peterson, S., Yilmaz, Z., & Ysasi, N. (2018). *Disability-related counseling competencies*. American Rehabilitation Counseling Association. https://www.counseling.org/docs/default-source/competencies/arca-disability-related-counseling-competencies-v51519.pdf

Commission on Rehabilitation Counselor Certification. (2023). *Code of professional ethics for certified rehabilitation counselors*. https://crccertification.com/wp-content/uploads/2023/04/2023-Code-of-Ethics.pdf

Council for Accreditation of Counseling and Related Educational Programs. (2023). *2024 CACREP standards*. https://www.cacrep.org/wp-content/uploads/2023/06/Combined-version-6.21.23.pdf

Davis, D. E., DeBlaere, C., Owen, J., Hook, J. N., Rivera, D. P., Choe, E., Van Tongeren, D. R., Worthington, E. L. Jr., & Placeres, V. (2018). The multicultural orientation framework: A narrative review. *Psychotherapy, 55*(1), 89–100. https://doi.org/10.1037/pst0000160

Dorans, N. J. (2017). Contributions to the quantitative assessment of item, test, and score fairness. In R. Bennett & M. von Davier (Eds.), *Advancing human assessment: The methodological, psychological and policy contributions of ETS* (pp. 201–230). Springer.

Drinane, J. M., Owen, J., Adelson, J. L., & Rodolfa, E. (2016). Multicultural competencies: What are we measuring? *Psychotherapy Research, 26*(3), 342–351. https://doi.org/10.1080/10503307.2014.983581

Duffy, M., Giordano, V. A., Farrell, J. B., Paneque, O. M., & Crump, G. B. (2009). No Child Left Behind: Values and research issues in high-stakes assessments. *Counseling and Values, 53*(1), 53–66. https://doi.org/10.1002/j.2161-007X.2009.tb00113.x

Durso, L. E., & Latner, J. D. (2008). Understanding self-directed stigma: Development of the weight bias internalization scale. *Obesity, 16*(S2), S80–S86. https://doi.org/10.1038/oby.2008.448

Emelianchik-Key, K., Glass, B., & Labarta, A. C. (2023). Teen dating violence: Examining counseling students' responses to gendered vignettes. *The Professional Counselor, 13*(2), 98–111. https://doi.org/10.15241/kek.13.2.98

Emir Öksüz, E., & Brubaker, M. D. (2020). Deconstructing disability training in counseling: A critical examination and call to the profession. *Journal of Counselor Leadership and Advocacy, 7*(2), 163–175. https://doi.org/10.1080/2326716X.2020.1820407

Folstein, M. F., Folstein, S. E., MuHugh, P. R., & Fanjiang, C. (2001). *Mini-Mental State Examination user's guide*. Psychological Assessment Resources.

Fruzzetti, A. E. (2017, October 3). *Why borderline personality disorder is misdiagnosed*. National Alliance on Mental Illness. https://www.nami.org/Blogs/NAMI-Blog/October-2017/Why-Borderline-Personality-Disorder-is-Misdiagnose

Fullen, M. C. (2018). Ageism and the counseling profession: Causes, consequences, and methods for counteraction. *The Professional Counselor, 8*(2), 104–114. https://doi.org/10.15241/mcf.8.2.104

Fullen, M. C. (2019). Defining wellness in older adulthood: Toward a comprehensive framework. *Journal of Counseling and Development, 97*(1), 62–74. https://doi.org/10.1002/jcad.12236

Garcia, J. G., DiNardo, J., Nuñez, M. I. L., Emmanuel, D., & Chan, C. D. (2020). The Integrated Acculturation Model: Expanding acculturation to cultural identities in addition to race and ethnicity. *Journal of Multicultural Counseling and Development, 48*(4), 271–287. https://doi.org/10.1002/jmcd.12199

Goodrich, K. M., Farmer, L. B., Watson, J. C., Davis, R. J., Luke, M., Dispenza, F., Akers, W., & Griffith, C. (2017). Standards of care in assessment of lesbian, gay, bisexual, transgender, gender expansive, and queer/questioning (LGBTGEQ+) persons. *Journal of LGBT Issues in Counseling, 11*(4), 203–211. https://doi.org/10.1080/15538605.2017.1380548

Harper, A., Finerty, P., Martinez, M., Brace, A., Crethar, H. C., Loos, B., Harper, B., Graham, S., Singh, A., Kocet, M., Travis, L., Travis, L., Lambert, S., Burnes, T., Dickey, L. M., & Hammer, T. (2013). Association for Lesbian, Gay, Bisexual, and Transgender Issues in Counseling competencies for counseling with lesbian, gay, bisexual, queer, questioning, intersex, and ally individuals. *Journal of LGBTQ Issues in Counseling, 7*(1), 2–43. https://doi.org/10.1080/15538605.2013.755444

Hays, D. G., Milliken, T. F., & Randall, J. (2014). Themes and future directions in multicultural counseling theory, ethics, practice, and research. In D. G. Hays & B. T. Erford (Eds.), *Developing multicultural counseling competence: A systems approach* (2nd ed., pp. 529–542). Pearson.

Helms, J. E. (2003). Racial identity and racial socialization as aspects of adolescents' identity development. In R. Lerner, F. Jacobs, & D. Wertlief (Eds.), *Handbook of applied developmental science: Promoting positive child, adolescent, and family development through research, policies, and programs* (Vol. 1, pp. 143–163). Sage.

Helms, J. E. (2006). Fairness is not validity or cultural bias in racial-group assessment: A quantitative perspective. *American Psychologist, 61*(8), 845–859. https://doi.org/10.1037/0003-066x.61.8.845

Human Rights Campaign. (n.d.). *Sexual orientation and gender identity definitions*. https://www.hrc.org/resources/sexual-orientation-and-gender-identity-terminology-and-definitions

International Association of Marriage and Family Counselors. (2017). *International Association of Marriage and Family Counselors code of ethics*. https://www.iamfconline.org/public/IAMFC-Ethical-Code-Final.pdf

Irwing, P., & Hughes, D. J. (2018). Test development. In P. Irwing, T. Booth, & D. J. Hughes (Eds.), *The Wiley handbook of psychometric testing: A multidisciplinary reference on survey, scale, and test development* (pp. 1–47). John Wiley & Sons.

Katsiaficas, D., Suárez-Orozco, C., Sirin, S. R., & Gupta, T. (2013). Mediators of the relationship between acculturative stress and internalization symptoms for immigrant origin youth. *Cultural Diversity & Ethnic Minority Psychology, 19*(1), 27–37. https://doi.org/10.1037/a0031094

Kerl-McClain, S. B., Dorn-Medeiros, C. M., & McMurray, K. (2022). Addressing anti-fat bias: A crash course for counselors and counselors-in-training. *Journal of Counselor Preparation and Supervision, 15*(4). https://research.library.kutztown.edu/jcps/vol15/iss4/3

Lenz, A. S., Ault, H., Balkin, R. S., Barrio Minton, C., Erford, B. T., Hays, D. G., Kim, B. S. K., & Li, C. (2022). Responsibilities of Users of Standardized Tests (RUST-4E): Prepared for the Association for Assessment and Research in Counseling. *Measurement and Evaluation in Counseling and Development, 55*(4), 227–235. https://doi.org/10.1080/07481756.2022.2052321

Lenz, A. S., Gómez Soler, I., Dell'Aquilla, J., & Uribe, P. M. (2017). Translation and cross-cultural adaptation of assessments for use in counseling research. *Measurement and Evaluation in Counseling and Development, 50*(4), 224–231. https://doi.org/10.1080/07481756.2017.1320947

Lewis, R. J., Cash, T. F., Jacobi, L., & Bubb-Lewis, C. (1997). Prejudice toward fat people: The development and validation of the Anti-Fat Attitudes Test. *Obesity Research, 5*, 297–307. https://doi.org/10.1002/j.1550-8528.1997.tb00555.x

Liang, J., Matheson, B. E., & Douglas, J. M. (2016). Mental health diagnostic considerations in racial/ethnic minority youth. *Journal of Child and Family Studies, 25*, 1926–1940. https://doi.org/10.1007/s10826-015-0351-z

McHugh, M. C., & Chrisler, J. C. (2019). Making space for every body: Ending sizeism in psychotherapy and training. *Women & Therapy, 42*(1–2), 7–21. https://doi.org/10.1080/02703149.2018.1524062

Meyer, I. H. (2003). Prejudice, social stress, and mental health in lesbian, gay, and bisexual populations: Conceptual issues and research evidence. *Psychological Bulletin, 129*(5), 674–697. https://doi.org/10.1037/0033-2909.129.5.674

Ng, R., Allore, H. G., Trentalange, M., Monin, J. K., & Levy, B. R. (2015). Increasing negativity of age stereotypes across 200 years: Evidence from a database of 400 million words. *PLoS One, 10*(2), e0117086. https://doi.org/10.1371/journal.pone.0117086

O'Hara, C., Clark, M., Hays, D. G., McDonald, C. P., Chang, C. Y., Crockett, S. A., Filmore, J., Portman, T., Spurgeon, S., & Wester, K. L. (2016). AARC standards for multicultural research. *Counseling Outcome Research and Evaluation, 7*(2), 67–72. https://doi.org/10.1177/2150137816657389

Paniagua, F. A. (2014). *Assessing and treating culturally diverse clients: A practical guide* (4th ed.). Sage Publications, Inc.

Penfield, R. D., & Camilli, G. (2006). 5 differential item functioning and item bias. *Handbook of Statistics, 26*, 125–167. http://doi.org/10.1016/S0169-7161(06)26005-X

Perrin, P. B., Sutter, M. E., Trujillo, M. A., Henry, R. S., & Pugh, M. (2020). The minority strengths model: Development and initial path analytic validation in racially/ethnically diverse LGBTQ individuals. *Journal of Clinical Psychology, 76*(1), 118–136. https://doi.org/10.1002/jclp.22850

Puckett, J. A., & Levitt, H. M. (2015). Internalized stigma within sexual and gender minorities: Change strategies and clinical implications. *Journal of LGBT Issues in Counseling, 9*(4), 329–349. https://doi.org/10.1080/15538605.2015.1112336

Ratts, M., Singh, A., Nassar-McMillan, S., Butler, S. K., & McCullough, J. R. (2016). Multicultural and social justice counseling competencies: Guidelines for the counseling profession. *Journal of Multicultural Counseling and Development, 44*(1), 28–48. https://doi.org/10.1002/jmcd.12035

Reynolds, C. R., & Bigler, E. D. (2000). *CASE/CASE-SF professional manual*. Psychological Assessment Resources.

Reynolds, C. R., & Suzuki, L. A. (2012). Bias in psychological assessment: An empirical review and recommendations. In I. B. Weiner, J. R. Graham, & J. A. Naglieri (Eds.), *Handbook of psychology: Vol. 10. Assessment psychology* (2nd ed.; pp. 82–113). Wiley.

Roever, C., & McNamara, T. (2006). Language testing: The social dimension. *International Journal of Applied Linguistics, 16*(2), 242–258. https://doi.org/10.1111/j.1473-4192.2006.00117.x

Sireci, S. G., & Randall, J. (2021). Evolving notions of fairness in testing in the United States. In B. E. Clauser & M. B. Bunch (Eds.), *The history of educational measurement: Key advancements in theory, policy, and practice* (pp. 111–135). Routledge. http://doi.org/10.4324/9780367815318-6

Substance Abuse and Mental Health Services Administration & Health Resources and Services Administration. (2016). *Growing older: Providing integrated care for an aging population*. HHS Publication No. (SMA) 16-4982. https://store.samhsa.gov/sites/default/files/d7/priv/sma16-4982.pdf

Testa, R. J., Habarth, J., Peta, J., Balsam, K., & Bockting, W. (2015). Development of the gender minority stress and resilience measure. *Psychology of Sexual Orientation and Gender Diversity, 2*(1), 65–77. https://doi.org/10.1037/sgd0000081

Thompson, J. R., Schalock, R. L., Shogren, K. A., Tassé, M. J., Wehmeyer, M. L., Craig, E. M., & Hughes, C. (2023). *Supports Intensity Scale — Adult Version®: User's manual* (2nd ed.). American Association on Intellectual and Developmental Disabilities.

Thompson, J. R., Wehmeyer, M. L., Hughes, C., Shogren, K. A., Seo, H., Little, T. D., Schalock, R. L., Realon, R. E., Copeland, S. R., Patton, J. R., Polloway, E. A., Shelden, D., Tanis, S., & Tassé, M. J. (2016). *Supports Intensity Scale - Children's Version®: User's manual*. American Association on Intellectual and Developmental Disabilities.

U.S. Census Bureau. (2020). *2020 Census: 1 in 6 people in the United States were 65 and over*. https://www.census.gov/library/stories/2023/05/2020-census-united-states-older-population-grew.html

U.S. Census Bureau. (2021). *Childhood disability in the United States: 2019*. https://www.census.gov/library/publications/2021/acs/acsbr-006.html

U.S. Census Bureau. (2022). *Children and youth with special health needs: National survey of children's health research brief*. https://mchb.hrsa.gov/sites/default/files/mchb/programs-impact/nsch-data-brief-children-youth-special-health-care-needs.pdf

U.S. Department of Education. (n.d.). *Every Student Succeeds Act (ESSA)*. https://www.ed.gov/essa?src=rn

Wong-Rieger, D., & Quintana, D. (1987). Comparative acculturation of Southeast Asian and Hispanic immigrants and sojourners. *Journal of Cross-Cultural Psychology, 18*(3), 345–362. https://doi.org/10.1177/0022002187018003005

Zea, M. C., Asner-Self, K. K., Birman, D., & Buki, L. P. (2003). The Abbreviated Multidimentional Acculturation Scale: Empirical validation with two Latino/Latina samples. *Cultural Diversity and Ethnic Minority Psychology, 9*(2), 107–126. https://doi.org/10.1037/1099-9809.9.2.107

Zhu, P., Luke, M. M., Liu, Y., & Wang, Q. (2023). Cultural humility and cultural competence in counseling: An exploratory mixed methods investigation. *Journal of Counseling and Development, 101*(3), 264–276. https://doi.org/10.1002/jcad.12469

Meaningful Methods for Collecting and Applying Assessment Data

4

Methods of Assessment

KELLY EMELIANCHIK-KEY, AYSE TORRES, AND CLARA BOSSIE

2024 CACREP STANDARDS

3.G.9. use of environmental assessments and systematic behavioral observations

3.G.16. procedures to identify client characteristics, protective factors, risk factors, and warning signs of mental health and behavioral disorders

Clinical Mental Health Counseling

5.C.4. intake interview, mental status evaluation, biopsychosocial history, mental health history, and psychological assessment for treatment planning and caseload management

Clinical Rehabilitation Counseling

5.D.9. intake interview, mental status evaluation, biopsychosocial history, mental health history, and psychological assessment for treatment planning and caseload management for people with disabilities

When I told my kids I was writing a textbook on assessments, my youngest son was brutally honest and replied with, "Tests are dumb and no one likes tests. Why would you write about something people don't like?" As I was explaining about tests and the importance of tests in counseling, my oldest son interjected, "There are so many kinds of tests and ways you take tests. You are tested everyday, but don't know it. If there were no tests, there would be a bunch of crazy drivers on the road who never took a road test to make sure they know how to drive." I laughed to myself, but he had a great point. We are all tested with various methods, and sometimes on a daily basis. Tests are not always scary and they are part of life.

DIRECT AND INDIRECT ASSESSMENT TECHNIQUES

Assessment is an important component of the counseling process that directly influences clinical recommendations and treatment planning goals. Such decision-making is achieved by understanding the emotions, behaviors, thoughts, and diagnostic indicators gleaned from a battery of assessments. When considering what assessments to include, counselors must first consider the many assessment methods available to assist in data-gathering. First and foremost, assessments are divided into two primary categories: direct and indirect assessment methods. *Direct assessments* will capture the immediate experiences of clients as reported by them. This firsthand account allows counselors to gain insight into a client's world while having opportunities to build rapport and establish a safe environment. In contrast, *indirect assessment* allows counselors to gather insights from sources other than the client, such as their family, friends, educators, or auxiliary providers. Capturing information from these indirect sources can reveal aspects of a client's life that might not be readily apparent during direct assessment interactions, thus broadening our perspective. There are many instances where indirect methods are useful, such as working with minors, those who cannot provide accurate self-reports, or when a client is not forthcoming.

Counselors may find that, in many cases, a comprehensive approach will include using both direct and indirect assessment methods. Using combined direct and indirect methods produces a more comprehensive picture and thus better understanding of the client's needs and goals. While assessment allows us to create a picture, it is important to be well-informed, recognizing the vast landscape of human experience, cultural nuances that may be unfamiliar, and potential biases that can arise. To this end, it is important to approach assessment with care, respect, and cultural humility for diverse abilities, backgrounds, and traditions. This section will review common direct and indirect assessment methods, emphasizing their importance, benefits, and special considerations, especially when engaging with diverse client groups.

Narrative Recording in Counseling: An Insight-Oriented Assessment Technique

As an assessment method, *narrative recordings* use stories to illuminate the intricacies of a client's history, challenges, aspirations, and underlying emotions (van Wessel et al., 2021). Narrative recording offers several benefits, including a comprehensive understanding and detailed insights of client concerns, and it builds a bridge for clients to feel heard. This narrative method centers around the counselor recording detailed accounts of a client's experiences and insights through an interview grounded in flexible open-ended questioning. The narratives ideally chronicle pivotal moments, often including uncomfortable and fluctuating emotions (i.e., fear, sadness, grief, and shame), uncertainty, and ever-evolving situations. The success of the narrative recording method hinges on the counselor and client piecing narratives together through an inquiry process that allows the counselor to grasp the causal links between past experiences and current behaviors or emotions (van Wessel, 2018). Inherent in this approach, narrative recordings honor the individuality and context of each client while also helping to tailor care plans that resonate with the client's uniqueness.

Narrative recordings can be categorized as both a direct and indirect assessment tool. In its direct form of counselor–client interaction, narratives capture a client's firsthand and immediate feelings, thoughts, and actions. However, as an indirect tool, such as counselor–other interactions, narratives can include stories shared by family or friends, offering a broader view of a client's life. Both direct and indirect approaches hold merit when considering narrative recording assessment methods. Although direct narrative recordings provide a firsthand account of clients' experiences, indirect narrative recordings can offer supplemental data when facing resistant clients, reserved clients, or where cultural nuances play a significant role. Ultimately, blending both methods will ensure a comprehensive understanding of the client. A balanced approach, emphasizing the client's unique needs, remains as a pillar in effective assessment practices.

The power of storytelling becomes evident when gathering narratives, whether directly from the client or from members of their family and social circles. Rather than limiting individuals within the strict parameters of structured assessments, the organic process of narratives flows naturally as the client's experiences and emotions take center stage. The model's strength hinges on authenticity, bringing warmth and intimacy to counseling assessment sessions. While every method provides valuable data, narrative recording through client-shared stories uniquely strengthens the working alliance and fosters trust.

Diversity plays a pivotal role in narrative recording for clients from varied cultural, linguistic, or socioeconomic backgrounds; their narratives are often deeply influenced by their unique experiences and contexts. Every story filled with personal moments must be recorded accurately; therefore, it is paramount for counselors to acknowledge and respect cultural nuances ensuring narratives are understood. To this end, it is vital to have tools that work across a diverse range of clients of various languages and cultures. Counselors can choose between several recording methods. Some prefer the personal touch of handwritten notes, whereas others prefer the efficiency that technology offers. As we move toward more digital methods, keeping data secure and maintaining client privacy is crucial; being able to discern which platforms are reliable safeguards both the data and the client's trust. Considerations for working with diverse clients include cultural sensitivity to recognize the impact of traditions, values, and societal norms on a client's story. Additionally, understand that clients who speak different languages or dialects must have accurate translation or interpretation. Avoid biases that impact client narratives.

Interval Recording in Counseling: A Behavioral Assessment Technique

Interval recording, a technique primarily grounded in behavioral assessments, offers a systematic method of capturing the frequency of specific behaviors within a predetermined time or interval (Green et al., 1982). Rather than noting every occurrence of a behavior, this method focuses on whether the behavior happened at all during that interval or window of time. Interval recording equips counselors with a quantitative perspective of clients' actions and reactions by presenting a snapshot of behavior patterns. The importance of interval recording is underscored by its precision and efficiency. Counselors can better manage their observation times by focusing on a set of intervals, ensuring they are attuned to the client during critical moments (Singh et al., 2023). This strategy is beneficial when dealing with frequent behaviors or when the entire session's observation might be overwhelming or impractical (Cook & Snyder, 2020).

Interval recording can resemble indirect assessment in instances where the counselor is not the primary observer. For instance, when a teacher or caregiver is tasked with monitoring and recording behaviors, their observations, though still grounded in real time, offer an external perspective on the client's behaviors. When requesting caregivers to provide interval recordings, it is essential to discuss and define the target behavior and understand recording forms and approaches to interval recording. Table 4.1 notes common approaches to interval recording.

Today's digital advancements offer unmatched precision, instant analysis, and streamlined data storage for interval recording. These digital platforms allow for tailored interval settings, timely notifications, and sophisticated data visualization, setting a benchmark for efficient recording. Once observations are made, translating this data into percentages can offer a clearer picture of how often specific behaviors manifest. Counselors should ensure they are not only digitally prepared but also culturally informed. This includes consistent training for all observers and planning observations across different contexts to capture a truly comprehensive understanding of behavior. Whether approaching interval recordings directly or indirectly, these approaches can bridge the gap between quantitative data and qualitative understanding.

TABLE 4.1 **COMMON APPROACHES TO INTERVAL RECORDING**

Approach	Description	Considerations
Whole Interval Recording	A data collection method where the behavior is marked as having occurred if it persists throughout the entire preset interval. If the behavior stops even momentarily before the interval ends, it is not recorded.	• Records behavior only if it lasts throughout the entire interval • Can underestimate behaviors of short duration or sporadic occurrence • Ideal for observing behaviors of longer duration where you want to confirm a behavior's continuous presence • Ideal for controlled environments or 1:1 therapeutic settings
Partial-Interval Recording	A recording approach where the behavior is noted as having occurred if it manifests at any moment within the preset interval, regardless of how long it lasts. The behavior is recorded even if it doesn't persist for the entire interval.	• Captures any occurrence, no matter how brief, within an interval • Helpful in observing behaviors that may occur briefly and sporadically • Can overestimate occurrence as it does not consider duration • Ideal for diverse settings where brief behaviors are significant, including group and individual
Momentary Time Sampling (MTS)	An observational method where, instead of continuously monitoring, the observer checks and records if the behavior is occurring at the exact end of each preset interval. It captures only the presence or absence of the behavior at that specific moment.	• Less labor-intensive • Provides a snapshot of behavior occurrence • Might miss sporadic short-duration behaviors • Ideal for busy settings where continuous observation is not feasible compared to periodic checks
Planned Activity Check (PLACHECK)	This is a variation of momentary time sampling and is used for group observations. The observer notes how many individuals in a group are engaging in the target behavior at the end of each interval.	• Allows for quick assessments of group behavior • Can assess for overall group dynamics • Might not capture individual variances; requires synchronized behavior occurrence • Ideal for group observations such as educational settings, group counseling, or similar scenarios

Self-Monitoring in Counseling: An Engaging Assessment Technique

Self-monitoring is an introspective technique where clients actively observe and record their behaviors, feelings, and thoughts. This may include daily thought records, mood charts, diaries, symptom trackers, nutrition logs, activity schedules, and so on. This method empowers individuals to become more aware of their internal and external responses, facilitating a deeper understanding of personal patterns and triggers (McCool et al., 2023). In counseling assessments, self-monitoring provides a bridge between sessions, transforming clients from passive recipients to active participants in their treatment.

Self-monitoring stands out as an insightful indirect assessment method in the counseling process. While the data are derived directly from the client to ensure authenticity and immediacy, it is gathered without the direct oversight of the counselor. This method provides a comprehensive and multidimensional understanding of the client's experiences. Self-monitoring plans are carefully thought out to reflect themes being addressed in the counseling process. Moreover, planning for self-monitoring with diverse populations requires keen sensitivity and cocreation. Cultural norms, for instance, might affect how individuals perceive and document their behaviors and emotions. Discussing specific feelings or actions in certain cultures might be taboo, challenging candid self-reporting. Likewise, language barriers or literacy levels can influence the accuracy and depth of self-recording. Counselors must remain attuned to these nuances, ensuring tools and guidelines are adapted to each client's background and comfort level.

The benefit of self-monitoring lies in its ability to foster client autonomy and self-awareness. The hope is that by taking charge of their observations, clients can recognize problematic behaviors or cognitive patterns and begin the process of self-regulation (Wood & McKay, 2021). An added value of self-monitoring is extending the treatment beyond the counseling session, as clients can assess and track behaviors outside the counseling room, capturing real-world experiences and challenges. The dialectical behavior therapy (DBT) diary card developed by Marsha Linehan (2018) is one example of a self-monitoring tool. The diary card tool, completed via pen to paper or with a digital application, encourages clients to record emotional experiences, distress, and the urge and use of target behaviors between counseling sessions. There are many versions of diary cards available online (see www.dbtselfhelp.com for examples).

Many tools are available to reinforce and support effective self-monitoring by clients. Traditional methods, such as journals or diaries, remain favored for their tactile and personal touch. However, the digital age has ushered in a slew of applications tailored for self-monitoring purposes. Some digital applications allow clients to track emotional states, whereas others offer platforms for recording behaviors and habits. These tools come with the advantage of reminders, data visualization, and, in some cases, encrypted security features to protect sensitive information.

Behavioral Interviews in Counseling: Technique for Change

Rooted in the principle that past behavior best predicts future behavior, *behavioral interviews* are a powerful tool in the counselor's assessment repertoire. Behavioral interviews focus on eliciting detailed accounts of situations, actions, and outcomes from an individual's past. By delving into specific experiences, counselors can unearth behavior patterns, decision-making tendencies, and adaptive coping mechanisms. Behavioral interviews are typically viewed as a direct assessment method. The counselor actively engages with the client, eliciting firsthand information through questions about past behaviors. Unlike some tools where responses might be interpreted or reported by a third party, the client's recollections and self-reports drive the data collection, ensuring authenticity. It is important to remember that cultural differences can influence how events are perceived or remembered. In some cultures, direct questioning might be viewed as confrontational, so adapting the interview style might be necessary. Furthermore, language barriers or differing societal norms can impact the narratives shared. Counselors must approach these interviews with cultural sensitivity, possibly employing interpreters or cultural liaisons when needed.

Behavioral interviews help counselors in establishing a client's baseline behavior. Having a baseline becomes crucial in measuring progress or the effectiveness of therapeutic interventions over time. Moreover, behavioral anecdotes can also validate or challenge other assessment results. For instance, a client might express high confidence in a self-report questionnaire, yet their behavioral interview narratives might reveal instances of self-doubt or hesitancy. One primary benefit of behavioral interviews is their specificity. For instance, instead of asking, "Do you handle stress well?" a counselor might ask, "Can you describe a specific time when you were under much stress and how you managed it?" Such detailed probing offers deeper insight and minimizes the potential for ambiguous responses. Various assessment tools and techniques can help counselors facilitate effective behavioral interviews, such as structured clinical interviews aligned with the *Diagnostic and Statistical Manual of Mental Disorders* (*DSM*), crisis intervention interviews to assess immediate threats, employing interview protocols to delve into maladaptive behaviors, or identifying strengths, skills, and resiliency. Linehan's (2018) DBT chain analysis is only one example of a behavioral interview tool. The chain analysis is a key component of DBT, offering a meticulous assessment of events and actions to identify factors leading to problematic behaviors. Through open dialogue and structured questioning, behavioral interviews offer a window into a client's lived experiences. This allows counselors to tailor interventions based on genuine insight. Such interviews bridge the gap between broad assessments and the intricate realities of a client's daily life. There are many DBT examples of chain analysis online (see www.dbtselfhelp.com for examples).

INITIAL INTERVIEWS IN COUNSELING

Many of the assessment methods covered in this chapter incorporate an interviewing component. This is not a coincidence; rather, it points to the evolution of counseling techniques grounded in the research and insight of early pioneers like Carl Rogers (1995), one of the founding figures of humanistic psychology, who emphasized the importance of empathetic listening during interviews. Rogers believed that nondirective client-centered interviews (a) provide clients with the space to express genuine feelings and experiences and (b) help counselors understand the client's inner world. The art of interviewing stands as a vital tool in assessment and counseling. As we go further into assessment methods, it is essential to recognize that interview methods are integral to the assessment process because they facilitate a deeper understanding of the client. Through interviews, counselors can validate, clarify, and expand upon the information gleaned from assessment tools, ensuring a comprehensive understanding of the client's experiences and concerns. It is important for counselors to understand the three methods of interviewing so that they may be intentional about which they employ with clients.

Structured, Semistructured, and Unstructured Interviews

Interview methods can be categorized based on their level of structure: structured, semistructured, and unstructured. Each type has its own characteristics and applications. *Structured interviews* are marked by a predetermined set of questions, ensuring that every client encounters a reliable, systematic, and standardizable approach. By offering uniformity, structured interviews are ideal for situations like initial screenings, diagnostic questionnaires validated for specific diagnostic categories, and research situations where uniformity is crucial. Semistructured interviews, on the other hand, represent the bridge between the structured world and the more client-centered, open-ended approaches of therapists like Carl Rogers. While *semistructured interviews* might begin with a set framework, there is room for impromptu investigation based on the client's feedback. This adaptable approach combines consistency with the flexibility to dive deeper, making it particularly suitable for diagnostic discussions, clinical evaluations, and intake sessions. In the *unstructured interview*, where there are no predetermined questions, the counselor allows the interview's direction to be shaped organically by the interviewee's responses. This method, echoing the psychoanalytic approaches of figures like Sigmund Freud and the broader psychodynamic theories of Alfred Adler, Erik Erikson, and Carl Jung, offers the utmost flexibility. Although an unstructured interview can be rich in depth, the inherent absence of structure might impede the incorporation of essential administrative tasks typical of initial counselor–client sessions. While unstructured interviews are an excellent option for in-depth exploration during follow-up counseling sessions and for use in case studies, they are not typically the best fit for initial intake interviews due to their unpredictability and lack of specificity.

The Biopsychosocial-Spiritual Interview to Gain Structure

To explore interview approaches further, we can look at a commonly used assessment like the biopsychosocial-spiritual (BPSS) interview (Engel, 1977, 1980). This assessment exemplifies the adaptability of interview tools, highlighting the importance of selecting the appropriate interview structure that aligns with both the counselor's objectives and the client's needs. The goal of the BPSS assessment is to provide a holistic view of a client's life, and it can be adapted to various interviewing formats. In a structured format (see Figure 4.1), the counselor might employ a predefined set of questions that comb

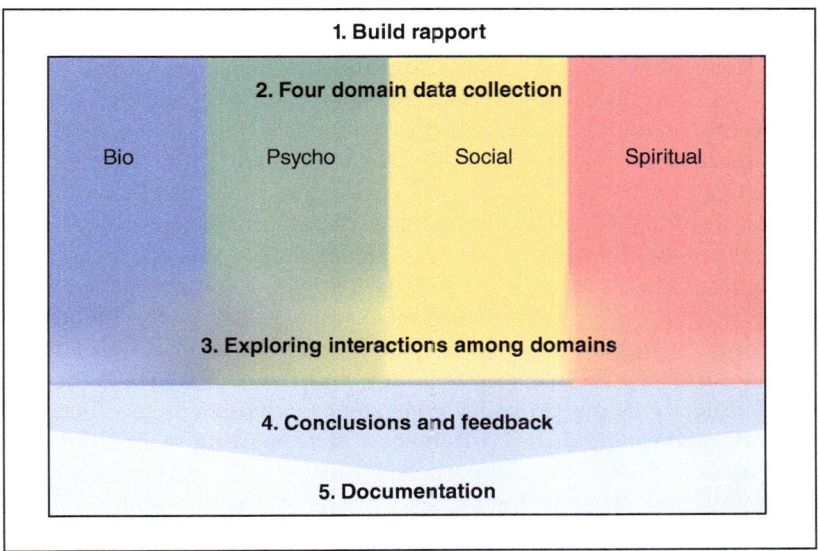

FIGURE 4.1. **Biopsychosocial-spiritual components.**

through each of the four domains: biological, psychologic, social, and spiritual. To do this, the counselor may prepare a variety of assessment questionnaires that provide more standardization. As discussed previously, this level of structure is most likely to be used when there is a need to collect data that can be standardized. In most settings, however, counselors will find that adopting a semistructured approach to the BPSS makes the most sense. Here, the counselor begins with a foundational framework while remaining open to exploration based on the client's feedback. This format is ideal for initial intakes where understanding the broad spectrum of a client's life is critical. As the semistructured BPSS interview unfolds, a counselor may find it helpful to incorporate additional interviewing strategies and self-reporting measures; again, this is a testimony to the flexibility of the approach.

As a practical tool, the BPSS interview allows counselors to develop tailor-made and effective intervention strategies while fostering the development of therapeutic alliance. The evolution of the BPSS model progressively elevates the human element in healthcare, fostering an environment of empowerment, personalization, and collaborative care (Borrell-Carrió et al., 2004). This is evident in adding the spiritual dimension over the last decade. In our modern, multilayered world, spirituality is a flexible and encompassing concept that stretches from nonreligious ideas, such as the power of positive thinking, to deeply profound religious experiences. In health sciences, spirituality is often seen as a journey or exploration toward deeper meaning and building relationships with various aspects of life such as oneself, family, community, nature, and even the divine. These relationships are expressed through a person's unique beliefs, values, traditions, and practices. As counselors utilize a BPSS assessment process, they acknowledge the invaluable role of spirituality as a fourth dimension, enhancing understanding beyond biological, psychologic, and social factors. By recognizing and incorporating these spiritual aspects into assessment, we foster a more comprehensive and holistic understanding of a client's well-being and health, honoring the complexity of the human experience.

Lastly, the BPSS assessment offers some inherent structure by providing specific domains for guiding the interview process. To this end, when we are using the BPSS it is not without structure. To approach an intake interview with an unstructured approach, the counselor will simply let the conversation evolve organically without guiding questions. In the subsequent section, we will discuss the historical evolution of the BPSS further, as well as walk through an intake assessment process centered around a semistructured BPSS interview emphasizing its versatility. It is important to note that the BPSS is just one of many interviewing methods that can benefit from a range of strategies. While each strategy has its advantages and challenges, the central task for clinicians is discerning and, if suitable, combining strategies depending on the client's unique needs, the setting, and the desired use of the assessment data. Table 4.2 lists common interviewing strategies that can be applied broadly, ensuring a comprehensive intake assessment interview, with the BPSS being a helpful example of one method where they can be applied. Selecting the right strategy for conducting an intake interview and assessment is essential to ensure its effectiveness, accuracy, and the counselor's ability to approach the client authentically. Some prioritize consistency, whereas others focus on building rapport or accommodating cultural differences. Incorporating technology undoubtedly brings convenience to the assessment process. However, it is also challenging, notably in maintaining safety and security standards. Understanding the range of strategies and their distinctions supports counselors in making informed decisions that are tailored to the task at hand.

TABLE 4.2 **COMMON INTERVIEWING STRATEGIES**

Strategy	Description	Strengths	Challenges
Experiential and Expressive Approaches	Using a multisensory approach to data collection that is often considered creative in nature (e.g., genograms, sand tray, psychodrama, family sculpting)	Accessible to various developmental levels and learners	Can require additional training, materials, and preparation
Narrative Approach	Clients share their life stories with clinician guidance	Yields rich data and builds rapport	Time-consuming
Checklist or Questionnaires	Structured forms where clients check off relevant items	Efficient and comprehensive	Might lack depth
Collateral Information Gathering	Data from other sources like family or records	Provides a fuller picture	Requires consent and has potential for bias
Technological Integration	Use of online tools, apps, or platforms	Convenience and accessibility	Confidentiality and accuracy concerns
Cultural and Contextual Tailoring	Modifying assessment for cultural relevance	Ensures cultural competence	Requires cultural humility and understanding of client's background
Iterative Process	Gathering information over multiple sessions	Builds rapport via thorough data collection	Extended process
Multidisciplinary Approach	Team-based assessment across specialties	Comprehensive	Requires coordination and collaboration
Incorporating Observation	Using observational data like behavior or nonverbal cues	Provides rounded view	Subjective interpretation
Use of Ancillary Tests	Using medical tests, scales, or diagnostic tools	Comprehensive and specific	Requires additional resources and expertise

GUIDELINES FOR INTERVIEWS: APPLYING THE INITIAL INTAKE ASSESSMENT

The initial intake assessment is more than just a procedural step. It is a series of carefully planned interactions that lay groundwork for the counseling process to come, setting its tone, guiding treatment planning, and fostering a positive working alliance. The initial intake assessment often incorporates interviewing strategies and both direct and indirect tools we will be introducing you to in Chapters 10 and 11. Such specialized tools offer precision, catering to the unique insights gained from the intake assessment. This section sheds light on how a counselor may apply assessment methods, tools, and processes that constitute the phases of intake by offering a guiding example. Specifically, we will highlight the core assessments integral to any counseling intake: the mental status exam (MSE) and the BPSS assessment. Though we will briefly introduce the diagnostic interview here, Chapter 5 is devoted to a comprehensive look at the history and applications of the diagnostic assessment process so that you may see how these initial tools and methods weave into a comprehensive diagnostic picture.

Phase 1: The Initial Contact and Intake Information

The initial intake assessment process begins with first contact, which is, in essence, the prescreening phase. Prescreening is much more than an introduction; it is an opportunity for the counselor or support staff to gain a first look into the client's world. Prescreening involves a variety of preparatory tasks that help determine the client's needs and assess immediate risks, among other things like intake documentation that may be relevant to the therapeutic setting. Often, how a client initiates counseling and manages these tasks will provide helpful diagnostic data.

While it may sound like a preliminary step, the prescreening phase accomplishes multiple crucial functions from the transparency of client rights to logistics like insurance verification. Moreover, secondary benefits of prescreening include the opportunity for clients to briefly share their motivation for seeking services, readiness, and potential resistance. These early conversations foster rapport building while easing clients into their first visit: the intake session. To clarify the sequence and nature of these tasks, consider Table 4.3, which outlines the key domains and tasks often covered during a prescreening call or visit.

Phase 2: The Clinical Intake Interview

To ensure a thorough diagnostic assessment, counselors must strategize for the clinical interview process to unfold across multiple encounters. The first of these is the initial intake session. Pashak and Heron beautifully describe the intake session, noting that "any psychological intervention must have a starting point, any therapy relationship must have a first

TABLE 4.3 **INITIAL CONTACT AND INTAKE INFORMATION**

1	Client's Request (prescreen phase)	Reason for reaching out, including a brief understanding of the client's goals and information about costs/insurance
2	Demographics	Name, date of birth, contact information, background information (education level, employment, cultural and spiritual considerations, relationship status, and ethical concerns), and presenting problems
3	Health History	Current or previous health concerns, including medications, diagnoses of mental and physical health problems, developmental milestones, and previous counseling experiences
4	Risk Assessment	Location of potential client, harm to self, harm to others, and crisis planning (knowledge of emergency services, crisis resources, immediate need for specialized services, or referrals)
5	Assess Level of Care	Motivation, readiness, appropriate level of care, and release of information for referral source
6	Logistics	Billing, insurance verification, and scheduling
7	Orientation	Informed consent, client rights and responsibilities, privacy policies, confidentiality, and intake documents

moment, and any assessment process must have an initiation—the intake is such a juncture" (2022, para. 3). The goal in this visit is to establish varying levels of therapeutic alliance and data collection, a variation that is influenced by a counselor's theoretical approach. The challenge of the intake interview is juggling the big three: accomplishing clinical tasks, building an alliance, and collecting clinical data. Clinical tasks are steps that must occur when providing ethical care, such as informed consent, MSE, and risk assessment. For example, counselors must provide informed consent to clients at the outset of the clinical interview. In the next sections, key clinical tasks are further explained. Of course, overarching is building an alliance that will foster information sharing and future participation in treatment. After all, who is to say the client will return for a follow-up without feeling some sense of safety and connection?

INFORMED CONSENT

Informed consent is a critical first step before any form of care, especially assessment practices. Informed consent ensures transparency and empowers clients to make well-informed decisions about their care. The American Counseling Association (ACA) Code of Ethics outlines key features of ethical consent. Similarly, organizations like the American Psychological Association (APA) and the National Board for Certified Counselors (NBCC) echo informed consent requirements. When securing informed consent for treatment and assessment, counselors must ensure that clients understand relevant information about the assessment and counseling process, potential risks and benefits, alternative options and methods, confidentiality, and client rights regarding the counseling relationship (Palmer & Burrows, 2021). Given the influx of telehealth, many practices use various software stacks. New inclusions to consider in the informed consent process are the utilization of technology from inquiry to treatment delivery, including client portals, digital signatures, secure messaging, electronic medical records, assessment tools, billing tools, and videoconferencing platforms. While clinics exert considerable effort to ensure that technology tools are compliant with Health Insurance Portability and Accountability Act (HIPAA) security requirements and furnish Business Associate Agreements (BAA) to affirm this compliance, they must also offer clients transparent information about the usage of these tools and explicitly communicate the inherent risks associated with potential privacy loss that may accompany the utilization of technology in counseling (Grundy et al., 2019). Whether counseling and assessment are digitally delivered, or face-to-face, informed consent must illuminate the many aspects of treatment. Informed consent is an ongoing process as treatment progresses, where the provider is responsible for ensuring transparency. In some settings, clients receive and sign consent documents before meeting their counselor for the intake interview. Regardless, counselors must review documentation, highlight important points, and answer questions before collecting intake interview data from the client.

THE MENTAL STATUS EXAM

The MSE has matured into an essential tool for assessment, gaining widespread use after the standardization in reference manuals like the *DSM* and the *International Classification of Diseases* (Donnelly et al., 1970). The MSE outlines key domains for briefly identifying symptoms, guiding treatment, monitoring progress, and evaluating risk. There are many schools of thought on which domains are to be recorded, which may depend heavily on the clinical setting and field of study (e.g., school counseling, mental health, rehabilitation counseling, healthcare, and medical). Table 4.4 outlines several of the most common domains in an MSE. Importantly, the MSE guides a timely snapshot of a client's mental condition. During an MSE, counselors assess several key areas through careful observation, and these findings form an integral part of the clinical record (Voss & Das, 2022).

TABLE 4.4 **COMMON DOMAINS OF THE MENTAL STATUS EXAM**

Appearance	Observing the client's physical presentation, grooming, and attire
Behavior	Noting any evident psychomotor agitation, retardation, or unusual mannerisms
Speech	Assessing rate, volume, and quantity of talk; also, noting any speech peculiarities
Mood and Affect	Understanding that, while mood is the client's self-reported emotional state, affect is the observed emotional expression
Thought Process and Content	Understanding the client's line of thinking and looking for any disturbances
Perceptions	Evaluating any hallucinations or false perceptions
Cognitions	Assessing the client's orientation, memory, and general knowledge
Insight and Judgment	Evaluating the client's understanding of their current situation and their capacity to make sound decisions

Given its concise nature, the MSE is used as the standard of care across diverse settings, from outpatient clinics to inpatient and emergency care units. The domains covered ensure a comprehensive review of the client's mental state, reducing the likelihood of an oversight. Ideally, impressions gained from the MSE are recorded at every visit. When reviewing impressions from varying points in the treatment process, invaluable insights shed light on the efficacy of interventions and highlight any emerging concerns. Counselors should remember that while the MSE is a powerful tool, it only reflects a snapshot in time. A client's mental state can fluctuate, and factors like fatigue, intoxication, or recent traumatic events can affect results. Therefore, counselors will need to contextualize the results of the MSE within the broader view of the client's history. The MSE stands out in clinical assessment as foundational and indispensable by offering a detailed yet concise overview of a client's mental state. As you progress in your counseling journey, mastering the nuances of the MSE and the various potential presentations of clients under duress will be an asset.

Phase 3: The Diagnostic Interview

Though a detailed exploration of diagnostic assessment will follow in Chapter 5, counselors must understand how a diagnostic interview is intertwined into the initial intake assessment process. The diagnostic interview is a crucial element in the intake assessment process, distinguished from the broader clinical interview where elements like the BPSS aspects are explored. While the clinical interview focuses on obtaining a comprehensive understanding of the client's life experiences, context, and presenting issues, the diagnostic interview will zero in on the identification of specific symptoms, levels of intensity, and patterns of behavior that align with established *DSM* diagnostic criteria. The overarching purpose of the diagnostic interview is to construct a clear diagnostic picture. By methodically exploring and evaluating a client's symptoms and behaviors, while considering context and history, the counselor can endorse a diagnosis. This focused approach is instrumental in tailoring interventions and predicting the course of a client's therapeutic journey, forming the basis for subsequent treatment planning. Incorporating a diagnostic interview in the intake assessment process will ensure that the counseling process is empathetic and holistic, as well as evidence based.

Phase 4: Synthesis

Initial assessments can be an intricate endeavor that starts with initial contact and continues with a tapestry of numerous intake elements such as the MSEs, clinical interviews, diagnostic interviews, and supplemental assessments, with each method contributing valuable threads to the overall picture of the client. The synthesis of these data points culminates into a comprehensive case conceptualization, weaving a narrative that captures the client's unique challenges and strengths. Several considerations are pivotal at this juncture to ensure that no aspect of the client's condition is overlooked. The aim is to create a robust and multidimensional portrait of the client's well-being, incorporating information from the counselor and, when possible, a multidisciplinary team of professionals. Multidisciplinary collaboration provides a holistic view, enabling the identification of optimal treatment paths. Counselors must become proficient in several key aspects of client assessment to best synthesize the data gleaned from the broad range of assessment methods employed. The capstone of the synthesis process is creating a collaborative treatment plan that aligns with the client's needs and goals. A collaborative treatment plan is not merely an administrative task but a crucial step in establishing a therapeutic relationship built on trust, clarity, and a shared mission for healing and growth.

ANALYZING THE DATA

Counselors should adopt a meticulous and systematic approach when analyzing a client's intake data and clinical assessments. This involves synthesizing the results from the MSE, clinical and diagnostic interviews, and supplemental diagnostic tools into an integrated case conceptualization. It is imperative to consider what is evident and what might be missing or ambiguous. Counselors must vigilantly explore discrepancies or inconsistencies across various data points that require further exploration or clarification. For example, contrasting narratives from self-reports and collateral information from family or other professionals could signify issues like denial, minimization, or potential dual diagnosis that otherwise go unnoticed. Attention must also be paid to cultural, educational, and developmental factors that may influence the client's responses or the interpretation of assessment results. Special heed must be given to standardized scores, their meaning, and their applicability to the individual client based on norms. Furthermore, assessing the readiness and motivational level of the client for treatment can offer invaluable insights into how to approach the therapeutic process. This thorough analysis culminates in a robust understanding of the client's unique challenges and strengths, providing a strong foundation for collaborative treatment planning and effective intervention.

TRANSLATING ASSESSMENT INTO ACTION: DOCUMENTATION AND OUTCOME REPORTING

When thinking about outcome reporting, it is important to understand how various forms of documentation work together. The intake report provides the groundwork by collecting essential initial information, while case conceptualization involves a more complex and nuanced understanding of the client's needs and treatment approach, often rooted in the therapist's theoretical orientation. Both are vital components in providing comprehensive, effective care in counseling settings. These initial steps result in a collaborative treatment plan strategically tailored to the client's current situation. This plan is cocreated with the client, considering the findings from initial intake assessments and the treatment recommendations. Chapter 12 will go further into depth on case conceptualization and treatment planning based on the intakes and interviews, as well as additional assessment data gathered.

Interviewing Children

Engaging in intake interviews and BPSS assessments with children can be a unqiue experience that is quite different from engaging in assessments with adults. The first step that always remains the same and at the core of the counseling process is esetablishing rapport. Establishing rapport is a critical step with children so trust is built and that they know you are there to support them and help them. The greatest challenges and differences that exist when interviewing children is tailoring the intake assessments to the child's appropriate level and making sure you are using words and language that the child will understand, but that is also clear and consistent. With children in clinical settings, there is always a conversation that takes place with a parent or someone who brings them to counseling that happens early on in the process. Often, minors may be frightened, unaware of what to expect in counseling, or feel that they have no voice in the counseling process. A great way to allow minors to open up and build rapport early on is to state something to the effect of, "I have heard a lot from your mom who brought you here today, but I would love to hear from you and understand your thoughts on why you are here and how I might be able to help you." Then explaining a bit regarding what the counseling process is about and stating confidentiality guidelines in clear and simple language will help to build rapport and make sure that everyone is on the same page.

Engaging in the interview process requires a lot of questions, so explaining why you have so many questions early on in the process is helpful. It can also be useful to take small breaks between the questions so minors can stay engaged when you are working with them and gathering information. Breaking the stigma that exists around counseling for minors is also helpful. While they may not call it stigma, depending on their families' experiences with counseling or things they have seen within media, they may have preconceived ideas that should be addressed. For school counselors, this is especially important as you are completely unaware of stigma or talk about therapy that takes place at home. It is often somewhat safer to assume that if a parent brings their child into counseling, that they are onboard with the process of therapy, but we can never be certain that there are not preconceived notions that are culturally based that have been shared with children.

Using creative techniques and evidence-based approaches is also recommended. Finding ways for children and teens to fully express themselves can be challenging. Think outside the box and use creative interventions. Many theoretical frameworks offer interventions, skills, and activities that might open up diaglogue with children during the interview process and allow them to be creative, while giving you insight. For example, the DBT house activity allows children or teens to visually represent their emotional experiences in a structured, organized manner. The construction of a "house," with various rooms, walls, foundation, and so on, represents different aspects of one's life and gives counselors insight into the child's important relationships, where they feel safe and supported, and their overall well-being.

Last, but not least important, is to make sure you are being culturally sensitive and working with minors through their lens. Being a teen is a culture of its own. There is different language and jargon, in addition to a teenage culture full of things we might not have experienced when we were of that age. Many children and teens may not have all the answers, and we need to ensure we are meeting them at their developmentally appropriate level, creating a safe and judgment-free environment, hearing them out, maintaining respect, and managing our own frustration if things do not go as planned. We must be encouraging and inviting to create an environment where minors feel comfortable opening up and sharing their stories.

OTHER METHODS OF ASSESSMENT

Assessment refers to the systematic process of gathering information about an individual to make informed decisions or inferences about them (Haynes & O'Brien, 2000). This process involves a wide range of formal and informal instruments. *Formal assessments* are rigorous instruments that follow standardized and systematic procedures. These instruments are grounded in extensive research and field testing, which provide compelling and reliable results. With structured and consistent test procedures, formal assessments employ predetermined scoring methods and encompass various test types, including achievement, aptitude, and ability tests. These assessments adhere to strict administration guidelines, ensuring their integrity and validity. Formal assessments are typically released by reputable companies that have conducted extensive research on the assessment's validity and reliability. Validity refers to the assessment's ability to accurately measure what it claims to measure, whereas reliability ensures consistent and dependable results.

Informal assessments are subjective and nonstandardized, but they play a unique role in the assessment process. They generally do not formally address reliability, validity, and cross-cultural issues. Although informal assessments can be valid and reliable, they do not carry the same authority as formal assessments, which have undergone extensive testing with a large sample size. Informal assessments can be either structured or unstructured. For example, an unstructured informal assessment could involve asking an individual to write in a journal, whereas a structured informal assessment may include a scored questionnaire. The term *informal* essentially means that it has not been rigorously tested by a large number of people, formalized, or standardized.

Formal and informal assessments serve as vital instruments in a counselor's arsenal, each offering unique advantages and limitations. Formal assessments, characterized by standardized measures, provide reliable and valid data due to their structured nature. They are often quantifiable, allowing for objective comparison and tracking of a client's progress over time. The use of norms can also facilitate the understanding of a client's performance relative to a specific population. Conversely, informal assessments prioritize flexibility and personalization over standardization. They offer a more holistic and individualized understanding of a client, capturing nuanced aspects of behavior or performance that might be overlooked in standardized testing. By focusing on observations, interviews, and case studies, informal assessments can offer insights into a client's experiences and feelings that a score on a standardized test cannot convey.

However, the choice between these two types of assessments is not mutually exclusive. In many cases, a combination of both can provide a comprehensive, accurate, and in-depth understanding of a client's unique needs and circumstances. For example, a counselor may use formal assessments to establish a baseline and track progress over time, while supplementing with informal assessments to gain a deeper understanding of the individual. Moreover, the context and goal of the evaluation should also be considered when choosing between formal and informal assessments. For diagnostic purposes, standardized measures are often preferred due to their reliability and validity. On the other hand, informal assessments may be more suitable for evaluating progress in therapy or as a tool for individualized treatment planning. When different assessment methods come together and show similar results (convergent validity), it adds validity to each method (Gresham, 2007). By combining data from different assessment methods, we can obtain a better and more accurate understanding of the client and their concerns. This approach not only reduces bias but also improves the overall assessment process. In this section, we examine various methods and types of assessments.

Standardized and Nonstandardized Assessments

Throughout history, the terms *assessment* and *testing* have often been used interchangeably, but they carry distinct meanings. According to Handler and Meyer (1998), testing is a relatively straightforward process that involves administering a specific test to obtain a particular score. In contrast, assessment is a broader concept that encompasses the integration of information about a client from various methods and sources, extending beyond the acquisition of a single test score. Standardized tests must adhere to specific standards and requirements throughout the testing process. This includes administering and scoring the test in a consistent manner for all test takers, using objective scoring methods, and incorporating representative norm groups for accurate test interpretation. Most standardized tests demonstrate clear reliability and value.

Standardized instruments in counseling, such as psychometric tests, provide counselors with reliable and objective ways to understand a client's mental health. Standardization in assessment refers to the consistent application of assessment tools and techniques. In a standardized assessment, each individual is evaluated using the same measures under the same conditions, ensuring consistency and fairness. This approach allows professionals to compare the results across individuals, groups, and at various points in time. Additionally, it minimizes bias and increases the reliability and validity of the evaluation. However, standardized instruments also have limitations. Their structured nature may not fully capture the complexity of a client's experience. They often focus on quantification, potentially overlooking important qualitative aspects of a client's life. Moreover, cultural bias within the instruments can misinterpret responses from diverse backgrounds, leading to inaccurate conclusions. Therefore, while standardized instruments are valuable to counseling, it is important to use them judiciously alongside other assessment methods.

Nonstandardized assessments in counseling refer to techniques and tools that do not follow a strict protocol or standardized scoring system. These assessments include qualitative methods. Qualitative assessments are verbal or written responses to open-ended questions, which can involve informal and flexible procedures. They are often tailored to meet the unique needs of each individual and can include methods such as interviews, observation, case histories, and projective techniques. Nonstandardized assessments in counseling present unique strengths and weaknesses. A significant strength lies in its flexibility and adaptability. Unlike standardized tests, nonstandardized assessments can be customized according to the client's unique needs, allowing for the inclusion of cultural, contextual, and individual factors. This adaptability often results in a more comprehensive understanding of the client's mental health state, which can inform personalized intervention strategies. These assessments also facilitate a relaxed and comfortable environment for open dialogue, which can lead to insightful revelations not possible through standardized methods. However, nonstandardized testing is not without its drawbacks. A significant weakness lies in the lack of standardization, which can lead to inconsistencies in the administration and interpretation of results. Without uniformity, it becomes difficult to compare results across different clients or over time, potentially impacting the reliability and validity of the data. Furthermore, these types of assessments often require a high level of professional judgment and expertise, which can increase the risk of bias. Additionally, they may lack the rigorous scientific testing that standardized assessments undergo, which can lead one to question their reliability and validity. Despite these concerns, when used in conjunction with other evaluation methods, nonstandardized testing can play a critical role in the holistic assessment of a client's mental health.

VERBAL AND NONVERBAL
Verbal assessments rely on the ability to effectively respond to questions presented in oral or written form. These assessments use letters and words and may encompass grammar, vocabulary, sentence completion, analogies, and the ability to follow verbal instructions. Due to the requirement for individuals to comprehend word meanings, language structure, and logical reasoning, verbal tests tend to favor native speakers of the language in which the test was developed. *Nonverbal* assessments employ visuals such as pictures and diagrams instead of words. They provide valuable insights into an individual's strengths and challenges, independent of language influence. Nonverbal assessments are particularly beneficial for children and young individuals who are nonverbal, have English as an additional language (EAL), experience delayed speech, struggle with comprehension or communication, or face difficulties in following instructions. These assessments offer valuable information about the underlying processes, providing a wide range of benefits. They aid in profiling strengths, accurately assessing individuals with EAL, accommodating nonverbal individuals, improving our understanding of their needs, guiding targeted interventions, and facilitating gifted and talented screening.

INDIVIDUAL AND GROUP ASSESSMENTS
Individual assessments are designed for one-on-one administration, to ensure focused attention for each individual. The personalized nature of individual assessments enables the assessment to be tailored to meet the unique needs of the examinee. This approach facilitates detailed observation of behaviors and is commonly utilized for in-depth diagnostic decision-making. It is essential that individual assessments are conducted by highly skilled examiners who possess a comprehensive understanding of the assessment materials and procedures.

Group assessments are designed to efficiently collect data from large groups of individuals. They offer a cost-effective approach, as they can be administered simultaneously to multiple examinees. Group assessments require less examiner skill and can often be scored objectively, reducing the likelihood of scoring errors. Technological advancements have further streamlined the administration of group assessments, resulting in reduced time and cost. However, group assessments cannot provide the same level of personalized experience as individual assessments, which are tailored to cater to the specific needs of each individual.

OBJECTIVE AND SUBJECTIVE ASSESSMENTS

Objective assessments, characterized by multiple-choice or true/false questions, provide consistent and unbiased results as they rely on predetermined answers. Their objectivity ensures that there are no scoring variations due to different examiners' judgments. This format is often favored because of its efficiency in assessing large groups and quick scoring process. Subjective assessments, on the other hand, encompass essay questions, performance tasks, or portfolios that necessitate nuanced judgment from examiners. The subjective nature of these assessments allows for the exploration of an examinee's depth of understanding, creativity, and critical thinking, which remain unassessed in objective assessments. However, they are more time-consuming to both administer and score, and there is a risk of scorer bias or inconsistency in grading.

ASSESSMENT FORMATS

Assessments can come in a variety of formats. There is no one format that is better than another, but there are some formats that are more conducive for certain client factors like age, culture, or disability status. We should always consider all relevant factors when selecting an assessment. In Chapter 6 we will detail the process for selecting appropriate assessments for your clients.

Screening Inventories

Screening inventories play a crucial role as the initial step in the counseling assessment process. These tools, often concise self-report questionnaires or checklists, are specifically designed to identify symptoms and concerns that may warrant further evaluation. With their broad scope, they cover a wide range of potential issues, ensuring that no aspect is overlooked. It's important to note that these inventories do not provide a diagnosis, but rather aid the counselor in developing a detailed and comprehensive understanding of the client's situation. Once clients' issues are identified, they can be further assessed through interviews and other assessment methods.

Rating Scales

Rating scales offer subjective estimations of different behaviors or characteristics. They are commonly used as a method of assessment based on the observer's observations. Essentially, a rating scale serves as a tool for individuals to evaluate and assess attributes or characteristics. Formal rating scales, such as standardized assessments, undergo an extensive validation process to ensure their reliability and accuracy. These scales are carefully crafted and rigorously tested to provide uniform, objective measurements that can be compared across different groups and populations. In contrast, informal rating scales are typically more subjective. The results of these assessments are based on the personal judgment of the rater, which can vary widely. Despite their relative simplicity to develop and administer, informal rating scales play a crucial role in assessing specific areas or attributes, offering a cost-effective alternative to more formalized methods.

There are several potential challenges associated with using rating scales, such as the halo effect, generosity error, drift, and decay. These factors can impact the accuracy and reliability of the ratings. The halo effect refers to the tendency of an evaluator to let their overall impression of a person, student, or employee positively or negatively influence their judgment on specific traits or abilities. Generosity error, on the other hand, is the inclination to provide lenient ratings for everyone, regardless of their actual performance. Drift is the deviation in an evaluator's criteria over time, leading to inconsistent ratings. Decay refers to the evaluator's potential to forget details over time, particularly in long assessment periods, which can negatively impact on the accuracy of the evaluation.

Commonly used rating scales in assessments present an efficient way to quantitatively measure subjective attributes such as attitudes, opinions, behaviors, or other defined variables. Rating scales come in various forms, such as Likert-type scales, numerical scales, rank-order scales, and semantic differential scales.

- *Likert-type scales* are another popular choice in psychologic research. These scales measure agreement or disagreement with a series of statements, with responses including options such as "strongly agree," "agree," "neutral," "disagree," and "strongly disagree."

- *Numerical scales*, often used in surveys, require respondents to select a number within a given range that best represents their response to a statement or question. The range typically extends from 1 to 5 or 1 to 7, with each end representing extreme responses.

- *Rank-order scales* are used when the goal is to compare items to each other. Participants are presented with several items and asked to rank them in order of preference or importance. This scale is particularly useful when distinct preferences among a list of options need to be identified.

    o *Q-sort tests*, which also use ranking, are a type of personality assessment method in which individuals rank or sort a set of items according to specific criteria, revealing their subjective views. It usually involves providing a client with a stack of cards detailing various characteristics (such as self-esteem, anxiety, family, etc.). The client is asked to sort these cards based on a broad set of stimuli into categories using a specific instruction set.

- Lastly, *semantic differential scales* evaluate a person's reaction to stimulus words or concepts along a continuum. Respondents are asked to choose between pairs of opposite adjectives (like "happy/unhappy") separated by a seven-point scale.

Checklists

Checklists serve to determine the presence or absence of specific attributes or characteristics, while rating scales are used to evaluate the magnitude of a particular attribute or characteristic. However, it is important to note that checklists may not capture the nuanced aspects of an individual's performance or behavior. Although intended as objective tools, the interpretation and application of checklists can be influenced by the assessor's bias, potentially resulting in inconsistent outcomes. Nevertheless, checklists are typically cost and time efficient.

Biological Measures

Biological measures seek to collect physiologic data, such as heart rate, brain activity, or hormone levels, to assess bodily functions. They are also used in clinical assessment and seek to assess nervous system–related behaviors such as reaction time, skin conductance (sweating), heart rate variability, breathing rate, and brain activity, to name a few. Electroencephalograms (EEGs) are common biological measures used to observe electrical activity patterns in the brain. They are a fundamental feature of therapeutic interventions like neurofeedback (also known as EEG biofeedback or neurotherapy). Neurofeedback is an evidence-based intervention used in the treatment of anxiety, depression, substance use, attention deficit hyperactivity disorder (ADHD), trauma, and other mood disorders that provides live feedback about brainwave activity to clients to help them learn to regulate their brain function. Similarly, biofeedback interventions that measure items like heart rate variability, temperature, respiration, blood pressure, and much more can be used in counseling to help clients develop regulation skills, reduce symptoms of stress and anxiety, improve mindfulness skills, and enhance overall well-being. These biological measures are often incorporated into a treatment plan and can be administered by trained/certified professionals.

Document Analysis

Document analysis is a form of assessment that requires reviewing personal records, such as journals, letters, diary cards, or other personal records. It can be an excellent source of information about personality and can be used to assess an individual across time (Friedman & Schustack, 2009). Document analysis can be especially helpful when accounting for the broader context of a client's life and how this impacts personality, emotions, thoughts, and behavior.

Projective Assessments

Projective assessments utilize ambiguous or unstructured stimuli to elicit responses. These stimuli may include inkblots, ambiguous pictures, or incomplete sentences. By purposefully presenting vague stimuli, individuals are prompted to interpret them, and their responses are believed to unveil concealed emotions, internal conflicts, and unconscious desires or impulses. Examples of common projective assessments include the Rorschach Inkblot Test, Thematic Apperception Test (TAT), and Sentence Completion Test. Although projective assessments have sometimes been under scrutiny due to their subjective nature, they can offer valuable insights into a client's internal world when used in conjunction with other assessment strategies. Projective assessments will be covered in detail in Chapter 10.

Observations

Observation is used from the very first moment an individual speaks to someone or meets someone. *Observation* is the informal judgment, inferences, or assumptions formed about a person based on the first interaction with that person or watching a person. Initial observations can be gathered visually or auditorily. Observations can come from a person's clothing, manner of speech, tone of voice, facial expressions, eye contact, and more. As counselors, observation is the most common and inexpensive form of assessment that we can utilize with clients to start making clinical inferences and judgments. Counselors are trained to make skilled observations that most others might not notice. For example, if a client arrives at the first session and does not make eye contact and looks down at the floor, the counselor might start to make clinical inferences. Some of these could include the client being shy or having low self-esteem, or maybe cultural background and norms could play a role in the lack of eye contact. This would be something for counselors to take note of as they continue in their work with the clients to make clinical interpretations and decisions. Observation can be a formal or an informal process. *Informal observations* are the judgments or interpretations that we make upon natural and nonprescribed encounters with a person, which are not planned observations. These types of observations may not utilize specific assessment tools or predefined criteria. Examples of informal observations include things like nonverbal signs, such as observing their body language, facial expressions, and tone of voice to understand how the client is feeling; verbal communication and observing what the client says and how they express themselves in order to identify recurring themes or patterns; and the quality of the therapeutic relationship, which also can be informally observed and allows for gauging trust and rapport between the client and therapist. Informal observations play a crucial role in counseling by fostering a strong therapeutic relationship and helping counselors gain deeper insights into their clients.

Formal observations are the judgments and interpretations we make based on a planned or prescribed activity. Formal observations are often made visually or audibly but can come along with a checklist or rating scale that coincides with the observation. Formal observations in counseling include standardized assessments, structured interviews, behavioral observations, and client feedback forms; these are important tools for evaluating specific concerns and measuring progress over time or between individuals. These formal observation methods allow counselors to gather reliable and consistent data regarding a client's mental health or well-being. They also assist in assessing the effectiveness of counseling interventions and identifying areas that can be improved upon. Additionally, formal observations help establish standardized policies and procedures necessary for delivering high-quality mental health. An example of this would be prescriptively watching a child client engage in play, or many counseling training programs have students engage in role-plays and watch the counselor trainee's eye contact, body language, and nonverbal-like facial expressions and give feedback or rate those behaviors on a scale, such as the Counselor Competencies Scale—Revised (CCS-R; Lambie et al., 2018).

TIME AND EVENT SAMPLING

Two forms of observation are *event sampling* and *time sampling*. Event sampling is watching and observing for a specific behavior without time constraints. The clinician or researcher would watch the subject and wait until the specific behavior is displayed and then make a formal or informal assessment of the behavior. An example of this would be a school counselor who shadows a child for the day in order to view anger outbursts reported by the teacher. The school counselor would note each occurrence, including the trigger, the client's response, and any subsequent behavior or coping strategies used. By collecting data on these specific events, the school counselor can gain insights into the frequency, triggers, and patterns of the child's anger-related behaviors. This information can inform the development of tailored interventions and strategies to manage and control anger effectively. The school counselor may also use checklists or rating scales when shadowing the event.

Time sampling is used similarly to event sampling, but the time frame is important. Many school counselors and clinicians do not have the entire day to shadow students and clients to observe behavior. The clinician or school counselor would gain as much information as possible about the behaviors and then work to narrow down certain time frames that might be best to witness the behaviors. In a school, a counselor might want to shadow a student in 15- to 20-minute time blocks at two or three specified points in the day when the student commonly exhibits the behavior. For example, a school counselor might observe the student at recess, lunch, and their elective class because the student tends to have anger outbursts when time is unstructured. Another example of time sampling in a different setting is a counselor working with a client dealing with anxiety. Time sampling can be used to assess the client's anxiety levels throughout a counseling session. The counselor might check in with the client's anxiety level at regular intervals (e.g., every 10 minutes). The goal is to monitor how anxiety levels fluctuate during the session and identify any specific moments or topics that seem to correlate with changes in anxiety. This information can guide the counselor in tailoring the session to address the client's anxiety as it arises and help the client develop coping strategies. Time and event sampling often take place in counseling when instructors ask students to time stamp certain skills being displayed in session. Then the instructor will listen to two or three portions of the tape in 5- to 10-minute intervals that display those specific skills being assessed.

Challenges With Observation

Even though observation is a great way to assess our clients, one of the biggest challenges that exists in all observations is subjectivity. *Subjectivity* in observational assessments is the variability that exists within the person assessing. This variability in the interpretations allows the potential for personal biases and judgments to influence observations. Subjectivity can introduce inaccuracies into the assessment process, as different observers may perceive and interpret the same behaviors differently based on their personal views. An example is if you were running groups with an inpatient population, and you observe sleepy clients stretching and moving all around. The observation was subjectively interpreted. If you ask the clients, they may note that many of them are on medications that make them tired and movement and stretching help them to stay awake and engaged. This is an example of subjective observational assessment information that was not accurate and needed to be coupled with another method to gather data.

To minimize subjectivity, clinicians and researchers often undergo training on standardized observation protocols when available. Through this protocol they can triangulate data with other data sources, use interrater reliability, and compare observations with other observers. Researchers and clinicians can engage in reflexivity practices to reflect and reduce chances of bias before working with someone, or technology can be used to assist in observational data analysis (Whiston, 2016).

General forms of measurement bias and those specifically related to culture are discussed in Chapters 3 and 6; these cause issues in the reliability and validity of tests. *Observation bias* can also cause reliability or consistency issues if different observers interpret behaviors differently. An example of observer bias would be if someone makes an assumption about a person's gender identity based on gender expression through clothing choices and personal gendered beliefs and values. This type of observation bias leads to systematic errors because the bias would cause the error to happen consistently and each time. Additionally, observation bias can include things that impact the observer for the time being. For example, if a counselor got a ticket driving to work, that person could be upset and distracted, and their observations of a client group might be harsh or critical. This type of error would be an unsystematic error because it is unlikely to happen each time (Whiston, 2016). These types of errors affect the reliability of observations.

Observations can also be biased due to the lack of context and time spent observing a situation, the limited scope of what can be directly observed, observer training, generalizability, representativeness (which impacts validity), and observer effects (the observer inadvertently affects the person's behavior), as well as the Hawthorne effect, in which the client's behaviors change to be more favorable because they know they are being observed (Merrett, 2006). Additionally, observer recall can become an issue in observational assessments. Clinicians may only recall things that are noteworthy from their own perspective and worldview and not remember everything. Selective attention from the observer can become problematic in observations. For example, a counselor who frequently works with nonsuicidal self-injury (NSSI) clients may see a client with marks on their arms and automatically think they are cuts and that the client engages in NSSI. They will selectively pay attention to the marks and may not notice that the client is jittery and unable to focus, which might suggest that the client could be a substance user and the marks are related to drug use. To enhance the validity and reliability of observational assessments and address some of these challenges, researchers and clinicians can utilize multiple methods of assessment, such as self-report questionnaires, interviews, or objective measures, to support their observations.

Direct and Indirect Observations

Direct observations entail gathering primary data by directly engaging with the subject of interest. Observations of this nature typically maintain objectivity, as they depend on firsthand sensory perception and quantifiable measurements. Direct observations are conducted to gather precise and unbiased data in real time. They are frequently employed to monitor behaviors, events, or activities. To illustrate, a counselor conducting in-home counseling may directly observe communication dynamics within a family system to assess their interaction styles. Researchers can also conduct direct observations in controlled experiments to observe participant behavior under specific conditions. Standardized measurement tools, checklists, or rating scales can be utilized throughout these observations to gather and document data systematically. For example, a therapist could employ a structured observation form to evaluate a client's anxiety levels during a counseling session.

Indirect observations involve data collection methods that do not require direct interaction or real-time monitoring. Instead, they rely on inferences, third-party reports, or preexisting information. Indirect observations are characterized by subjectivity and the use of self-reported data from individuals through questionnaires. They also involve interviews with those who have observed the behaviors or experiences as third-party reports and utilize preexisting data from historical documents or records. Psychologic assessments like projective tests or self-report questionnaires regarding a person's thoughts may also be used in indirect observations. When direct observations are not able to be obtained or subjectivity is needed, indirect observations are useful. However, they are more likely to be subject to biases, inaccuracies, or limitations due to the self-report nature. Researchers often use a combination of both types of observations to gain a comprehensive understanding of a subject or phenomenon.

Other Nontraditional Methods

Graphic assessment methods in counseling are the various approaches that utilize visual portrayals to assist in the assessment of psychologic well-being with clients. These techniques visually represent data, progress, and patterns related to clients' emotional, behavioral, and cognitive states. These methods are inclusive of scales, charts, diaries, genograms or diagrams for monitoring and communicating such things as changes in mood, behavior, or symptom severity over time. With advances in technology there are tools that can be used with clients to help depict graphic assessment measures, and many outcomes of standardized assessments are able to provide visual feedback to both therapists and clients, allowing for collaboration with counselors and clients.

Art-based assessment methods in counseling settings use methods of artistic experiences or materials to gain unique insights into individuals' psychologic states. These methods incorporate visual, auditory, or kinesthetic forms of expression to assess and understand individuals' emotions, thoughts, and behaviors. Art-based assessment tools may include projective drawings, visual tests, and art therapy techniques, which are carefully selected by professionals to assess individuals' functioning, strengths, and treatment objectives. Body mapping is a common example of an expressive arts therapy technique. Body mapping involves painting a life-size representation of one's body onto a large surface and using colors, pictures, symbols, and words to represent experiences within the body. This creative therapeutic tool brings together bodily experience and visual artistic expression, providing a safe space for clients to rediscover their bodies as a source of strength and healing. This strengths-based approach can be used with eating disorder clients or those who have experienced traumas, such as intimate partner violence. These approaches provide valuable understanding of individuals' experiences and promote holistic assessment and intervention strategies.

Autobiographical methods of assessing data in counseling encompass the use of autobiographical writing and narratives as a tool for self-understanding and change. Autobiographic methods facilitate a process to bring up issues in a different format, which can reveal things about the writer, challenge the story, make experiences reality, and honor a client's life. Autobiographical writing in counseling provides a unique opportunity for individuals to explore and express their experiences, emotions, and perceptions, ultimately contributing to self-understanding and personal growth. These methods offer valuable insights into the individual's experiences and psychologic well-being, contributing to a comprehensive understanding of the client's narrative and aiding in the therapeutic process. Some examples include assessing records, evaluating written narratives, and constructing timelines.

CHECKING IN WITH ARTURO

Let's think back to the case of Arturo in Chapters 1 and 2. Arturo comes from a strong spiritual background, but recently has not been connected to his faith and feels disenfranchised regarding his faith.

1. How would the biopsychosocial-spiritual assessment be useful with Arturo?

2. What additional information not present in the case vignette would you want to gather from Arturo in his initial intake assessment? How would these additional pieces of information be helpful in your work with Arturo?

3. What assessment method or approach would be a good fit for Arturo and why?

END-OF-CHAPTER RESOURCES

DISCUSSION QUESTIONS

1. Imagine you are conducting an intake interview with a new client seeking counseling services. Based on the information provided in the resources, develop a set of open-ended questions that you would ask during the intake interview to gather relevant information about the client's presenting concerns, background, and goals for counseling. Why did you select each question and how do they align with the goals of the intake interview? Consider the importance of building rapport, understanding the client's perspective, and identifying areas for further exploration in the counseling process. Share your insights on the significance of these questions in establishing a strong foundation for the counseling relationship and treatment planning.

2. Understanding a client's worldview and problems can be facilitated through the use of observational assessments. Cultural diversity plays a large role in client observations and must be considered. What are some ways counselors can ensure cultural competence when conducting observational assessments? Discuss the key considerations and challenges in maintaining cultural competence during observational assessments and provide examples of culturally sensitive observational practices that align with ethical guidelines and respect the diversity of clients' backgrounds and experiences.

CLASS ACTIVITIES

1. Complete a review of counseling intake forms from sources, such as the PDF Filler, Jotform, and Cedarville University forms. Analyze the structure, content, and purpose of these forms, along with the information presented in this chapter.

    a. Identify the essential information that you would want in a comprehensive counseling intake form. This may include personal details, presenting concerns, medical history, previous counseling experience, and consent information.

    b. Based on this identified essential information, draft your own form. Be sure to consider things like language, formatting, ease of use, methods to capture the information, and organization of the form.

    c. Exchange your draft intake forms with classmates for feedback and compare with their forms. Provide each other constructive feedback on the clarity, relevance, and sensitivity of the form content.

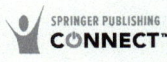

A robust set of instructor resources designed to supplement this text is located at http://connect.springerpub.com/content/book/978-0-8261-8913-4. Qualifying instructors may request access by emailing textbook@springerpub.com.

REFERENCES

Borrell-Carrió, F., Suchman, A. L., & Epstein, R. M. (2004). The biopsychosocial model 25 years later: Principles, practice, and scientific inquiry. *Annals of Family Medicine, 2*(6), 576–582. https://doi.org/10.1370/afm.245

Cook, K. B., & Snyder, S. M. (2020). Minimizing and reporting momentary time-sampling measurement error in single-case research. *Behavior Analysis in Practice, 13,* 247–252. https://doi.org/10.1007/s40617-018-00325-2

Council for Accreditation of Counseling and Related Educational Programs. (2023). *2024 CACREP standards.* https://www.cacrep.org/wp-content/uploads/2023/06/Combined-version-6.21.23.pdf

Donnelly, J., Rosenberg, M., & Fleeson, W. P. (1970). The evolution of the mental status–past and future. *The American Journal of Psychiatry, 126*(7), 997–1002. https://doi.org/10.1176/ajp.126.7.997

Engel, G. L. (1977). The need for a new medical model: A challenge for biomedicine. *Science (New York, N.Y.), 196*(4286), 129–136. https://doi.org/10.1126/science.847460

Engel, G. L. (1980). The clinical application of the biopsychosocial model. *The American Journal of Psychiatry, 137*(5), 535–544. https://doi.org/10.1176/ajp.137.5.535

Friedman, H. S., & Schustack, M. W. (2009). *Personality: Classic theories and modern research* (M. Limoges, Ed.). Pearson Education.

Green, S. B., McCoy, J. F., Burns, K. P., & Smith, A. C. (1982). Accuracy of observational data with whole interval, partial interval, and momentary time-sampling recording techniques. *Journal of Behavioral Assessment, 4,* 103–118. https://doi.org/10.1007/BF01321385

Gresham, F. (2007). Response to intervention and emotional and behavioral disorders: Best practices in assessment for intervention. *Assessment for Effective Intervention, 32,* 214–222. https://doi.org/10.1177/15345084070320040301

Grundy, Q., Chiu, K., Held, F., Continella, A., Bero, L., & Holz, R. (2019). Data sharing practices of medicines related apps and the mobile ecosystem: Traffic, content, and network analysis. *BMJ, 364,* l920. https://doi.org/10.1136/bmj.l920

Handler, L., & Meyer, G. J. (1998). The importance of teaching and learning personality assessment. In L. Handler & M. J. Hilsenroth (Eds.), *Teaching and learning personality assessment* (pp. 3–30). Lawrence Erlbaum Associates.

Haynes, S., & O'Brien, W. (2000). *Principles and practice of behavioral assessment.* Kluwer Academic/Plenum Publishers.

Lambie, G. W., Mullen, P. R., Swank, J. M., & Blount, A. (2018). The Counseling Competencies Scale: Validation and refinement. *Measurement and Evaluation in Counseling and Development, 51*(1), 1–15. http://doi.org/10.1080/07481756.2017.1358964

Linehan, M. M. (2018). *Cognitive-behavioral treatment of borderline personality disorder.* Guilford Publications.

McCool, M. W., Mochrie, K. D., Lothes, J. E., Guendner, E., St. John, J., & Noel, N. E. (2023). Dialectical behavior therapy skills and urges to use alcohol and substances: An examination of diary cards. *Substance Use & Misuse, 58*(11), 1409–1417. https://doi.org/10.1080/10826084.2023.2223283

Merrett, F. (2006). Reflections on the Hawthorne effect. *Educational Psychology, 26*(1), 143–146. http://doi.org/10.1080/01443410500341080

Palmer, K. M., & Burrows, V. (2021). Ethical and safety concerns regarding the use of mental health–related apps in counseling: Considerations for counselors. *Journal of Technology in Behavioral Science, 6,* 137–150. https://doi.org/10.1007/s41347-020-00160-9

Pashak, T. J., & Heron, M. R. (2022). Build rapport and collect data: A teaching resource on the clinical interviewing intake. *Discovery in Psychology, 2,* 20. https://doi.org/10.1007/s44202-022-00019-5

Rogers, C. R. (1995). *On becoming a person: A therapist's view of psychotherapy.* Houghton Mifflin Harcourt.

Singh, N. N., Lancioni, G. E., Felver, J. C., Myers, R. E., Hwang, Y. S., Chan, J., & Medvedev, O. N. (2023). Effects of mindful engagement and attention on reciprocal caregiver and client interactions: A behavioral analysis of moment-to-moment changes during mindfulness practice. *Mindfulness, 14*(8), 1893–1907. http://doi.org/10.1007/s12671-023-02190-9

van Wessel, M. (2018). Narrative assessment: A new approach to evaluation of advocacy for development. *Evaluation, 24*(4), 400–418. http://doi.org/10.1177/1356389018796021

van Wessel, M. G. J., Ho, W. W. S., & Tamas, P. A. (2021). *Narrative assessment: A new method for monitoring, evaluating, learning and communicating about advocacy.* WUR/Hivos.

Voss, R. M., & Das, J. M. (2022). Mental status examination. *StatPearls.* Accessed January 30, 2024. https://www.statpearls.com/point-of-care/24998

Whiston, S. C. (2016). *Principles and applications of assessment in counseling.* Cengage Learning.

Wood, J. C., & McKay, M. (2021). *The dialectical behavior therapy diary: Monitoring your emotional regulation day by day.* New Harbinger Publications.

5

Assessment and Diagnosis in Counseling

CLARA BOSSIE AND CARMAN S. GILL

2024 CACREP STANDARDS

3.G.7. use of culturally sustaining and developmentally appropriate assessments for diagnostic and intervention planning purposes

3.G.11. diagnostic processes, including differential diagnosis and the use of current diagnostic classification systems

I continued to specialize in addiction care for many years, and I realized how often clients are (a) misdiagnosed based on the symptoms of detoxing or becoming sober and (b) the incredible number of diagnoses one may receive when stuck in a chronic relapse cycle. I often requested a comprehensive list of previous diagnoses from clients, highlighting those they found to be accurate and any suspected conditions that had never been formally assessed. I recall a young man who had been living with undiagnosed obsessive-compulsive disorder (OCD), though he had been previously labeled with various mood disorders and narcissism. Another poignant example was a woman in her later years, misidentified as having avoidant personality disorder when, in reality, she had been coping with undiagnosed autism. Moreover, numerous individuals diagnosed with both addiction and mood disorders revealed, upon deeper exploration, a lifelong struggle with unrecognized learning disabilities. Clients rely on us to see them in context and understand how they move through the world. The truly rewarding aspect of diagnostic assessments lies in supporting that process and embracing the opportunity to "be curious" as we peel back the layers of our client's life. This involves remembering always to ask ourselves what is being left out before we decide how to move forward.

HISTORY OF DIAGNOSIS AND THE COUNSELING FIELD

In Chapter 1, we covered terminology related to assessment, evaluation, and testing. In this chapter, we build upon some of those definitions, delineating and describing the process of diagnostic testing and assessment. The word *diagnosis* comes from the Greek *dia* (apart) and *gnosis* (to perceive or to know) and at its core implies an objective assessment of the individual and process (Neukrug & Fawcett, 2010). Symptoms of mental problems and disorders are referred to throughout human history. The book of Job in the Bible seems to describe Job suffering mental symptoms after his horrific experiences. The Greek historian Herotodus referred to mental issues that appeared related to battle. These early references to traumatic stress were not the only noteworthy mentions of symptoms of mental struggles. In 1918, the psychiatric profession attempted to capture these symptoms in a way that could be standardized. This attempt ultimately resulted in the *Statistical Manual for the Use of Institutions for the Insane*, a predecessor of the *Diagnostic and Statistical Manual of Mental*

Disorders (*DSM*; Kawa & Giordano, 2012). The naming of this nosology reflects not only a psychiatric practice that at the time was based primarily in mental asylums but also the fluid and culturally based nature of diagnosis.

As noted earlier in our text, Frank Parsons was credited with detailing the first counseling processes, which included research, evaluation, and testing. In the United States, the original centers were called "counseling and testing" centers (National Board of Forensic Evaluators [NBFE], 2022). However, the focus for counselors remained on guidance and holistic wellness. Differing from this, psychiatry as a discipline focuses on the treatment of mental disorders from a medical perspective. Psychiatrists introduced the primary U.S. system for classifying these disorders in their 1952 publication of the *DSM* (American Psychiatric Association, 1952). Understanding the philosophical underpinnings of counseling and psychiatry, as well as their differences and similarities (see Box 5.1), provides greater insights into the current issues related to the *DSM*, diagnosis, and the role of the counselor.

History and Philosophy of This Nosology

The original *DSM* was published in 1952 by the American Psychiatric Association in response to the sixth edition of the *International Classification of Diseases* (*ICD-6*; World Health Organization [WHO], 1949), which, for the first time, covered mental disorders (Dailey et al., 2014). Representing psychiatry's first attempt at standardizing mental health symptoms, at that time, the *DSM* was based largely on psychodynamic formulations and on Adolf Meyer's psychobiological view. Meyer believed that mental disorders were primarily "reactions" of the personality to biological, psychologic, or social aspects of client functioning (Gill et al., 2024). Totaling 106 pages, the *DSM-I* included three categories of psychopathology, specifically organic brain syndromes, functional disorders, and mental deficiency (American Psychiatric Association, 1952). This nosology differed in substantial ways from the *ICD-6*.

The second edition of the *DSM* coincided once again with a new edition of the *ICD* (*ICD-8*; WHO, 1965) but moved away from Meyer's theories. This edition, the *DSM-II*, was published in 1968 and included 11 categories with 182 diagnoses (American Psychiatric

---

BOX 5.1 PSYCHIATRY VERSUS COUNSELING

Different Disciplines

Counseling is a discipline that approaches client care from a strengths-based, holistic wellness approach. Keep in mind that psychiatry is a medically based discipline and those who practice psychiatry hold medical doctorates (MDs). Because of the medically based nature of this discipline, the publications they produce, including the Diagnostic and Statistical Manual of Mental Disorders (DSM), *will have a different focus than does counseling.*

1. What are the commonalities between counselors and psychiatrists?
2. What do "strengths-based" and "holistic" mean to you?
3. How does this distinguish counseling from a medically based mental health approach?
4. Identify the ways in which counselors will approach a client that vary from those of psychiatric practice.

Association, 1968; Gill et al., 2024). The noteworthy shift in this nosology was toward psychoanalysis, as evidenced by the removal of "reactions" in favor of neuroses and psychophysiological disorders. Additionally, milder diagnoses were added, which were intended to be more reflective of the public (i.e., "Conditions Without Manifest Psychiatric Disorder" and "Transient Situational Disturbances"). Whereas diagnoses that lacked verification were removed, this edition did provide 76 additional diagnoses, expanding the manual significantly and making it more consistent with the *ICD* (Kawa & Giordano, 2012).

The *DSM-III* was revised in 1980 and was heavily influenced by the acceptance of the medical model and the rise of managed care. The edition reflected a move toward well-defined symptomology based on positivistic science with descriptive checklists or diagnostic criteria as we know them. Due in part to the rise of rating scales and psychometric instruments, this publication represented psychiatry's attempt to operationalize, measure, and identify medically based treatments for mental disorders (Kawa & Giordano, 2012). In a controversial move at the time, homosexuality as a category was permanently removed from this edition. Totaling 265 pages, the version introduced the multiaxial system and integrated demographic information into diagnostic classifications (American Psychiatric Association, 1980). It also fully embraced a research-based, medical model approach to mental illness, relying heavily on a biological view of symptoms and psychopharmacology as treatment.

The *DSM-III* was criticized for lacking a holistic approach to mental health, which could easily result in inaccurately viewing the individual as solely responsible for their symptomology. For counselors, focusing only on a medical treatment model directly contradicts our distinct emphasis on prevention, wellness, and social justice (Gill et al., 2024). Noteworthy is that, following the release of this nosology, the federal government and pharmaceutical companies committed billions of dollars to psychopharmacological research. With 292 pages, the following version, the *DSM-III-R* (American Psychiatric Association, 1987), was intended to represent minor changes while increasing the reliability of diagnosis using the information gathered through diagnostic interviews and field trials. However, criticism of the nosology continued and included questions surrounding the functionality of the multiaxial system.

The publication of the *DSM-IV* (American Psychiatric Association, 1994) represented minor changes to diagnosis. The steering committee associated with this version focused on the clinical utility of the manual and included 365 diagnoses for a total of 886 pages. The major change was the increased inclusion of empirically based information, which was also the major change for the *DSM-IV-TR* published in 2000. This version also attempted to align diagnostic codes with the *ICD* and introduce less pathologizing language (Gill et al., 2024). Although the authors of the nosology attempted to use field trials and diagnostic interviews to improve the reliability and utility of this manual, the *DSM* continued to receive heavy criticism for questionable reliability, comorbidity of diagnosis, bias, and the multiaxial system.

Intended to be the most radical change yet, the *DSM-5* task force proposed major alterations to the nosology, including a philosophical shift in how diagnoses are viewed from categorial to dimensional, lowering of the diagnostic threshold for key disorders, a new system for understanding and diagnosing personality disorders, and the removal of the controversial multiaxial system. Many of these proposed changes were met with a firestorm of resistance, particularly the restructuring of substance use disorders and the proposed lowering of diagnostic thresholds for substance use disorders. As diagnostic codes in the *DSM* received more widespread use due to insurance and other reimbursement, mental health professionals working in disciplines other than psychiatry relied heavily on this manual. These professionals voiced concerns regarding the change process, the lowering of diagnostic thresholds, using the multiaxial system, and other changes. Representing the second largest group to use this manual, counselors employed the *DSM* for diagnosis, when needed, and as part of a holistic client conceptualization. However, counselors were not invited to participate in the task force. Counselors were involved, however, in the field trials, and ACA created a task force that provided the organization with education and recommendations related to the new nosology. These recommendations also included two open letters from different American Counseling Association (ACA) presidents to the American Psychiatric Association focusing on the major concerns regarding changes. Ultimately, some changes were retained, such as the removal of the multiaxial system and the philosophical move to dimensional thinking in terms of symptomology, and others were not included, such as the proposed changes to personality disorders (American Psychiatric Association, 2013).

The current edition of the *DSM*, the *DSM-5-TR*, was released in 2022. This publication was intended to be a true text revision, with a focus on clarity and providing guidance. Therefore, minor changes, corrections, and updates were provided. The authors intended to remove stigmatizing language throughout and highlight the risk factors associated with systemic racism, oppression, and discrimination (American Psychiatric Association, 2022a). The *DSM-5-TR* incorporated updated empirical research to inform text sections such as Diagnostic Prevalence, Risk Factors, Comorbidity, and others. The authors added associations with suicidal ideation or attempt as information was available and included Prolonged Grief Disorder as a new diagnosis. Following the publication, the American Psychiatric Association released three supplemental documents. The first supplement removed Suicidal Behavior Disorder from "Conditions for Further Study" and changed the language around suicidal ideation to reduce stigma (American Psychiatric Association, 2022c) while also updating specific codes. The second supplement only focused on updating codes for specific diagnoses. The final supplement, released in September 2023, addressed coding changes for two disorders and text updates for differential diagnoses for three disorders. It also included a statement regarding clinical judgment and warning clinicians not to use the manual in a "rigid cookbook fashion" (American Psychiatric Association, 2022b, p. 3).

The history and development of the *DSM* underscores the notion that diagnosis and diagnostic categories are "constructed concepts" (Kawa & Giordano, 2012, p. 8). Diagnostic systems are culturally bound and subject to clinical scrutiny and modification. Evidence of this is clearly available in the removal of homosexuality from the *DSM-III* (American Psychiatric Association, 1980). A diagnosis such as Gender Dysphoria reflects the controversial nature of what we consider to be pathological. The idea that an individual suffers from a mental disorder because they are transitioning is inaccurate, at the very least. Because of the difficulty accessing medical and other care without a formal diagnosis, however, counselors may, with the client's fully informed consent, use a diagnosis like Gender Dysphoria as circumstances and health insurance barriers warrant to ensure the client is able to receive the appropriate care. Moreover, information from the Trevor Project, which focuses on eliminating suicidality among LGBTQ young people, indicates that transgender youth experience suicidal ideation at much higher rates than their heterosexual peers (The Trevor Project, 2021). They also note that gender-affirming health does result in lower suicide rates and point to a recent study in which gender-affirming hormone therapy was associated with lower rates of depression and suicidality (Green et al., 2021). Further, the standards of care of the Society for Sexual, Affectional, Intersex, and Gender Expansive Identities (Goodrich et al., 2017) state that the counselor understands that "the diagnosis of gender dysphoria is only relevant when a client wishes to access medical treatments related to the transition process and is required by insurance. They also explore with the client the systemic oppression related to the medical requirement to have the diagnosis to obtain access to the requested treatment" (Goodrich et al., 2017, p. 5).

Questions surrounding the etiology of disorders continue as well. Whereas the medical model relies on the idea that the issue originates with the brain or body, as counselors, we note that some depressive symptoms and/or disorders may flow from the environment. Factors such as systemic discrimination and racism are at the core of this acute emotional pain. Therefore, as you continue through this chapter, it is essential to understand that the reliability of diagnostic assessments across cultural groups can vary. Engaging in culturally appropriate diagnostic procedures is crucial to accurately identify client characteristics, protective factors, risk factors, and warning signs of mental health and behavioral disorders. This nuanced approach paves the way for more effective and empathic counseling practices by ensuring that assessments are tools for diagnosis and instruments for understanding clients' diverse experiences and needs.

DIAGNOSTIC ASSESSMENTS IN COUNSELING: A MULTIFACETED LENS

Diagnostic assessments multifacetedly influence therapeutic intervention, serving roles far beyond symptom identification. The utility of a *DSM* diagnosis extends from shaping a structured treatment framework to practical matters like insurance billing, thereby ensuring the sustainability of care. However, assigning a diagnostic label demands cautious deliberation. Ethical considerations arise, necessitating a balance between the benefits of targeted treatment protocols and the inherent risks of stigmatization or oversimplification of complex mental health issues. Our ethical obligation as counselors is to be precise in our diagnostic efforts. Reaching an accurate diagnosis is a professional standard and the ethical foundation for effective treatment and seamless continuity of care (ACA, 2014). As we delve into the diagnostic assessment in this section, we explore its diverse roles in modern counseling practice. Whether charting the course of treatment, safeguarding client well-being, streamlining resource allocation, or continually adapting strategies based on measurable outcomes, using diagnostic tools is integral to delivering high-quality, evidence-based care (Jensen-Doss & Hawley, 2011). Each of the following subsections will unpack the various applications of diagnostic assessments, providing you with a comprehensive understanding that will enhance your skills as an emerging counselor.

The Universal Language: Continuity of Care and Interdisciplinary Communication

As the therapeutic journey unfolds, diagnostic assessments serve as invaluable tools. Several key reasons are given as a rationale for the use of diagnosis in counseling. One such rationale is the idea of using the same language, or consistency, across mental health and medical disciplines. These objective metrics also provide essential data for communicating with multidisciplinary teams, especially when standardized diagnostic labels and codes, such as those from the *DSM-5-TR* (American Psychiatric Association, 2022a) or *ICD-11* (WHO, 2019), are involved. Such common terminology ensures cohesive and effective treatment when multiple healthcare providers are engaged in a client's care. When a general practitioner is told that their patient has a history of bipolar I disorder, that doctor has a general idea of what to expect in terms of symptomology. When a counselor sees a referral for a client who is experiencing posttraumatic stress disorder (PTSD), that counselor may begin to consider trauma-focused diagnostic assessments such as the Posttraumatic Stress Disorder Symptom Scale Interview (PSSI-5; Foa et al., 2016) and corresponding treatments that include eye movement desensitization and reprocessing (EMDR) or prolonged exposure for PTSD. Moreover, a standardized diagnostic language facilitates seamless continuity of care for clients, whether they relocate, pursue complementary therapies, or need to transition to a new counselor.

Uniform terminology fosters seamless continuity of care, benefiting clients who may relocate, opt for complementary therapies, or transition to another counselor. This chapter highlights accurate diagnosis as the cornerstone for effective treatment and the continuity of care as a crucial link between a client's well-being and a clinician's efficacy. Following the ACA's (2014) guidelines, it is an ethical imperative that counselors be meticulous in their diagnostic efforts.

From Blueprint to Roadmap: The Role of Diagnostic Assessments in Treatment Planning

Diagnostic assessments are the foundation for any therapeutic journey, often comprising the initial intake evaluation and case conceptualization. These preliminary steps enable counselors to make sense of a client's presenting issues, psychosocial history, and potential diagnostic categories. They offer clinicians a structured understanding of the client's situation and set the stage for focused, evidence-based interventions (Patel et al., 2022). Here, an integrated review of psychometric properties, cultural considerations, and coexisting conditions provides the scaffold upon which treatment is built. Upon gaining a foundational understanding of the client, the application of diagnostic assessments directly informs the treatment planning process. This includes determining suitable interventions, therapeutic modalities, and potential referrals. These assessments offer a roadmap for therapeutic strategies and interventions aligning with the client's needs. Transparent discussion of diagnostic findings can foster a collaborative relationship where the client is more actively involved in treatment planning. Diagnostic data allow the client and counselor to collaborate effectively in crafting a tailored, evolving treatment plan that is realistic, achievable, and measurable. Moreover, diagnostic results and treatment plans can be disseminated to the client, caregivers, and the multidisciplinary care team (i.e., medical professionals, occupational and physical therapists, educators, dieticians, and integrative care providers).

Safety Nets and Ethical Foundations: Risk Management and Ongoing Monitoring

Risk assessment and ongoing monitoring using client-reported outcomes and measurement-based care are essential safety nets in comprehensive treatment. By utilizing standardized measures such as symptom checklists, counselors can quantify changes in clients' symptom severity, functional status, and overall well-being while fine-tuning treatment plans. This measurement-based care offers the utility of detecting the deteriorating wellness of clients; however, Lewis et al. (2019) found that less than 20% of behavioral healthcare workers are taking advantage of such diagnostic tools within their practice. Diagnostic assessments offer invaluable data that pinpoint potential risk areas, such as suicidality, substance misuse, or self-harm behaviors. Here, diagnostic data do more than guide initial interventions; the data become longitudinal markers for tracking client progress and mitigating risk over time. Repeated diagnostic assessments offer quantifiable data, furnishing a basis for the continual refinement of treatment plans; thus, the goal is to inform changes in the care plan. Such ongoing scrutiny ensures that treatment interventions remain timely, targeted, and effective. Thus, diagnostic data equip counselors with the empirical support needed for making immediate and long-term judgments in a field fraught with complex ethical and clinical challenges.

In the exciting and complex realm of measurement-based care, the ongoing use of diagnostic assessments is not just about monitoring numbers on a chart; it is a dynamic dialogue between clinician and client. Counselors must comprehend both the rationale for selecting a particular measurement and the art of interpreting the results (Brundage et al., 2020). Think of it as a two-way street where data-driven insights fuel the therapeutic journey. However, the road isn't always smooth. Some common roadblocks in this approach involve the client's uncertainty about how to wield this newfound data for self-improvement. They might wonder, "How do I use this information to boost my self-care strategies or better manage my mental health?" On the other hand, counselors are not immune to stumbling blocks either. Many professionals need a better grasp on how to apply diagnostic assessment data in a therapeutic context (Brundage et al., 2020). The silver lining? The academic community is buzzing with solutions. Recommendations are increasingly pointing toward robust training programs that empower clinicians to use evidence-based diagnostic assessments effectively at the outset and throughout the therapeutic journey (Brundage et al., 2020; Lewis et al., 2019). Technological advancements facilitate the risk and outcome monitoring process, allowing for more streamlined and efficient monitoring (Barbera & Moody, 2019; Brundage et al., 2020).

Navigating Logistical Considerations: Resource Allocation and Regulatory Compliance

Beyond direct clinical applications, diagnostic assessments perform crucial roles in the systemic aspects of mental healthcare. One often-overlooked application lies in resource allocation, particularly in community mental health and hospital settings. Diagnostic categorizations inform counselors about the intensity and types of services clients require. For instance, a diagnosis of borderline personality disorder necessitates more intensive treatments like dialectical behavior therapy (DBT), guiding the allocation of resources to such modalities. Similarly, a diagnosis of OCD often calls for staff training in evidence-based interventions like exposure response prevention (ERP) therapy. Resource allocation aims to provide effective treatment economically and sustainably, thereby extending the reach of community services.

Furthermore, diagnostic data fulfill documentation and billing requirements, especially where third-party payers are involved. These logistical aspects significantly influence the quality and sustainability of care. Healthcare systems and community mental health agencies frequently operate at their limits; thus, accurate diagnoses become essential in utilizing resources effectively and efficiently. In parallel, diagnostic assessments maintain regulatory compliance. Healthcare providers must present diagnostic data to meet an ethical standard of care, insurance billing requirements, and quality assurance protocols. Compliance is not only administrative; it also safeguards the integrity of care, ensures transparency, and protects both the client and provider. In totality, diagnostic assessments function as a multifaceted tool bolstering the resilience and effectiveness of mental healthcare systems clinically, economically, and ethically.

CONDUCTING A DIAGNOSTIC ASSESSMENT

Although a clinical interview (i.e., biopsychosocial-spiritual) will often uncover diagnostic features, the diagnostic assessment is more direct and focused on the data needed to understand the etiology and presentation of a potential diagnosis. Moreover, data may lead to referrals to other allied healthcare professionals as potential medical health concerns arise. The use of diagnostic interviews requires extensive knowledge and experience in mental health assessment, as well as the ability to interpret the information gathered in the context of relevant diagnostic criteria, such as those found in the *DSM* or the *ICD*. In treatment planning, a diagnostic interview is a critical tool to assess clients' suitability for certain therapeutic interventions and tailor the treatment to their needs and symptoms. The significance of reaching a precise diagnosis cannot be overstated. As such, accurate diagnosing is a key player in unlocking a tailored and effective treatment plan that supports the entire structure of a client's therapeutic journey. Without completing the critical step of a diagnostic assessment, the counseling process is at risk of becoming a directionless endeavor, potentially ineffective, or even counterproductive. The benefits of a precise diagnosis are numerous, including the guidance of risk management, the assurance of proper resource allocation, and the facilitation of treatment progress measurement, as discussed earlier in the chapter. Furthermore, counselors who engage in evidence-based diagnostic assessment practices maintain a high standard of professional care and demonstrate accountability. Clearly, diagnostic assessment is not just about labels; it is a pivotal step in mapping out a path to recovery and fostering understanding, autonomy, and client well-being. Counselors must consistently evaluate clients, particularly at the onset of services. In Chapter 4, we provided an example of an initial intake assessment process that includes a diagnostic assessment phase. Key to evidence-based evaluative practices, a comprehensive diagnostic assessment allows for ethical treatment decisions, eligibility decisions for resources, and distribution of services. *The diagnostic assessment is a process of evaluation that is achieved by acquiring the necessary insights to develop a comprehensive understanding of a client and their issues.* A thorough diagnostic assessment will include a variety of methods and produce a holistic view of a client's past, present, and future potential in the process. There are many ways to approach a diagnostic assessment. The treatment setting, population, and salient concerns must be considered to meet client needs. For example, diagnostic assessments with clients seeking addiction counseling or eating disorder treatment must include additional data to assess medical risk and safety.

Moreover, in outpatient and private practice settings, a counselor's approach to diagnostic assessment can be largely influenced by their preferred theoretical framework. Each approach brings a unique perspective and varying emphasis on a client's history, present symptoms, environment, systemic factors, and goals. For example, cognitive behavioral therapy (CBT) and DBT are more likely to focus on reaching a diagnosis during assessment. These therapies, particularly CBT, often use structured diagnostic assessments and standardized tools to identify specific psychologic disorders or issues, aligning with a more medical model approach. DBT, a third-wave CBT model developed initially for borderline personality disorder, also involves assessing for specific diagnoses, especially related to emotional regulation and interpersonal issues. In contrast, Adlerian, humanistic, and systems therapies focus less on diagnostic labels and more on understanding clients' experiences, relationships, and behavior patterns. These approaches are more inclined toward exploring broader aspects of a person's life and experiences rather than fitting their issues into a specific diagnostic category. Counselors will find common factors when exploring various diagnostic assessment approaches, regardless of the reasons one seeks counseling or a counselor's theoretical approach. Drawing from common factors included in a diagnostic assessment, we offer an overarching process for the diagnostic assessment with utility in a variety of settings (see Table 5.1).

The diagnostic assessment process goes hand in hand with the initial intake and assessment process, commonly intertwined, as demonstrated in Chapter 4. Still, because diagnostic data can evolve, these assessments are useful at various phases in the treatment process.

TABLE 5.1 **THEORETICAL PERSPECTIVES OF DIAGNOSTIC ASSESSMENTS**

Theoretical Approach	View of Assessment	Emphasis	Features
CBT	CBT therapists conceptualize assessment as a structured process to identify and understand the interrelationships among a client's thoughts, feelings, and behaviors, guiding targeted interventions.	The emphasis is on understanding the relationships between thoughts, feelings, and behaviors, and how these contribute to the clients' issues or underlying diagnosis.	• Use of structured tools like self-report questionnaires • Thought records to track cognitions in response to specific events • Behavioral assessments to identify patterns and triggers of maladaptive behaviors
DBT	DBT therapists conceptualize assessment to evaluate and monitor a client's emotional regulation, distress tolerance, interpersonal effectiveness, and mindfulness skills, guiding the therapy's focus and interventions.	The emphasis is on identifying a client's life worth living, adaptive skills, maladaptive behaviors, and understanding a client's diagnosis from a biosocial model.	• Use of self-monitoring diary cards to track daily emotions, thoughts, behaviors, and skills use • Assessing progress in learning and applying DBT skills • Use of diagnosis-specific diagnostic assessments
Adlerian	Adlerian therapists conceptualize assessment as a holistic exploration of an individual's lifestyle, family history, and social context to understand their unique motivations, perceptions, and behavior patterns.	The emphasis is on exploring family history, early childhood experiences, and social context.	• Use of techniques like lifestyle assessment and early recollections • Exploration of family constellations and personal narratives • Understanding the individual's logic and goal orientation
Humanistic	Humanistic therapists conceptualize assessment as an empathetic and client-centered process focused on understanding the individual's subjective experience and promoting self-awareness and personal growth.	The emphasis is on the client's current experience, feelings, and self-perception.	• Nondirective, empathetic listening, and unconditional positive regard • Less reliance on structured assessment tools • Focus on creating a supportive environment for self-exploration
Systems Therapy	Systemic therapists conceptualize assessment as a process to understand and analyze the patterns, roles, and dynamics within a client's relational system, such as a family or social group, to address and transform dysfunctional interactions.	The emphasis is on the interactions and communication patterns within the family or system.	• Use of genograms to map family relationships and histories • Observational assessment of family interactions • Family interviews to understand roles and dynamics within the system

CBT, cognitive behavioral therapy; DBT, dialectical behavior therapy.

Regardless of which point in time the diagnostic assessment process is initiated, counselors must complete preassessment tasks to determine the needed measures, orient clients to the assessment process, provide transparency, and secure consent.

Breaking Down the *DSM-5-TR* Diagnostic Assessment

Whether delivered in an interview or self-reporting format, diagnostic assessments will often follow a standardized protocol, employing various questionnaires or checklists to accurately assess and identify any underlying mental health disorders or concerns. Additionally, counselors will synthesize this data with information and observations from the initial contact, clinical intake interviews, and diagnostic criteria, such as those in the *DSM-5-TR*, to evaluate possible diagnoses. This is a tentative process, as diagnoses may change or be refined as more information is gathered and treatment unfolds. Counselors will find it necessary to explore differential diagnoses, further screen maladaptive behaviors more closely, and appraise personal strengths. Using supplementary diagnostic strategies enables counselors to address gaps left after the intake session for either supporting or ruling out initial diagnostic considerations.

CROSS-CUTTING SYMPTOM MEASURES

Numerous diagnostic assessments are available for any one diagnosis listed in the *DSM*; familiarity in choosing an appropriate measure that is valid, reliable, and appropriate for your client is key. Ideally, counselors will begin to uncover diagnoses they may want to rule out through the initial interviewing process, thereby narrowing down the choices of diagnostic assessments. Cross-cutting measures have emerged as a widely accepted model in modern diagnostic assessment, serving as a versatile tool to identify key symptom domains across various disorders. This approach not only streamlines the diagnostic process but also aids in exploring a broad spectrum of symptoms efficiently, ensuring a comprehensive and targeted assessment for each client.

The *DSM-5-TR* encompasses over 70 disorders (American Psychiatric Association, 2022a), presenting a complex challenge in the assessment and diagnosis of clients. Given the extensive nature of the content, there is a need for a more efficient method to apply this information to client cases. To address this complexity, the *Diagnostic and Statistical Manual Cross-Cutting Symptom Measures* (*DSM-XC*) were introduced in the *DSM-5* in 2013, providing a structured framework for counselors to identify domains most relevant to a client's specific presentation and symptoms during the diagnostic assessment (American Psychiatric Association, 2013). This two-level process encourages a more comprehensive clinical evaluation by helping counselors pinpoint additional areas of concern that might not be captured during an initial assessment.

The systematic two-level cross-cutting process first identifies pertinent domains through a self- or informant-rated *DSM-XC* measurement. Counselors can access the adult and childhood versions of the *DSM-XC* Level 1 assessment measure online at www.psychiatry.org/psychiatrists/practice/dsm/educational-resources/assessment-measures and in print via the *DSM-5-TR* (American Psychiatric Association, 2022a, pp. 843–851). Level 1 serves as a gateway to a more complex diagnostic pathway. In Level 2 of the *DSM-XC*, counselors will explore these identified domains using additional measures to understand symptomology better. The authors of the *DSM-5-TR* offer many Level 2 measurement options to enhance clinical decision-making, which can be found via the manual's resource site; however, the list is not exhaustive. Many assessment measures are available, and new technology makes administration more accessible to counselors and clients. By utilizing diverse diagnostic tools, including contemporary software such as Blueprint, Proem Behavioral Health, PsychSurveys, and similar behavioral health assessment platforms, counselors can delve into diagnosis-specific symptom severity and enhance clinical decision-making.

As with any approach to client care, *DSM-XC* requires careful adherence to best practices and ethical guidelines, considering the client's unique needs, such as culture, age, and specific circumstances. While the list of tools and methodologies within the field of mental health diagnostics is extensive and continues to grow, the *DSM-XC* stands as a practical addition to the toolkit. It symbolizes a step forward in mental health diagnostics and signifies a broader trend toward integrating varied assessment measures to create more tailored, client-centered care.

SUPPLEMENTAL DIAGNOSTIC TOOLS

In the dynamic field of counseling, understanding the unique aspects of an individual's condition, such as disabilities or trauma, necessitates a comprehensive and multifaceted approach. While standard diagnostic tools are crucial for providing foundational insights, they may not capture the full complexity of certain conditions or individual experiences. Hence, clinicians often rely on supplemental diagnostic tools to enhance the precision and effectiveness of their assessments. These specialized instruments are tailored to meet clients' diverse needs, enriching the counselors' understanding and treatment planning. In the forthcoming sections, we explore several essential factors to consider when selecting supplemental diagnostic tools. These include discussions on comprehensiveness, cultural sensitivity, risk, and other ethical considerations, ensuring a more nuanced, personalized, and ethically grounded approach to counseling.

Comprehensiveness: Navigating Depth and Detail. Comprehensiveness is a key factor when selecting supplemental diagnostic tools. Standard diagnostic tools, while essential, may not encompass all facets of certain conditions or experiences. Supplemental tools, therefore, play a pivotal role in providing a more detailed and nuanced understanding of a client's unique situation. Comprehensiveness refers to the tool's ability to cover a broad spectrum of symptoms and behaviors, thereby offering a rounded view of the client's condition. Tools offering subscales, for instance, provide a layered analysis that can go beyond a general overview to reveal intricate patterns and specificities. These subscales are invaluable for facilitating more accurate diagnoses and informed treatment planning, as they offer insights into various dimensions of a client's experience. When contemplating the comprehensiveness of a tool, counselors might ponder several questions regarding scope, depth, and utility to gauge its suitability. Does the tool cover the breadth of symptoms and behaviors relevant to the client's condition? For example, does it address only the general symptoms of anxiety, or does it differentiate between subtypes like social phobia, PTSD, and generalized anxiety disorder? Can the tool provide in-depth insights into specific aspects of the condition? How well does it delve into underlying causes, triggers, and behavior patterns? How effectively can this tool be combined with other standard and supplemental assessments to create a comprehensive diagnostic picture? In essence, comprehensiveness in supplemental diagnostic tools is about striking the right balance between breadth and depth. To this end, those using the tool must ensure the tool is wide-ranging in its scope and detailed in its analysis. This balanced approach allows for a more accurate and personalized assessment process, which is crucial in developing effective treatment plans.

Adaptability: Tailoring to Unique Abilities and Needs. The principle of adaptability is essential when selecting supplemental diagnostic tools in counseling. This aspect of assessment is particularly pertinent when working with clients with varying abilities, where a one-size-fits-all approach is insufficient. It focuses on customizing the diagnostic process to align with each client's unique learning, language, functioning, and developmental profiles. Counselors considering adaptable tools can ponder questions like: How does the tool accommodate different cognitive abilities and developmental stages? Can it be adjusted (accommodated) or fundamentally altered (modified) to suit specific disabilities or learning styles?

Discerning between accommodations and modifications within the assessment process is important. Accommodations refer to adjustments in the administration of a tool to make it accessible, whereas modifications involve changes to the tool's content, which may impact its validity. Key considerations include evaluating whether the tool allows the necessary adjustments to meet client's needs and how effectively it captures the intricacies of individual client presentations. The aim is to select tools offering a personalized assessment experience, reflecting each client's challenges and strengths. Ultimately, adaptability in supplemental diagnostic tools is about understanding and meeting each client's needs, ensuring that the assessment process is as inclusive and accurate as possible.

Multidisciplinary: Harnessing Diverse Expertise. The multidisciplinary approach in supplemental diagnostic assessments is invaluable when addressing complex conditions. This approach leverages the expertise of various professionals from disciplines like healthcare, medicine, dietetics, occupational therapy, speech-language pathology, physical therapy, and holistic health providers. Counselors can better understand a client's needs by incorporating a wide range of perspectives, leading to more effective treatment strategies.

When choosing supplemental diagnostic tools, a factor to consider is their applicability and compatibility within a multidisciplinary framework. Questions to consider may include: Are the tools designed to be easily interpreted and used by professionals from different disciplines? How effectively can these tools integrate information from various sources to provide a cohesive understanding of the client's condition? Does the tool facilitate communication and collaboration among professionals from different fields? Integrating supplemental tools from multidisciplinary team members fosters an environment where distinct professional insights converge, offering a richer, more complete picture of the client's health and well-being. This approach enhances the quality of the assessment and promotes a shared understanding among the team. To this end, multidisciplinary assessments can reveal interconnected aspects of a client's presentation that might be overlooked in a single-discipline approach. For example, a speech-language pathologist's evaluation might uncover communication barriers that affect a client's mental health, whereas a dietitian's assessment could reveal nutritional deficiencies impacting cognitive function. Ultimately, employing multidisciplinary supplemental tools encourages the integration of diverse expertise, enriching the therapeutic journey and ensuring that client care is approached from every necessary angle. This holistic view is crucial in crafting tailored, effective interventions that address the full spectrum of a client's needs.

Risk: Proactive Identification and Management. Incorporating specialized diagnostic tools to identify risks or concerns offers a significant advantage in clinical assessments. These tools can pinpoint potential issues that standard assessments might miss, facilitating early intervention and crisis management. This proactive approach is particularly important in mitigating risks that, if not addressed, could lead to severe complications or heightened distress for the client. When selecting supplemental tools focusing on risk assessment, consider questions like: Does the tool effectively identify early signs of deterioration or emerging issues in the client's condition? How sensitive and specific is the tool at detecting risks or concerns relevant to the client's profile? Can the tool provide guidance on the urgency and type of intervention required? Often, we may think of risk in terms of suicidal risk, though risk can present in many ways across the life span. In counseling, assessing risk is a multifaceted process that goes beyond identifying immediate dangers like suicidal tendencies. It involves understanding a broad spectrum of potential risks that clients may face, each requiring a tailored approach for intervention and management. Table 5.2 provides examples of common risk areas to consider.

Like the examples in Table 5.2, employing risk-focused supplemental tools allows us to provide acute care and cope with potential challenges in a client's therapeutic journey. Early detection of risks empowers counselors to take timely and appropriate actions, potentially altering the course of treatment for better outcomes. These tools enhance clients' safety and well-being while contributing to a more informed and responsive counseling practice.

TABLE 5.2 UNDERSTANDING THE SPECTRUM OF RISK IN COUNSELING

Suicidal Ideation and Self-Harm: A critical area of risk assessment, focusing on clients who exhibit signs of self-harm or express suicidal thoughts. Immediate and specialized intervention is crucial. • Beck Scale for Suicide Ideation (BSS; Beck & Steer, 1991) • Linehan Suicide Attempt Self-Injury Interview (SASII; Linehan et al., 2006)
Trauma and PTSD: Clients with a history of trauma or PTSD may engage in behaviors such as dissociation, self-harm, or substance abuse as coping mechanisms. Recognizing and addressing these issues is vital for effective treatment and preventing retraumatization. • Clinician-Administered PTSD Scale (CAPS; Blake et al., 1995) • PTSD Checklist for *DSM-5* (PCL-5; Weathers et al., 2013)
Co-Occurring Disorders: Dual diagnoses, such as a combination of substance abuse and mental health disorders, increase the complexity of treatment due to higher symptom severity and challenges in treatment adherence. • Dual Diagnosis Screening Instrument (DDSI; Mestre-Pintó et al., 2013) • Psychiatric Research Interview for Substance and Mental Disorders (PRISM; Hasin et al., 1996)
Impulsivity and Risky Behaviors in Youth: Adolescents and young adults may engage in risky behaviors like substance use or reckless driving due to impulsivity or peer influence. Identifying these behaviors is essential for early intervention. • Youth Self Report (YSR; Achenbach & Rescorla, 2001) • Behavior Assessment System for Children (BASC; Reynolds & Kamphaus, 2004)
Domestic Violence and Abuse: Identifying signs of abuse in clients and providing necessary support is critical for their safety and psychologic well-being. • Conflict Tactics Scales (CTS2; Straus et al., 1996) • The Propensity for Abusive Scale (Dutton, 1995)
Social and Environmental Factors: Factors like homelessness or unemployment can exacerbate mental health issues. Understanding these social determinants is essential for holistic client care. • Quality of Life Enjoyment and Satisfaction Questionnaire–Short Form (Q-LES-Q-SF; Riendeau et al., 2018) • The Adjustment Disorder–New Module 20 (ADNM-20; Lorenz et al., 2016)

(continued)

TABLE 5.2 **UNDERSTANDING THE SPECTRUM OF RISK IN COUNSELING** (*continued*)

Special Populations: Vulnerable groups, such as children, older adults, or individuals with disabilities, may face unique risks, including neglect, exploitation, or age-related cognitive decline. • Geriatric Depression Scale (GDS; Yesavage et al., 1982) • Pediatric Quality of Life Enjoyment and Satisfaction Questionnaire (PQ-LES-Q; Endicott et al., 2006) • Maltreatment and Abuse Chronology of Exposure (MACE) Scale (Teicher & Parigger, 2015)
Medical and Physical Health Risks: Conditions like eating disorders or substance abuse can lead to serious medical complications. Identifying these risks, like heart complications from purging or malnutrition, is crucial for comprehensive care. • Eating Disorder Inventory (EDI; Garner et al., 1983) • Alcohol Use Disorders Identification Test (AUDIT; Babor et al., 2001)
Behavioral and Psychologic Risks: These include the potential for relapse in addiction care or managing hypomania to prevent manic episodes. Proper assessment can guide crisis planning and preventive strategies. • Beck Depression Inventory (BDI; Beck et al., 1961) • Young Mania Rating Scale (YMRS; Young et al., 1978)

DSM-5, Diagnostic and Statistical Manual of Mental Disorders, Fifth Edition; PCL-5, PTSD Checklist for *DSM-5*; PTSD, posttraumatic stress disorder.

Alliance: Enhancing Therapeutic Relationships. Thoughtfully chosen supplemental diagnostic tools can transform the counseling assessment process into an engaging, client-involved process. When tools resonate with a client's personal narrative, they serve more than a diagnostic purpose; they validate the client's experiences and emotions and foster a deeper connection to the therapy process. As you may recall, several assessment methods that offer such flexibility were discussed in Chapter 4. In review, assessments that allow for counselor-led interviews are particularly ripe for deepening rapport. They allow for empathetic engagement and validating responses that can create a safe and trusting environment. Such interactions are data-gathering exercises and opportunities to solidify the counselor–client bond, laying the groundwork for effective therapy in the future.

When selecting a tool, a crucial consideration is acknowledging and honoring the client's preferences and comfort levels regarding assessment methods. This understanding guides our decisions to employ introspective self-report measures or more interactive counselor-led assessments. Catering to a client's preferences reflects the counselor's commitment to respecting agency and comfort within the therapeutic setting. Moreover, our approach in introducing and employing supplemental diagnostic tools is pivotal in reducing stigma and promoting openness. To this end, normalizing the assessment process encourages clients to share openly and engage actively. Such an approach demystifies the process, creating a nonjudgmental and accepting atmosphere. It goes without saying that cultural sensitivity is a subject in its own right; its brief mention here as we discuss the factor of alliance underscores its significance in choosing supplemental assessment tools. Tools that acknowledge and respect the client's cultural and individual background significantly influence their perception of the therapeutic alliance. Lastly, the alliance is built as much in the feedback process as in the administration phase, if not more. The value of seeking and incorporating client feedback about the assessment process cannot be overstated. To this end, it is essential that as counselors, we understand the diagnostic tools we employ and are prepared to discuss them at length with our clients in the feedback process. This may include discussing the assessment and administration process where clients feel their input is valued and their experiences are integral to shaping their therapeutic journey.

The selection and utilization of supplemental diagnostic tools within counseling are not just about their technical merit. Selection is also deeply intertwined with how the tool is perceived and experienced by clients. Counselors can significantly enhance the therapeutic alliance by choosing supplemental diagnostic tools that resonate with clients, acknowledging their preferences, employing assessments in a stigma-reducing manner, and valuing client feedback. This, in turn, facilitates a more effective, empathetic, and client-centered counseling experience, laying a solid foundation for successful therapy outcomes.

Legalities: Playing by the Rules. The legal landscape for mental health practitioners varies by region and sets specific requirements for administering certain assessments. For instance, formalized and standardized diagnostic tools might require specialized credentialing. Neglecting these stipulations could lead to legal repercussions, especially if a counselor, lacking the necessary credentials and training, employs an assessment tool inappropriately. This highlights the importance of understanding the scope of practice and training requirements associated with various diagnostic tools. Assessment manuals outline the credentials required to administer tools and note how these tools may be utilized and distributed. Utilizing diagnostic tools involves respecting intellectual property rights, purchasing legitimate copies of assessments, and avoiding unauthorized use. For instance, photocopying a copyrighted assessment measure without permission constitutes copyright infringement, necessitating the acquisition of necessary licenses for legal and ethical usage. In the digital age, usage may look like employing electronic tools for diagnostic purposes, adding another layer of legal consideration when selecting and administering supplemental diagnostic tools. Compliance with laws like the Health Insurance Portability and Accountability Act (HIPAA) is nonnegotiable. For example, if a counselor uses an online assessment platform, it must have robust encryption and security measures to safeguard client data against breaches, aligning with legal standards for confidentiality. Chapter 13 delves deeper into technology as we navigate new digital tools and look ahead to the future of assessment.

When selecting supplemental diagnostic assessments for special populations, such as minors or individuals with disabilities, heightened legal responsibilities must be considered. This includes considering if legal mandates require specific assessments, as in court-ordered evaluations or as stipulated by the Americans with Disabilities Act (ADA), which demands reasonable accommodations. This could involve modifying tools to meet diverse needs and selecting diagnostic tools that are legally defensible and nondiscriminatory. For example, using tools not validated for specific cultural groups should be avoided to prevent biased outcomes and legal violations against antidiscrimination laws. Navigating these legal considerations, counselors manage the complexities of assessment selection and reinforce their commitment to ethical practice. By staying informed and vigilant, counselors ensure their selection of diagnostic tools aligns with legal requirements, safeguarding their professional practice and clients' rights.

Ethics: Upholding Integrity and Professionalism. Ethical responsibility is paramount, especially when selecting supplemental diagnostic tools. Ethical considerations in tool selection extend beyond compliance with guidelines. It includes being critically aware of the potential impact of these tools on clients. This involves assessing whether a tool is scientifically valid, reliable, appropriate, and sensitive to the client's unique context, including cultural, social, and personal factors. For example, employing a heavily biased assessment toward a particular cultural or socioeconomic group could lead to misdiagnosis or misinterpretation, ultimately harming the client. Furthermore, ethical tool selection demands transparency and informed consent. Clients have the right to understand the nature of their assessments, including their purpose, process, and how their results will be used. This transparency builds trust and empowers clients, allowing them to participate actively in their therapeutic journey. For transparency to occur, the counselor's competence in using the chosen tool is paramount. This means ensuring you have the training and understanding to discuss, administer, score, and interpret results accurately. Misapplication of a tool due to a lack of understanding can lead to ethical dilemmas and potentially harm the client. As mentioned in the previous section, the legal requirement for informed consent and privacy is also an ethical standard. It is crucial to ensure that any information gathered through these tools is securely stored and shared only with the client's consent, except in cases where there is a legal or ethical obligation to disclose. When selecting supplemental diagnostic tools, ethical considerations, as well as all the others previously mentioned, are integral to ensuring that the counseling process is respectful, informed, and centered around the client's well-being. By considering these factors, counselors uphold their professional integrity and enhance their interventions' therapeutic alliance and efficacy.

INCORPORATING DIVERSITY, EQUITY, AND INCLUSION INTO DIAGNOSTIC PRACTICES

The need for culturally appropriate diagnostic assessment is magnified in a society that is increasingly diverse and complex (Sue et al., 2022). Not only does this promote equitable care, but it also enhances the diagnostic validity and reliability of assessments. To ensure diagnostic assessment practices honor diversity equitably and inclusively, it is paramount to look beyond traditional psychometric tools and delve into supplemental assessments that allow an individual's cultural fabric to inform their well-being. As discussed in Chapter 4, narratives are an emerging method used to bring forth a nuanced view of the individual's lived experience, thereby enriching the diagnostic process. Numerous factors must be considered in this context, from the language employed in assessments to how data are interpreted, all of which are deeply influenced by the cultural context in which the assessment tools were originally developed and validated. To this end, it is imperative that counselors ensure that the diagnostic assessments they use are validated for and resonate with the client's cultural background. It is not just a matter of accuracy but also of delivering respectful and effective mental healthcare.

Protective Factors, Risk Factors, and Warning Signs

Understanding protective factors within specific cultural contexts can significantly enhance the diagnostic assessment and overall counseling process by identifying resources that can be activated during treatment. For example, collectivist cultures often derive significant strength and support from family systems. In such cultures, integrating family-oriented assessment interventions might be beneficial and essential for effective treatment (Sperry, 2019; Ungar, 2011). Additionally, facets of culture such as religion and spirituality often serve as significant protective factors. They offer a framework for meaning-making, coping, and resilience and must be considered in the treatment-planning process (Lucchetti et al., 2021). Contrastingly, unique cultural risk factors can significantly impact the mental health of individuals. These risk factors include experiences of racial or ethnic discrimination, minority stress, and challenges related to acculturation and assimilation (Williams et al., 2019). Several tools are available (see Table 5.3), and more are on the horizon that will help illuminate

TABLE 5.3 **CULTURE-RELEVANT ASSESSMENT TOOLS**

Tool	Target
Cultural Formulation Interview (CFI)	Designed to help clinicians obtain clinically useful, culturally relevant information from clients during mental health assessments.
Ethnic Identity Scale (EIS)	Assesses how individuals relate to their own ethnic backgrounds as a potential source of stigma or discrimination.
Multigroup Ethnic Identity Measure (MEIM)	Assesses ethnic identity and can help to understand cultural risk factors.
Discrimination and Stigma Scale (DISC)	Used in interviews to measure unfair treatment or discrimination due to mental health in key life areas like work, marriage, parenting, housing, and social activities.

cultural considerations during the diagnostic assessment process. It is not enough to select culturally sensitive diagnostic tools. Counselors must employ methods of increasing cultural understanding of risk factors if the goal is to integrate them into treatment planning and risk assessment (Brohan et al., 2013). Further, recognizing culturally specific expressions of psychologic distress is an art that requires specialized skills and awareness. In some cultures, for instance, psychologic suffering may be communicated through somatic symptoms rather than overt emotional expression. Similarly, standard Western diagnostic criteria may not readily capture the language used to describe psychologic states. Therefore, counselors must be versed in these diverse modes of expression to conduct accurate and humane assessments.

CHECKING IN WITH SARAH

Sarah was referred by her school counselor to an outpatient counselor specializing in childhood and adolescent care. As part of the assessment process, the counselor's support staff completed a brief phone screening with one of Sarah's parents. The parents and Sarah were scheduled for several assessment appointments that included a parent intake, a teen intake, and a feedback session. The parents signed a release of information allowing the counselor to collect data from the school and cheer coach. During their meeting with the counselor, Sarah's parents provided a detailed history, expressed their concerns, and discussed their family system. The counselor employed a genogram to systematically gather and analyze information about Sarah and her family. At this juncture, the counselor has gained indirect data (persons other than Sarah) to start forming a direction that the diagnostic assessment will take. Sarah's counselor then conducted a comprehensive biopsychosocial-spiritual clinical interview with Sarah, followed by a diagnostic assessment interview. The initial findings from the cross-cutting diagnostic assessment, based on parent and child screeners, revealed areas needing further exploration, including sleep disturbances, inattention, depression, anger, irritability, and risks associated with suicidality and nonsuicidal self-injury (NSSI). In addition to the Level 2 diagnostic screeners recommended by the cross-cutting assessment, Sarah's counselor sees a need for supplemental diagnostic tools that address areas not included in the cross-cutting measure. The current challenge is selecting the most appropriate supplemental diagnostic tools that will assist in developing a comprehensive diagnostic picture, ultimately guiding the treatment planning process.

1. Given Sarah's presentation as described in Chapter 1, what diagnoses would you suppose her counselor is wanting to rule out and what supplemental diagnostic tools would be ideal?

2. When choosing tools, the counselor must keep in mind several factors, one of which is the age level the assessments are validated for; what other factors might Sarah's counselor consider when choosing supplemental diagnostic tools?

3. The counselor is concerned about the risk to Sarah's health and safety. Recognizing that Sarah can benefit from a multidisciplinary team approach, what other types of health professionals would the counselor want to refer to for further assessment and evaluation?

INDIVIDUALIZING CARE AND UNDERSTANDING VARYING ABILITIES

The prevalence of treatment failures and client frustration underscores the urgency to recognize and address the unique learning needs of clients. Failure to consider underlying developmental and educational disabilities may inadvertently lead to ill-fitting treatment approaches, contributing to a client's struggle and subsequent withdrawal from therapy. Therefore, it is not enough to consider supplemental assessments for overall functioning and abilities as a recommended practice; rather, they should be integrated into every intake process and regarded as a standard of care. By identifying these specific challenges from the outset, counselors can individualize treatment, fostering a therapeutic relationship where clients feel understood and supported. This shift toward a more client-centered approach is vital in reducing treatment failures, improving outcomes, and building collaboration within the therapeutic process. To this end, we explore the use of the World Health Organization Disability Assessment Schedule (WHODAS) 2.0, a general screening tool for ability assessment (Üstün et al., 2010).

Understanding the World Health Organization Disability Assessment Schedule 2.0

In previous editions of the *DSM*, the Global Assessment of Functioning (GAF) scale was used to assess a person's overall level of functioning, but it was removed in the transition to *DSM-5* (American Psychiatric Association, 2013). The removal of the GAF in the 2013 *DSM-5* publication was due to various concerns, including lack of conceptual clarity, difficulty in consistent scoring across raters, and a need to provide a more detailed and multidimensional understanding of a person's functioning and disability. Instead, current recommendations include using the WHODAS 2.0 for a more comprehensive evaluation of disability and functioning (see Table 5.4). The WHODAS 2.0, a tool developed by WHO, is a versatile instrument in disability and functioning measurement with applications across diverse contexts and populations (Üstün et al., 2010). Built on an extensive global study across 19 countries, the WHODAS 2.0 represents an inclusive and cultural advancement in disability measures. The development process includes a multifaceted exploration of health assessment across diverse cultures. Researchers tapped into various methods such as analyzing linguistic nuances in health-related terms, conducting in-depth interviews,

TABLE 5.4 **WHODAS 2.0 DOMAINS**

Domain 1	Cognition	Understanding and communicating
Domain 2	Mobility	Moving and getting around
Domain 3	Self-care	Attending to hygiene, dressing, eating, and staying alone
Domain 4	Getting along	Interacting with others
Domain 5	Life activities	Domestic responsibilities, leisure, work, and school
Domain 6	Participation	Joining in community activities, participating in society

WHODAS 2.0, World Health Organization Disability Assessment Schedule 2.0.
Source: Adapted from Üstün, T. B., Kostanjsek, N., Chatterji, S., & Rehm, J. (Eds.). (2010). *Measuring health and disability: Manual for WHO Disability Assessment Schedule WHODAS 2.0.* World Health Organization. https://www.who.int/standards/classifications/international-classification-of-functioning-disability-and-health/who-disability-assessment-schedule

and utilizing innovative qualitative techniques like pile sorting and concept mapping. The result is a universally applicable and sensitive tool, demonstrating a promising ability to transcend sociodemographic boundaries, adapt to various cultural settings, and respond to change. The goal is to provide a standardized method for assessing health, disability, and overall well-being while aligning with the *International Classification of Functioning, Disability, and Health* (ICF; WHO, 2021). The WHODAS 2.0 is a general tool, so unlike disease-specific measures, it provides a broader lens, offering insights into a person's daily life capabilities and participation in their community through various domains, from cognition to mobility and interpersonal interactions. Its wide applicability makes it an asset in clinical practice and research, opening avenues for data comparison and aggregation across different settings. Though general, the WHODAS 2.0's comprehensive approach ensures that it resonates with the core essence of a functional assessment, making it an essential tool for professionals aiming to gauge disability and foster client-centered care.

APPLICATIONS

The WHODAS 2.0 has been used in various research and clinical settings to evaluate interventions' effectiveness, assess specific populations' needs, and contribute to policy and planning. The measure can be used with adults aged 18 and older who have temporary or permanent disabilities, chronic health conditions, or other health-related issues that impact their daily functioning. There are limitations in the application of the measure to minors and to adults with intellectual delays. There is a growing body of research on administering the WHODAS 2.0 by proxy, an approach specifically tailored for assessing disability and functioning in children, adolescents, and in instances where adults are not able to participate independently (Ferro et al., 2022; Hernández et al., 2023). The utility of the WHODAS 2.0 in direct assessment with adults or by proxy with diverse populations underscores its utility in providing a comprehensive understanding of functional impairment. Scorza et al. (2013) adapted the WHODAS 2.0, delivering the World Health Organization Disability Assessment Schedule for Children (WHODAS-Child) for children in Rwanda. Since 2013, other translations have emerged; however, more research and development are needed to validate specialized versions specifically for children and adolescents to ensure the instrument's efficacy across all age groups and cultures (Federici et al., 2023; Hamdani et al., 2020). Ongoing exploration in this direction can lead to broader application of the WHODAS 2.0 and WHODAS-Child, leading to even more versatile tools in the mental health assessment repertoire.

PSYCHOMETRICS

There are different versions and translations of the 36-item WHODAS 2.0 to fit a variety of research and clinical needs, including a shorter 12-item version as well as the WHODAS-Child adaptation. The WHODAS 2.0 demonstrates high reliability, with test-retest consistency (intra-class coefficient from 0.69 to 0.98) and exceptional internal consistency (Cronbach's alpha values ranging from 0.88 to 0.98; Üstün et al., 2010). The instrument features a hierarchical structure, encompassing a general disability factor that informs six domains consistent across different study sites and populations (Üstün et al., 2010). Additionally, WHODAS 2.0 has been proven sensitive to changes in social functioning, showcasing responsiveness across various health contexts. These factors, combined with high face and concurrent validity, make WHODAS 2.0 a valuable tool for counseling professionals. It is important to note that psychometric properties can vary based on the population and context; thus, counselors and researchers must consider validation studies specific to the target group being assessed. By using a standardized measure like the WHODAS 2.0, health professionals, researchers, and policy makers can consistently understand and assess disability across different contexts and populations.

ENDORSING A DIAGNOSIS

Chapter 4 included guidelines for completing initial intake assessments, including capturing data with diagnostic assessment methods. Most importantly, these guidelines highlight the importance of synthesizing the diagnostic assessment data with additional information from various methods and sources (e.g., mental status exams, biopsychosocial-spiritual interviews, indirect sources, self-monitoring, etc.). Synthesizing diagnostic data with multiple sources will improve the accuracy of diagnostic endorsements. But what does it mean to endorse a diagnosis? The practice of diagnosing, though grounded in science, is very much an art. It requires counselors to understand human development and pathology, understand the client's experience, and uncover the etiology of symptoms while considering external vulnerabilities and common factors. Thus, endorsing a diagnosis means that given a culmination of multiple data sources, the symptoms can be best described by a specific diagnosis. To this end, a single diagnostic assessment tool cannot definitively point to a diagnosis with exactness because one tool cannot account for the multitude of internal-external vulnerabilities, cultural differences, and similar factors. In essence, endorsing a diagnosis is not about ticking boxes based on symptoms observed or reported; rather, it is about drawing from a well of knowledge, interpreting the relationship of various data streams, and using that insight to guide the treatment. Diagnosing is both an art and a science, a balancing act of intuition grounded in evidence-based knowledge.

Over the decades, the diagnostic assessment process has become more refined through research and development. Today's *DSM*, an evolving tool, reflects our best understanding of mental health, yet it is imperative to remember that it is not definitive. Some diagnoses, like OCD, attention deficit hyperactivity disorder (ADHD), and schizophrenia, are chronic and might persist throughout a person's life. However, numerous other disorders, such as certain personality or eating disorders, may change over time, especially with intervention. Consider the case of PTSD and depression: A client presenting with these diagnoses at the outset might, with the right interventions, show significant progress. Perhaps, upon reevaluation, their symptoms might align more with generalized anxiety disorder. Moreover, as therapeutic engagement continues, they might eventually not qualify for any diagnosis. This dynamic nature underscores the importance of viewing diagnosis not as a static label but as a tool in the therapeutic journey.

END-OF-CHAPTER RESOURCES

DISCUSSION QUESTIONS

1. What are the pivotal roles that diagnostic assessments play in the counseling process? Discuss specific examples to illustrate your points.

2. Considering the historical evolution of the *DSM*, how has the medical model influenced the field of counseling? As a counselor, how would you reconcile this medicalized approach when conducting a diagnostic assessment, especially given the discipline's strengths-based approach?

3. What are the risks of not properly assessing varying abilities in a client?

4. What ethical considerations should counselors keep in mind when implementing the WHODAS 2.0, particularly when adapting it for specific populations or cultures?

5. How do culturally sensitive assessments break down barriers in the global counseling landscape?

CLASS ACTIVITIES

1. **Role-Play Activity:** Students pair up and assume the roles of counselor and client. With one student playing the counselor role and the other playing the client role, conduct a diagnostic interview using an example case with symptoms suggesting multiple possible diagnoses. Halfway through the role-play, the "counselor" receives new information that could alter the diagnosis (e.g., a "new symptom" card handed out by the instructor). After the role-play, discuss how new information can refine or change initial diagnostic impressions and the importance of being open to evolving diagnoses. See the diagnostic interview video in Chapter 14 as an example.

2. Given a 4-week time frame, ask students to visit various community mental health centers, clinics, or online platforms to identify what types of diagnostic interviews and supplemental tools are available. Students should ask for permission and respect privacy guidelines. Students will then present their findings in the next class, discussing the diversity of diagnostic approaches and tools they discovered.

3. Using the resources provided, students create art pieces that express how they perceive assessment and the diagnostic process. This could include expressing how certain disorders may be oversimplified or stigmatized through conventional diagnostic criteria and assessment. Students present their artwork and discuss how it highlights gaps, challenges, or opportunities when conducting a diagnostic assessment.

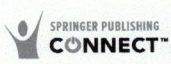

A robust set of instructor resources designed to supplement this text is located at http://connect.springerpub.com/content/book/978-0-8261-8913-4. Qualifying instructors may request access by emailing textbook@springerpub.com.

REFERENCES

Achenbach, T. M., & Rescorla, L. A. (2001). *Manual for the ASEBA school-age forms & profiles*. University of Vermont, Research Center for Children, Youth, & Families.

American Counseling Association. (2014). *2014 ACA code of ethics*. https://www.counseling.org/docs/default-source/default-document-library/ethics/2014-aca-code-of-ethics.pdf.

American Psychiatric Association. (1952). *Diagnostic and statistical manual of mental disorders* (1st ed.). Author.

American Psychiatric Association. (1968). *Diagnostic and statistical manual of mental disorders* (2nd ed.). Author.

American Psychiatric Association. (1980). *Diagnostic and statistical manual of mental disorders* (3rd ed.). Author.

American Psychiatric Association. (1987). *Diagnostic and statistical manual of mental disorders* (3rd ed., rev.). Author.

American Psychiatric Association. (1994). *Diagnostic and statistical manual of mental disorders* (4th ed.). Author.

American Psychiatric Association. (2000). *Diagnostic and statistical manual of mental disorders* (4th ed., text rev.). Author.

American Psychiatric Association. (2013). *Diagnostic and statistical manual of mental disorders* (5th ed.). https://doi.org/10.1176/appi.books.9780890425596

American Psychiatric Association. (2022a). *Diagnostic and statistical manual of mental disorders* (5th ed., text rev.). https://doi.org/10.1176/appi.books.9780890425787

American Psychiatric Association. (2022b). DSM-5-TR *neurocognitive disorders supplement: Updated excerpts for delirium codes major and mild neurocognitive disorders*. https://psychiatryonline.org/pb-assets/dsm/update/DSM-5-TR_Neurocognitive-Disorders-Supplement_2022_APA_Publishing.pdf

American Psychiatric Association. (2022c). DSM-5-TR *update: Supplement to the diagnostic and statistical manual of mental disorders* (5th ed., text rev.). https://www.psychiatry.org/getmedia/34c43e15-2618-4d2b-9f67-6bef5c40f75a/APA-DSM5TR-Update-September-2022.pdf

Babor, T. F., Higgins-Biddle, J. C., Saunders, J. B., Monteiro, M. G., & World Health Organization. (2001). *AUDIT: The alcohol use disorders identification test: Guidelines for use in primary health care* (No. WHO/MSD/MSB/01.6 a). World Health Organization.

Barbera, L., & Moody, L. (2019). A decade in review: Cancer Care Ontario's approach to symptom assessment and management. *Medical Care, 57*(Suppl. 1), S80–S84. https://doi.org/10.1097/MLR.0000000000001084

Beck, A. T., & Steer, R. A. (1991). *Manual for the Beck Scale for Suicide Ideation*. Psychological Corporation.

Beck, A. T., Ward, C. H., Mendelson, M., Mock, J., & Erbaugh, J. (1961). An inventory for measuring depression. *Archives of General Psychiatry, 4*(6), 561–571. https://doi.org/10.1001/archpsyc.1961.01710120031004

Blake, D. D., Weathers, F. W., Nagy, L. M., Kaloupek, D. G., Gusman, F. D., Charney, D. S., & Keane, T. M. (1995). The development of a clinician-administered PTSD scale. *Journal of Traumatic Stress, 8*(1), 75–90. https://doi.org/10.1002/jts.2490080106

Brohan, E., Clement, S., Rose, D., Sartorius, N., Slade, M., & Thornicroft, G. (2013). Development and psychometric evaluation of the Discrimination and Stigma Scale (DISC). *Psychiatry Research, 208*(1), 33–40. https://doi.org/10.1016/j.psychres.2013.03.007

Brundage, M. D., Wu, A. W., Rivera, Y. M., & Snyder, C. (2020). Promoting effective use of patient-reported outcomes in clinical practice: Themes from a "Methods Tool kit" paper series. *Journal of Clinical Epidemiology, 122*, 153–159. https://doi.org/10.1016/j.jclinepi.2020.01.022

Council for Accreditation of Counseling and Related Educational Programs. (2023). *2024 CACREP standards*. https://www.cacrep.org/wp-content/uploads/2023/06/Combined-version-6.21.23.pdf

Dailey, S. F., Gill, C. S., Karl, S., & Barrio Minton, C. (2014). DSM-5 *learning companion for counselors*. American Counseling Association.

Dutton, D. G. (1995). A scale for measuring propensity for abusiveness. *Journal of Family Violence, 10*(2), 203–221. https://doi.org/10.1007/bf02110600

Endicott, J., Nee, J., Yang, R., & Wohlberg, C. (2006). Pediatric Quality of Life Enjoyment and Satisfaction Questionnaire (PQ-LES-Q): Reliability and validity. *Journal of the American Academy of Child and Adolescent Psychiatry, 45*(4), 401–407. https://doi.org/10.1097/01.chi.0000198590.38325.81

Federici, S., Balboni, G., Buracchi, A., Barbanera, F., & Pierini, A. (2023). WHODAS-Child: Psychometric properties of the WHODAS 2.0 for children and youth among Italian children with autism spectrum disorder. *Disability and Rehabilitation, 45*(10), 1713–1719. https://doi.org/10.1080/09638288.2022.2071481

Ferro, M. A., Basque, D., Elgie, M., & Dol, M. (2022). Agreement of the 12-item World Health Organization Disability Assessment Schedule (WHODAS) 2.0 in parents and youth with physical illness living in Canada. *Disability and Rehabilitation, 45*(19), 3125–3134. https://doi.org/10.1080/09638288.2022.2120095

Foa, E. B., McLean, C. P., Zang, Y., Zong, J., Rauch, S., Porter, K., Knowles, K., Powers, M. B., & Kauffman, B. (2016). Psychometric properties of the Posttraumatic Stress Disorder Symptoms Scale Interview for *DSM-5* (PSSI-5). *Psychological Assessment, 28*(10), 1159–1165. https://doi.org/10.1037/pas0000259

Garner, D. M., Olmstead, M. P., & Polivy, J. (1983). Development and validation of a multidimensional eating disorder inventory for anorexia nervosa and bulimia. *International Journal of Eating Disorders, 2*(2), 15–34. https://doi.org/10.1002/1098-108X(198321)2:2<15::AID-EAT2260020203>3.0.CO;2-6

Gill, C. S., Dailey, S. F., Karl, S., & Barrio Minton, C. (2024). *DSM-5-TR learning companion for counselors* (2nd ed.). American Counseling Association.

Green, A. E., DeChants, J. P., Price, M. N., & Davis, C. K. (2021). Association of gender-affirming hormone therapy with depression, thoughts of suicide, and attempted suicide among transgender and nonbinary youth. *Journal of Adolescent Health, 70*(4), 643–649. https://doi.org/10.1016/j.jadohealth.2021.10.036

Goodrich, K. M., Farmer, L. B., Watson, J. C., Davis, R. J., Luke, M., Dispenza, F., Akers, W., & Griffith, C. (2017). Standards of care in assessment of lesbian, gay, bisexual, transgender, gender expansive, and queer/questioning (LGBTGEQ+) persons. *Journal of LGBT Issues in Counseling, 11*(4), 203–211. https://doi.org/10.1080/15538605.2017.1380548

Hamdani, S., Huma, Z., Wissow, L., Rahman, A., & Gladstone, M. (2020). Measuring functional disability in children with developmental disorders in low-resource settings: Validation of Developmental Disorders-Children Disability Assessment Schedule (DD-CDAS) in rural Pakistan. *Global Mental Health, 7*, E17. https://doi.org/10.1017/gmh.2020.10

Hasin, D. S., Trautman, K. D., Miele, G. M., Samet, S., Smith, M., & Endicott, J. (1996). Psychiatric Research Interview for Substance and Mental Disorders (PRISM): Reliability for substance abusers. *American Journal of Psychiatry, 153*(9), 1195–1201. https://doi.org/10.1176/ajp.153.9.1195

Hernández, J. D., Spir, M. A., Payares, K., Posada, A. M., Salinas, F. A., Garcia, H. I., & Lugo-Agudelo, L. H. (2023). Assessment by proxy of the SF-36 and WHO-DAS 2.0. A systematic review. *Journal of Rehabilitation Medicine, 55*, jrm4493. https://doi.org/10.2340/jrm.v55.4493

Jensen-Doss, A., & Hawley, K. M. (2011). Understanding clinicians' diagnostic practices: Attitudes toward the utility of diagnosis and standardized diagnostic tools. *Administration and Policy in Mental Health and Mental Health Services Research, 38*, 476–485. https://doi.org/10.1007/s10488-011-0334-3

Kawa, S., & Giordano, J. (2012). A brief historicity of the *Diagnostic and Statistical Manual of Mental Disorders*: Issues and implications for the future of psychiatric canon and practice. *Philosophy, Ethics, and Humanities in Medicine, 13*(7), 2. https://doi.org/10.1186/1747-5341-7-2

Lewis, C. C., Boyd, M., Puspitasari, A., Navarro, E., Howard, J., Kassab, H., Hoffman, M., Scott, K., Lyon, A., Douglas, S., Simon, G., & Kroenke, K. (2019). Implementing measurement-based care in behavioral health: A review. *JAMA Psychiatry (Chicago, Ill.), 76*(3), 324–335. https://doi.org/10.1001/jamapsychiatry.2018.3329

Linehan, M. M., Comtois, K. A., Brown, M. Z., Heard, H. L., & Wagner, A. (2006). Suicide Attempt Self-Injury Interview (SASII): Development, reliability, and validity of a scale to assess suicide attempts and intentional self-injury. *Psychological Assessment, 18*(3), 303–312. https://doi.org/10.1037/1040-3590.18.3.303

Lorenz, L., Bachem, R. C., & Maercker, A. (2016). The adjustment disorder--new module 20 as a screening instrument: Cluster analysis and cut-off values. *The International Journal of Occupational and Environmental Medicine, 7*(4), 215–220. https://doi.org/10.15171/ijoem.2016.775

Lucchetti, G., Koenig, H. G., & Lucchetti, A. L. G. (2021). Spirituality, religiousness, and mental health: A review of the current scientific evidence. *World Journal of Clinical Cases, 9*(26), 7620–7631. https://doi.org/10.12998/wjcc.v9.i26.7620

Mestre-Pintó, J. I., Domingo-Salvany, A., Martín-Santos, R., Torrens, M., & PsyCoBarcelona Group (see Appendix). (2013). Dual diagnosis screening interview to identify psychiatric comorbidity in substance users: Development and validation of a brief instrument. *European Addiction Research, 20*(1), 41–48. https://doi.org/10.1159/000351519

National Board of Forensic Evaluators. (2022). *Can licensed mental health counselors administer and interpret psychological tests* https://www.nbfe.net/resources/Documents/Can%20Counselors%20Test.pdf

Neukrug, E. S., & Fawcett, R. C. (2010). *Essentials of testing and assessment: A practical guide for counselors, social workers, and psychologists* (2nd ed.). Brooks/Cole Cengage Learning.

Patel, Z. S., Jensen-Doss, A., & Lewis, C. C. (2022). MFA and ASA-MF: A psychometric analysis of attitudes towards measurement-based care. *Administration and Policy in Mental Health and Mental Health Services Research, 49*(1), 13–28. https://doi.org/10.1007/s10488-021-01138-2

Reynolds, C. R., & Kamphaus, R. W. (2004). *Behavior assessment system for children (BASC-2)*. American Guidance Service.

Riendeau, R. P., Sullivan, J. L., Meterko, M., Stolzmann, K., Williamson, A. K., Miller, C. J., Kim, B., & Bauer, M. S. (2018). Factor structure of the Q-LES-Q short form in an enrolled mental health clinic population. *Quality of Life Research: An International Journal of Quality of Life Aspects of Treatment, Care, and Rehabilitation, 27*(11), 2953–2964. https://doi.org/10.1007/s11136-018-1963-8

Scorza, P., Stevenson, A., Canino, G., Mushashi, C., Kanyanganzi, F., Munyanah, M., & Betancourt, T. (2013). Validation of the "World Health Organization Disability Assessment Schedule for Children, WHODAS-Child" in Rwanda. *PLoS One, 8*(3), e57725. https://doi.org/10.1371/journal.pone.0057725

Sperry, L. (2019). *Couple and family assessment: Contemporary and cutting-edge strategies*. Routledge.

Straus, M. A., Hamby, S. L., Boney-McCoy, S. U. E., & Sugarman, D. B. (1996). The revised conflict tactics scales (CTS2) development and preliminary psychometric data. *Journal of Family Issues, 17*(3), 283–316. https://doi.org/10.1177/019251396017003001

Sue, D. W., Sue, D., Neville, H. A., & Smith, L. (2022). *Counseling the culturally diverse: Theory and practice*. John Wiley & Sons.

Teicher, M. H., & Parigger, A. (2015). The 'Maltreatment and Abuse Chronology of Exposure' (MACE) scale for the retrospective assessment of abuse and neglect during development. *PLoS One, 10*(2), e0117423. https://doi.org/10.1371%2Fjournal.pone.0117423

The Trevor Project. (2021). *Estimate of how often LGBTQ youth attempt suicide in the U.S.* https://www.thetrevorproject.org/research-briefs/estimate-of-how-often-lgbtq-youth-attempt-suicide-in-the-u-s

Ungar, M. (2011). The social ecology of resilience: Addressing contextual and cultural ambiguity of a nascent construct. *American Journal of Orthopsychiatry, 81*(1), 1–17. https://doi.org/10.1111/j.1939-0025.2010.01067.x

Ustün,, T. B., Kostanjsek, N., Chatterji, S., & Rehm, J. (Eds.). (2010). Measuring health and disability: *Manual for WHO Disability Assessment Schedule WHODAS 2.0*. World Health Organization. https://iris.who.int/bitstream/handle/10665/43974/9789241547598_eng.pdf?sequence=1&isAllowed=y

Weathers, F. W., Litz, B. T., Keane, T. M., Palmieri, P. A., Marx, B. P., & Schnurr, P. P. (2013). *The PTSD checklist for DSM-5 (PCL-5)*. National Center for PTSD. https://www.ptsd.va.gov

Williams, D. R., Lawrence, J. A., & Davis, B. A. (2019). Racism and health: Evidence and needed research. *Annual Review of Public Health, 40*, 105–125. https://doi.org/10.1146/annurev-publhealth-040218-043750

World Health Organization. (1949). *International statistical classification of diseases and related health problems* (6th ed.). Author.

World Health Organization. (1965). *International statistical classification of diseases and related health problems* (8th ed.). Author.

World Health Organization. (2019). *International statistical classification of diseases and related health problems* (11th rev.). https://icd.who.int

World Health Organization. (2021). *International classification of functioning, disability, and health*. https://www.who.int/standards/classifications/international-classification-of-functioning-disability-and-health

Yesavage, J. A., Brink, T. L., Rose, T. L., Lum, O., Huang, V., Adey, M., & Leirer, V. O. (1982). Development and validation of a geriatric depression screening scale: A preliminary report. *Journal of Psychiatric Research, 17*(1), 37–49. https://doi.org/10.1016/0022-3956(82)90033-4

Young, R. C., Biggs, J. T., Ziegler, V. E., & Meyer, D. A. (1978). A rating scale for mania: Reliability, validity and sensitivity. *The British Journal of Psychiatry, 133*(5), 429–435. https://doi.org/10.1192/bjp.133.5.429

6

Test Selection, Scoring, and Statistics

HALEY R. AULT AND KELLY EMELIANCHIK-KEY

2024 CACREP STANDARDS

3.G.2. basic concepts of standardized and nonstandardized testing, norm-referenced and criterion-referenced assessments, and group and individual assessments

3.G.3. statistical concepts, including scales of measurement, measures of central tendency, indices of variability, shapes and types of distributions, and correlations

While I was in the process of writing this textbook, my son came home from school one day with all of his state test scores. They had taken them weeks prior, so I assumed no news was good news since I had not heard from the teacher. To my surprise, he said he failed all of them. I told him not to panic and asked to see his test scores. I looked up each test and the scores were in a raw form. I helped him to understand that his score (although appearing low by looking at the number) was actually really good and he scored in the 90% percentile compared to other kids his age and in his grade. Needless to say, he told me the scoring was "ridiculous" and someone should have just told him that in the first place. This was a great reminder to me about making sense out of scores for clients, especially children.

SELECTING THE APPROPRIATE TESTS

There is a great deal of information to understand before starting to think about test selection. Statistics, albeit dreaded by many, are necessary to understand before diving into test selection and administration. *Statistics* is all about gathering, studying, and making sense of patterns and trends in data. Statistics can be used for analyzing data, making predictions about future events and behaviors, and drawing conclusions from it. Counselors use statistics to track client progress, monitor changes, analyze problems, and measure behaviors. Statistics also play an important role in research, where they are used to test hypotheses and draw conclusions. *Descriptive statistics* describe the properties of sample and population data, whereas inferential statistics use those properties to test hypotheses and draw conclusions. In statistics, variables are classified into two main types: quantitative and qualitative. *Quantitative variables* are variables whose values are counted or measured in a numerical form. They are divided into two types: discrete and continuous. *Discrete quantitative* variables are variables whose values are obtained by counting, whereas continuous quantitative variables are variables whose values are obtained by measuring. In counseling, discrete variables are variables that can only take on specific, distinct values. Examples of discrete variables in counseling may include the number of therapy sessions attended, the number of previous mental health diagnoses, or the number of coping skills learned in therapy. These variables are counted and represented in a numerical form. On the other hand, *continuous variables* in counseling are variables that can take on any value within a range. Examples of continuous variables in counseling may include the length of time in therapy, age of the client, or severity of symptoms. *Qualitative variables*, also known as categorical variables, are variables that fit into categories and descriptions instead of numbers and measurements. Their values do not result from counting. Examples of qualitative variables include gender, religion, political affiliation, preferences, feelings, and relationship status. When selecting assessments, we must ensure that we are aware of the variables we are attempting to measure, and we must be sure that those variables on the scale we are using are psychometrically sound.

As discussed in Chapter 2 of this text, counselors have an ethical obligation to select appropriate tests and possess the competence and knowledge to administer, score, and interpret these tests. Yet, this still leaves us questioning how we select the appropriate tests for our clients. This is an enormous responsibility, as making these decisions takes careful consideration and evaluation. The following steps need to be taken to ensure we select the appropriate tests for our clients.

1. **Gathering information and understanding needs**
   The primary source of information to understand what assessments are needed will always come from the individual in counseling. You must understand your clients' presenting problems, goals for treatment, and developmental history. Best practice recommendations advocate for multiple assessments and methods of gathering data (Heilbrun et al., 2008; Riccio & Rodriguez, 2007; Rudy & Levinson, 2008). When needed, supplementary sources of data to help make assessment determinations can come from family members, spouses/partners, educators, and medical professionals (Drummond & Jones, 2010), as well as documentation and records such as medical records, school records, court documents, or previous evaluations. All of this additional information can also be helpful once you interpret the results. As you gather all of this information and feel that you know the client's goals, the directions to take regarding the type of assessment needed will become clearer. For example, you are working with a first-year college student who is struggling in their classes. The student reports that everything is fine and is just a typical setback for a new college student. The student reports going out more often, making new friends, joining a fraternity, and having a great social life in college. He wants to improve his grades while maintaining his fun and social life. The student's academic record shows that they were required to seek counseling services by the dean and are on academic probation after arriving at class intoxicated. After compiling all of this information, you determine that the client might have a substance abuse problem and should be screened. In addition to a substance abuse screening or questionnaire, you decide to also do an unstructured interview to build rapport and trust while also checking for social desirability bias in responses on the formal assessment. Social desirability bias is when test takers respond based on what they think is socially acceptable and not their actual opinion.

2. **Determining methods and accessing information**
   Now that you have narrowed down the needed assessment type, you will need to decide on the methods you will use to assess the client. If you remember back to Chapter 4, this includes formal and informal assessment methods. For the client in the previous example, you could use a standardized and formal assessment such as the Substance Abuse Subtle Screening Inventory-4 (SASSI-4; Lazowski & Geary, 2019), and you could also pair it with an informal method, like an unstructured interview, that would help build rapport while gaining additional information. The interview may also assist in checking for social desirability bias that could be present in the results of the SASSI. The thing to keep in mind is that there are many standardized substance abuse assessments available. For the purpose of the example, I selected the SASSI, but if I were a counselor in the field and did not have

knowledge or experience with a specific substance abuse assessment, I would need to start researching available instruments, which would lead us to the next step.

3. **Examining available instruments**

   As counselors, there is no way we can know about or keep track of all the available assessment tools that exist to aid us in working with our clients. Once we have determined the necessary assessment type, we might explore resources for learning about the wide range of available counseling assessments. Further, it is important to consider culturally appropriate and normed instruments for our client. There are probably tens of thousands of standardized and unstandardized assessments, but searching through each separately would take forever. However, many resources are available for counselors to sort through large sets of assessments with more speed and detail. Each source will differ in the type of information and level of detail provided about the assessment, but Table 6.1 is a list (which is not exhaustive) of some common ways to search for assessment information.

TABLE 6.1 COMMON FORMATS FOR ACCESSING ASSESSMENT INFORMATION

Type or Name	Information Provided	Location of This Resource
Mental Measurement Yearbook (MMY)	The MMY contains consumer-oriented test reviews. It provides comprehensive, critical, and unbiased reviews of published tests and assessments. It is an invaluable resource to assist in selecting and using appropriate tests for various purposes, such as clinical assessments, educational evaluations, and research studies.	Buros Center for Testing: https://buros.org/mental-measurements-yearbook
Tests in Print (TIP)	The complementary source to the MMY is TIP. TIP contains a comprehensive bibliography of commercially available tests in the English language. TIP helps users quickly locate basic information about available tests, making it easier to make informed decisions. This information includes test purpose, intended population, administration times, scores generated, price, test publisher, in-print status, test acronym, publication date(s), and test author(s).	Buros Center for Testing: https://buros.org/tests-print
Publisher catalogs and manuals	Suppose you know of a specific type of assessment. In that case, you can look on a test publisher's website and find offerings about various assessments that might be available in any given content area. You can also find the specific assessment of interest and then explore any available test developer's manuals for more information.	Some publishers include: • Psychological Assessment Resources, Inc.: www.parinc.com • Association of Test Publishers: www.testpublishers.org • Pearson (formerly Harcourt Assessment): www.pearsonassessments.com Manuals would be dependent on the availability of the selected instrument.

(continued)

TABLE 6.1 **COMMON FORMATS FOR ACCESSING ASSESSMENT INFORMATION** (*continued*)

Type or Name	Information Provided	Location of This Resource
Professional associations—journals, books, and websites	Professional associations often provide assessment information, specifically through their journals, books, and websites. Textbooks and books created by experts in the field of testing and assessment often detail critically and widely used assessments. In addition, publishers and test developers often have websites and internet resources that detail their specific assessment and provide information. Something to keep in mind is the level of detail in all of these sources will vary and could be biased.	Dependent on your specific needs. Some example resources include: Association of Assessment in Research and Counseling (AARC) • Journal: *Measurement and Evaluation in Counseling and Development* • Database of available assessment reviews • https://aarc-counseling.org/resources American Psychological Association (APA) • Textbook and journal offerings focused on the assessment of various issues. • Journal: *Psychological Assessments* • www.apa.org/pubs/books

4. **Narrowing down**

   After all of the information you need has been gathered about both your client and available assessments, it is time to narrow down to make a selection. There are various components to be considered before selecting an assessment. Of most importance is ensuring the assessment meets your purpose and establishes the goal of learning more about the individual. Additionally, you would consider the psychometric properties of the assessment, such as reliability and validity information, norming groups, and cultural considerations and limitations. You may also consider the availability of the technical manual and guidance around administration, scoring, and interpretation. The last consideration (which could be considered a priority for many clinicians) addresses the practical components of selecting the assessment. This includes the cost(s) for training, purchase, and administration of the test; the time it takes to complete; the available languages; the necessary test taker education level; available formats (i.e., pen-and-paper, electronic); and your ability to score and interpret the results without additional training. As noted in Chapter 2, competency and training to provide assessments are part of our ethical codes and guidelines.

5. **Selection and Implementation**

   The last step is the obvious one: selecting the instrument that checks the most boxes you are looking for in an assessment for your client. When in doubt, it is recommended that you consult with a supervisor or even your client. For example, if there is an assessment tool that is available and far superior to others, but it costs a small fee or takes a much longer amount of time, you could consult with your client and provide them with the pros and cons of each to see which one they prefer. They may want to spend the money or take the extra time to take a far superior and more appropriate assessment.

TEST ADMINISTRATION

Many counselors are responsible for administering assessments in their place of employment. School counselors commonly perform assessments, some of which include the Scholastic Aptitude Test (SAT), career testing, and gifted testing. Administering tests, whether psychologic assessments or educational evaluations, requires careful planning and adherence to standardized procedures to ensure accuracy and fairness. There are many methods of test administration, which the test manual and publisher should specify. Some of those methods include group, computer, video, audio, nonverbal, and sign language administration. The most common administration types we use as counselors are group administration, when tests like the SAT are provided in school settings, and computer administration, where each person takes the assessment on the computer, and the computer presents the directions. To prepare, counselors should thoroughly review the administration guidelines provided by the test publisher to understand the test's purpose, administration procedures, scoring, and interpretation guidelines.

Test administrators are responsible for gathering all necessary materials, including test booklets, answer sheets, pencils, scoring guides, timers, and other required equipment to set up the testing environment. The test publishers often have specific guidelines for registration and administration, especially for aptitude or achievement tests like the Graduate Record Examination (GRE) or SAT. For example, many of these types of tests require adherence to guidelines around required identification and administration procedures. For instance, when completing the GRE, individuals must provide documentation of identification and adhere to guidelines about bringing personal items into the testing room. In all cases, test administrators should strive to create a comfortable and nonthreatening atmosphere. Still, many publishers have restrictions on who can proctor and administer a test as well as the degree of familiarization the administrator can have with the test taker. For example, the Counselors Preparation Comprehensive Examination (CPCE) is a widely used exit examination for counselor education programs that has an option to be provided by the school, but according to the Center for Credentialing & Education (2024), "the proctor must be employed by the school. However, staff, faculty, students, and graduate assistants associated with the school's counseling or psychology departments are strictly prohibited from proctoring the CPCE" (para. 8).

The administrator should clearly explain the purpose of the assessment, what it involves, and how the test taker will use the results. Informed consent should always be obtained. The test developer often details instructions for those administering and taking the assessments and should be carefully followed. These instructions include things like time limits, ways to address questions, and other guidelines that are critical for the test taker and administrator of the assessment. If there are technical issues with equipment, materials, or the test takers themselves, the administrator should address them promptly and fairly. Additionally, many test protocols often have an area for test administrators to note any irregularities during the test-taking process. For example, a former student was taking the National Counselor Examination when the fire alarm went off in the testing facility, requiring an evacuation of the building and leaving all of the test takers short of time. Even once they were let in, the alarms could not be turned off for an additional period of time. This was all documented, and eventually the students received an email offering them the chance to retake the test at no cost.

Test administrators also need to be aware of deviations or changes that are allowable and must occur to accommodate those living with a disability and young or aging clients. Many of the major group-administered tests, like GREs and SATs, require proof of the situation ahead of time, documenting the disability so specific accommodations can be laid out for the test taker and the administrator. However, some accommodations are not foreseeable and need to be made immediately; for example, if a client has an auditory impairment and does not realize that the test has an auditory component. The counselor may need to provide headphones to the client, identify a separate space where the computer volume can be turned up, or toggle on a closed captioning function (if available). The administrator would need to document these modifications that may impact the test taker's ability to perform to the fullest potential. Some formal group tests also have forms that ask the administrators to rate test taker behaviors.

Many of the previously noted test administration directions are for standardized tests, which are often provided in a group setting. Many counselors often provide assessments in individual counseling within agencies and community-based settings. Many of the same requirements apply, but for one-to-one administration of tests and scales that may not have strict administration requirements, a more personal touch can be added, and rapport can be built with the client. Many individual assessments that do not have strict administration procedures allow test administrators to take a more therapeutic approach that meets their client's needs.

SCORING ASSESSMENTS

Various ways exist to score an assessment depending on the publisher's requirements and available scoring options, which should have been found during the assessment selection steps. Some scoring methods include hand scoring, computer-based scoring, publisher scoring, or self-scoring. Each method has advantages and disadvantages, which are outlined in Table 6.2. Scoring errors are common in all methods of assessment scoring, regardless of who scores the assessments. Scoring errors could lead to misinterpretation of results, which could alter a client's treatment plan in a counseling setting. Errors can take place in various ways. There are human errors, which are mistakes in scoring made by scorers, such as misreading responses, applying scoring criteria inconsistently, or entering scores incorrectly. There can be errors due to unclear or poorly designed scoring guidelines. Hopefully, this will not be the case if the counselor or assessment administrator does their due diligence in following the steps for selecting assessments. A lack of scoring or clear guidelines would be a great reason for not using an assessment. Additional sources of error could be the scorer's personal biases that influence their judgments, leading to scoring errors. A recent study examining Wechsler protocols completed by graduate students and new school psychologists found that mistakes are common and the norm, not the exception. The errors included failure to administer sample items, incorrect calculation of raw scores, failure to record responses verbatim, and failure to query. The study strongly recommended training programs to provide ample feedback when students are learning about the administration of assessments. Best practices should include refresher lessons and continuing education regarding assessments (Oak et al., 2019).

Performance assessments and authentic assessments are both methods of evaluating a person's skills and abilities, but they have distinct characteristics and purposes. *Performance assessments* emphasize representing precise predetermined skills or tasks (Whiston, 2016). They often involve tasks or activities that can be observed, measured, and evaluated. Performance assessment is more about instruction and does not have multiple-choice responses. It emphasizes observed performance, which serves as a positive way to facilitate instruction and student learning. Scoring performance assessments is often based on predetermined rubrics or criteria that outline expected performance standards. These criteria are typically objective and clear (Palm, 2008). An example of performance-based tests would be if a school counseling intern did a classroom demonstration in front of their fellow students

TABLE 6.2 **ADVANTAGES AND DISADVANTAGES OF SCORING METHODS**

Method	Description	Pros.	Cons.
Hand Scoring	Hand scoring involves a person (usually the counselor or maybe an intern) manually evaluating and scoring the responses based on predefined criteria, rubrics, or guidelines.	Allows for nuanced assessment of open-ended or subjective questions. Provides opportunities for human judgment and expertise. Can be adapted easily for different types of assessments.	Time-consuming. Not cost-effective. Prone to scorer bias or variability in grading. May lack consistency or interrater reliability in scoring.
Computer-Based Scoring	Computer scoring, often referred to as automated or machine scoring, uses algorithms and computer programs to evaluate and assign scores to assessments.	Rapid and consistent scoring. Less time-consuming Reduces the potential for human bias or subjectivity. Can provide immediate feedback and even interpret results at times. Less training and experience are needed.	Limited in assessing complex or creative responses. Requires well-designed algorithms and training data for accuracy. May not capture all aspects of performance. Does not consider test irregularities.
Publisher Scoring	Educational publishers or testing organizations employ procedures for scoring to evaluate and assess their tests.	Less time-consuming for the administrator. Accurate and consistent results. Less training is required.	The time it takes to get scores back. Costs involved or the cost of the tests could be more.
Self-Scoring	Individuals assess and score their own performance on a test.	Saves the test administrator time. Provides fast results to the test taker. Promotes autonomy and could be insight-provoking. Client empowerment and confidentiality.	Anxiety and distress due to the score or understanding of how to score the test. Higher chances for error due to a lack of expertise, and the administrator may need to recheck. Bias or possible cheating.

and course instructor. Another example would be if a mental health counseling student did a mock counseling session with a prescribed client and standardized intervention. Both situations would require a rubric or way to observe and assess (with some degree of professional judgment) the student completing the performance-based assessment. *Authentic assessments* emphasize applying knowledge and skills in real-world contexts and situations. They aim to assess how well learners can transfer their learning to practical, authentic scenarios. Scoring authentic assessments can be more holistic and less structured than performance assessments. Authentic assessments often involve subjective judgments and require rubrics, but they also value the richness and complexity of the response (Palm, 2008). An example of authentic assessments could be if a student were at their internship site doing a session while we observe them with a two-way mirror. Alternatively, a school counselor might do an actual classroom lesson in front of elementary students in a classroom setting while we observed them. These situations differ from the ones noted previously because they are in real-life contexts, and rubrics cannot fully account for things that may happen within the real-life context.

Interpreting Test Scores

Counselors who administer tests are also responsible for interpreting the results. Interpreting assessments effectively is crucial for making informed decisions based on assessment results. Those interpreting test results should be up to date and knowledgeable on the various methods for interpretation of test results. While there are no universal standards for interpreting all assessments, there are general principles and guidelines provided by many organizations, such as the American Educational Research Association (AERA), the American Psychological Association (APA), the Association of Assessment in Research and Counseling (AARC), and others, that should be followed to ensure accurate and meaningful interpretation. Additionally, the *Code of Fair Testing Practices in Education* (Joint Committee on Testing Practices, 2004), the American Counseling Association's Code of Ethics (2014), and the *Diagnostic and Statistical Manual of Mental Disorders* (5th ed., text revision; *DSM-5-TR*; American Psychiatric Association, 2022) urge that no decisions about a client are made solely from one assessment or piece of information.

With that said, there are different ways to analyze test scores, and they can be categorized into either interindividual or intraindividual approaches. Interindividual approaches evaluate an individual's performance on specific test constructs or scales by comparing them to a reference group or the general population. On the other hand, intraindividual scoring assesses variations within an individual across different scales or subscales of the same test, examining inconsistencies within that individual's performance on the same test.

The most common ways of interpreting test scores are through norm-referenced or criterion-referenced tests. *Norm-referenced* tests are those where the performance of a sample population has been determined and it serves as a way to determine performance by comparisons to others in the same sample population. Norm-referenced tests typically have higher reliability and validity since norms are established with large sample populations (Ornstein, 1993). Norm-referenced tests are those that commonly use developmental stages or periods to compare to a peer group in the same period or stage. Examples of norm-referenced tests would be an intelligence test like the Wechsler Adult Intelligence Scale, the GRE, or the SAT. *Criterion-referenced* tests report how well someone does on a test relative to a predetermined performance level on a specified set of outcomes or criteria (Ornstein, 1993). The objective of criterion-referenced tests is not about comparing to the population or others but whether the person is performing to a certain level or standard. In counseling, criterion-referenced tests assess if a person has learned specific knowledge sets or mastered certain skills. Success on a criterion-referenced test means the person met the established performance standard and has demonstrated an acceptable level of skill. An example of a criterion-referenced test would be a driver's license exam or the National Counselor Examination. After you take the National Counselor Examination, you will know your score, but whether you passed or failed would not yet be determined until the scores were compared with your group taking the test.

Measurement Scales

Measurement scales play a significant role in helping counselors make meaning of an individual's score on a given assessment. There are four primary scales of measurement used for explaining score data: nominal, ordinal, interval, and ratio. Each of these types of scales has distinct properties and applications in counseling assessment; it is essential for counselors to understand the nuances for accurate interpretation and decision-making. *Nominal scales* are the simplest of the four scales and primarily describe characteristic or categorical data. Social and cultural demographic data are often described as nominal because the different categories do not have any order or numerical significance. Additionally, if we surveyed a group of counselors on their preferred counseling theory, we could describe our findings based on the number of individuals who indicated humanistic, cognitive behavioral therapy (CBT), Gestalt, solution-focused, and so forth. However, these scales are mostly descriptive and do not give us information about how individuals compare to one another.

Ordinal scales provide information about ordered categories where the order is significant, but not defined. Ordinal scales are often used in counseling assessment for self-reporting around questions of preference, agreement, or satisfaction. For instance, we might ask an individual, "In the last week, how often have you felt like crying?" with the answer options of "Never," "Sometimes," "Often," and "Always." While we know that an answer of "Always" would indicate more frequent crying than "Often," it does not provide us specifics about *how much* more frequent. This is especially confusing when we consider the difference between "Often" and "Sometimes."

In comparison, *interval scales* demonstrate ordered categories that consist of equal, meaningful intervals. Simply, the distance between the data points has a consistent meaning, so a score of 10 would be five points higher than a score of 5 and 10 points lower than a score of 20. One thing to note is that interval scales do not have a true absolute zero point. In other words, there is no point on the scale where a score of zero indicates a true absence of the construct. Let's imagine a personality assessment that measures the Big 5 Personality Traits (i.e., openness, conscientiousness, extroversion, agreeableness, and neuroticism). While individual scores will range across the various subscales, it is highly unlikely that we would identify an individual with an absolute lack of conscientiousness or agreeableness. A lack of a true zero indicates this scale is likely an interval scale.

Similar to the interval scale, the numbers in *ratio scales* are spread across a consistent, meaningful distance; however, the ratio scale includes a true zero point that indicates the absence of a quality or characteristic. The true zero allows for more meaningful calculations to occur between scores. For instance, we can now suggest that a score of 20 is twice as much as a score of 10 and four times as much as a score of 5. Ratio scales tend to be measures of countable quantities, like age, years of education, or frequency of behaviors.

UNDERSTANDING RAW SCORES

Counselors across settings play a critical role in helping clients, students, and families understand the meaning behind their assessment scores. We talk more about how to communicate these results to our clients in Chapter 11, but first, you need to learn more about the importance of scores. Given that most of our clients have limited exposure to concepts like scores and scales, counselors help provide additional information about their results so individuals can understand them within the context of their own well-being.

A score without any context of how it is calculated, how it compares to other scores, or how it relates to the larger scale is meaningless. *Raw scores* are the most basic calculation of a test score. Without any additional information about the instrument, scales, or distribution, it is difficult to understand what a raw score means for your performance or results on a given assessment. To better understand the meaning behind scores, let's use a sample data set from a fictional assessment, the Ethical Counseling Competence Scale (ECCS). A cohort of 10 counseling graduate students completed the 100-item ECCS, measuring their ability to apply ethical standards to complex counseling situations. Of the 10 students, we focus on the raw scores, or the number of items answered correctly, of the subsample displayed in Table 6.3.

TABLE 6.3 **RAW SCORES ON THE ETHICAL COUNSELING COMPETENCE SCALE**

Student	Raw Score
Maria	73
Frank	90
Aisha	89
Olivia	96
Malik	80
Elijah	91
Elizabeth	89
Diego	91
Jackson	76
Jewel	93

TABLE 6.4 **FREQUENCY DISTRIBUTIONS**

Raw Score	Frequency	Percentage	Cumulative Percentage
73	1	10.0%	10.0%
76	1	10.0%	20.0%
80	1	10.0%	30.0%
89	2	20.0%	50.0%
90	1	10.0%	60.0%
91	2	20.0%	80.0%
93	1	10.0%	90.0%
96	1	10.0%	100.0%

To further understand raw data and gain more information, we can use frequency distributions to organize the scores. Frequency distribution is a way to represent scores and summarize how often different scores are distributed within a sample. See Table 6.4 for a frequency distribution using our ECCS data from the previous example. In the first column, we list the raw scores. In the second column, we list the frequency of each raw score. To calculate frequency, count the number of times a score appears in a data set. In the third column, we list the percentage of each raw score. In the fourth column, we list the cumulative percentage of each raw score. We can see that the cumulative percentage of each raw score is the sum of the percentages of all the raw scores up to and including the current raw score. Frequency distributions help to compare scores.

Intervals are ranges or sections that data points are divided into. Intervals are used to group continuous data into discrete, manageable categories. When creating a frequency distribution, the data can be divided into intervals and the frequency of occurrences within each interval is recorded. This is particularly useful when dealing with large data sets. Histograms and frequency polygons are both graphical representations of continuous frequency distribution data, but histograms are the most common. Frequency polygons are multidimensional, whereas histograms are two dimensional. Histograms are best for displaying the form and gaps in data distributions, whereas frequency polygons are better to show trends and patterns. See Figure 6.1 for a histogram and Figure 6.2 for a polygon displaying the same data points within one table.

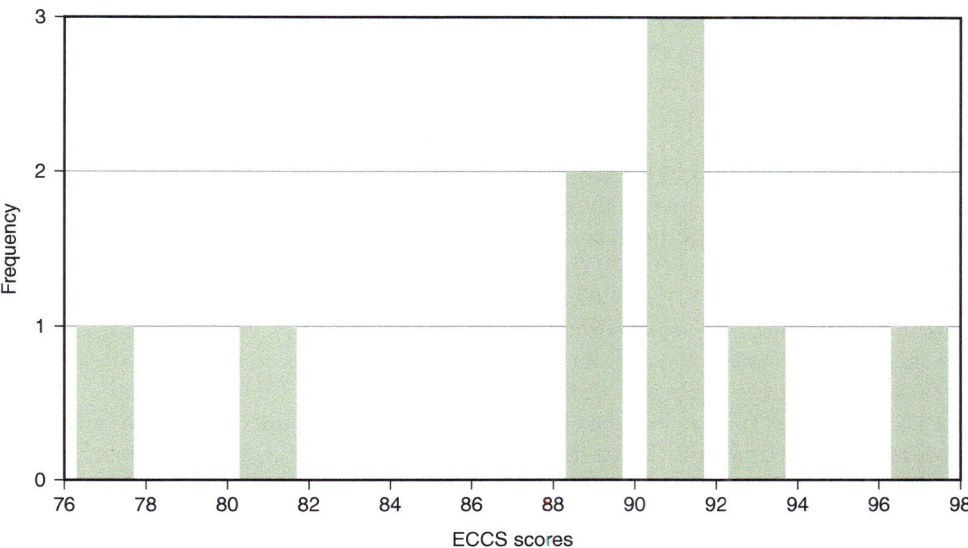

FIGURE 6.1. **Sample histogram of student raw scores.**
ECCS, Ethical Counseling Competence Scale.

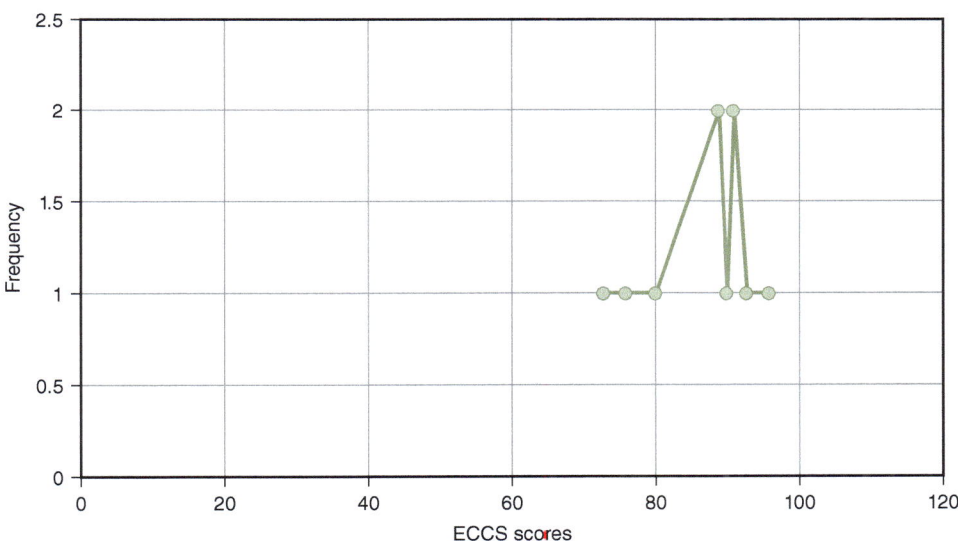

FIGURE 6.2. **Sample frequency polygon of student raw scores.**
ECCS, Ethical Counseling Competence Scale.

Measures of Central Tendency

When examining a set of raw scores, *measures of central tendency* provide information about the typically expected score or average. The first measure of central tendency is the *mean*. The mean is described as the arithmetic average because it is calculated using basic algebraic functions. To find the mean, sum all of the raw scores within the data set and divide the sum by the number of individual data points. In the ECCS example, we can calculate the mean by adding 73 + 90 + 89 + 96 + 80 + 91 + 89 + 91 + 76 + 93 to receive a total of 868. Then, we can divide by the number of students or data points (10) to receive a mean of $M = 86.8$. The table at the end of the chapter contains all of the formulas you will read about, including the mean.

The next measure of central tendency is the *median,* which describes the score that falls in the "middle" of the data set when the raw scores are ordered from smallest to largest. The median describes the point in the data set where 50% of the raw scores fall above and 50% fall below. To compute the median of the ECCS scores, we would first need to order them from smallest to largest (73, 76, 80, 89, 89, 90, 91, 91, 93, 96). Then, we would identify the value that falls in the middle of the set of numbers. Since we have an even number of values, there are two numbers that fall in the middle (89 and 90). To find the true median, we add these numbers and divide by 2 to provide a median of $Mdn = 89.5$.

The last measure of central tendency is the *mode.* This is a measure that describes the score that is presented most frequently in the data set. The mode is a useful indicator when working with outliers or extreme values in the data, a nonnormal distribution, or categorical data. In the ECCS example, there are two modes, 89 and 91, since both scores appear two times in the data set. This can be clearly seen when you refer back to our frequency distribution in Table 6.4.

Measures of Variability

In comparison, *measures of variability* are descriptors that provide information about how a given set of raw scores are distributed with respect to various measures of central tendency. *Variance* is a measure of how far or spread a set of data is from its mean. In other terms, it is the average amount of variability. Variance is usually used as a calculation in other statistics, such as analysis of variance (see the table at the end of the chapter). The two types of variances are population variance, which is a group of people that belong to a particular population, and sample variance, which is a subset of the population when the data set gets too large. The simplest measure of variability is the *range*. This describes the difference between the highest and lowest scores. To calculate the range, we would simply identify the maximum score (96) and the minimum score (73) and subtract them to receive a range of 23. The range as an indicator of variability alone does not provide us with much information about our data, but it can be helpful in our initial attempts to make sense of our data.

A more informative measure of variability is the *interquartile range (IQR)*. Similar to range, IQR describes the spread or distribution of a set of scores. However, IQR describes the range of the middle 50% of scores to provide a more accurate representation of the central distribution of scores. To find IQR, we first need to determine the values in the first quartile (Q1), or lowest 25% of the data, and the third quartile (Q3), or the lowest 75% of the data. In the ECCS data set, Q1 is 80 and Q3 is 91. IQR is calculated by subtracting Q1 from Q3. The IQR of the ECCS data is 11.

IQR is often displayed in a box and whisker plot or box plot (Figure 6.3). Understanding IQR is helpful when comparing scores across groups on the same assessment. Imagine we administered the ECCS to another cohort of counseling students. Calculating the IQR of each cohort allows us to make comparisons between groups around their performance within a specified range.

Another helpful measure of variability is the *standard deviation (SD)*, which demonstrates the spread of data by calculating the average distance between individual data points and the mean. Understanding how the scores fall relative to the mean provides context to how accurately the mean represents the raw scores in the data set. With both IQR and *SD*, a

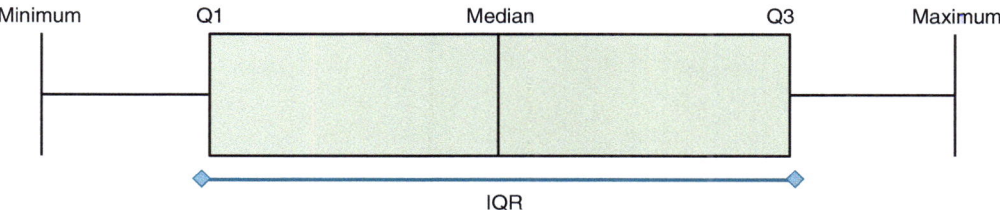

FIGURE 6.3. **Box plot.**
IQR, interquartile range.

smaller measure of variability indicates a more condensed cluster of scores near the mean, whereas a larger measure would indicate further spread from the mean.

DATA DISTRIBUTIONS AND CURVES

So far, we've discussed different ways of describing a set of scores, also known as a *data distribution*. Often, we think of data being distributed around a measure of central tendency, like the mean, with data points falling on either side. We would describe the data as *normally distributed* when all three measures of central tendency are equal, data points fall equally on either side of the mean, and the distribution curve is a symmetrical mirror image of itself (also known as a "bell curve"). In a normal distribution (see Figure 6.4), the *SD* is used to divide the data into approximately six primary ranges around the mean. For normal curves, 34.1% of the data fall within one *SD* above the mean and 34.1% of the data fall within one *SD* below the mean. Alternatively, we can suggest that approximately 68% of the raw data fall within one *SD* of the mean. Between the first and second *SD*, there is approximately 14% of the data, and approximately 2% of the data reside between the second and third *SD*.

Data that falls beyond the third *SD*, or in the tails of the bell curve, may be an indication of an extreme value or outlier given that the score does not fall within the majority of the data (within three *SD*). Although many data distributions may not be a perfect normal distribution, it is hypothesized that a sufficiently large sample size, or number of data points,

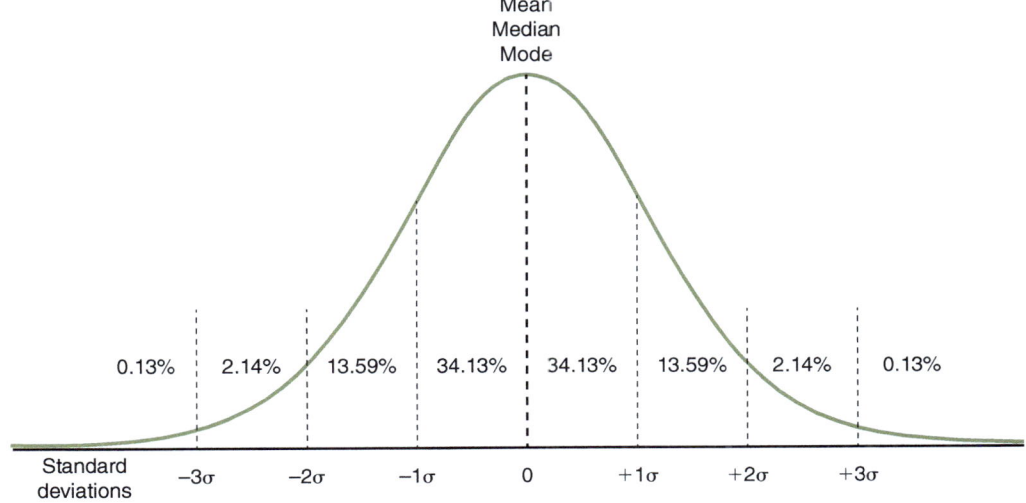

FIGURE 6.4. **Normal distribution with standard deviations.**

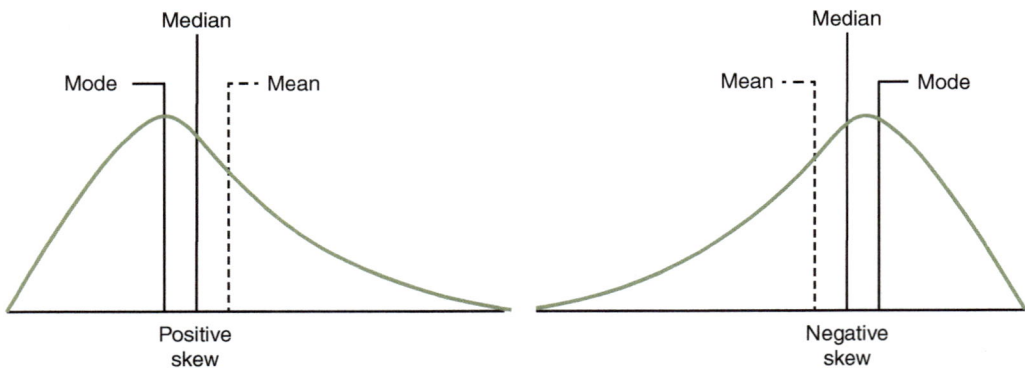

FIGURE 6.5. **Skewed curves.**

would likely produce a bell-shaped curve. In the previous ECCS example, our distribution would likely become more normal if we were to continue to assess another 100 or even 1,000 counseling students.

At times the curve can be asymmetrical, or a *skewed* curve. Measures of central tendency play a significant role in determining the direction and degree of skewness, as they can tell you whether extreme values or a concentration of data are pulling the distribution in one direction. A positive skew indicates that the data are concentrated on the left side with the tail extending to the right, whereas a negative skew indicates concentration on the right side with the tail extending to the left (see Figure 6.5).

Comparing Scores

Up to this point, we've discussed ways of describing a set of scores. Now, let's consider ways to further make meaning of individual scores in comparison to the larger data set.

PERCENTILE SCORES

The easiest method of score comparison that is widely used is percentiles. Each student's score on the ECCS individually could be described as a *percentage*. Since we know the highest score someone could receive on the ECCS is 100, we could say Aisha answered 89% of the answers correctly, or Maria scored 73%. In contrast, *percentile scores* or *percentile ranks* provide information about how a raw score is situated in comparison to other test takers. Percentile ranks or percentiles can explain how data points from the larger sample were above or below one specified data point. For example, we might communicate a child's physical characteristics (i.e., height, weight) or academic abilities in comparison to other children their age by using percentile ranks.

In the example of the ECCS, we want to know more information about Frank's score of 90 and how it compares to the other ECCS test takers. To find a specific percentile rank, first determine the number, or frequency, of test takers who scored a given score. Then, calculate the cumulative frequency to determine the total number of data points below a certain score. As you see in Table 6.3, five students scored below Frank's score (90). Then, calculate percentiles using the formula: $100*((B+0.5E)/n)$ where B is the number of values below X, E is the frequency of values equal to X, and N is the total number of values. Using this formula, we identify that Frank's score is in the 55th percentile or 55% higher than the scores of the other test takers. We

TABLE 6.5 **PERCENTILE SCORES FOR THE ETHICAL COUNSELING COMPETENCE SCALE**

Score (X)	73	76	80	89	90	91	93	96
Frequency (E)	1	1	1	2	1	2	1	1
Cumulative Frequency	1	2	3	5	6	8	9	10
Percentile	5th	15th	25th	40th	55th	70th	85th	95th

could infer that Frank scored slightly above average in comparison to this group of students. In another sample of test takers, Frank's score of 90 could rank in a different percentile depending on the scores of the other students. All percentile scores are shown in Table 6.5.

Standard Scores

Another way of comparing a singular data point to a larger group or norming group is through the use of *standard* or *standardized scores*. Standard scores describe how far a raw score deviates from the mean, or average of the reference group. Transforming data points from raw scores to standard scores allows for comparisons to be made across assessments. This is beneficial when looking at an individual's results across a group of assessments and how they perform compared to the mean on various constructs. Standard scores come in many forms such as Z-scores, T-scores, stanines, sten scores, and deviation IQs. The standard scores and their equivalents are all placed on a normal curve in Figure 6.6.

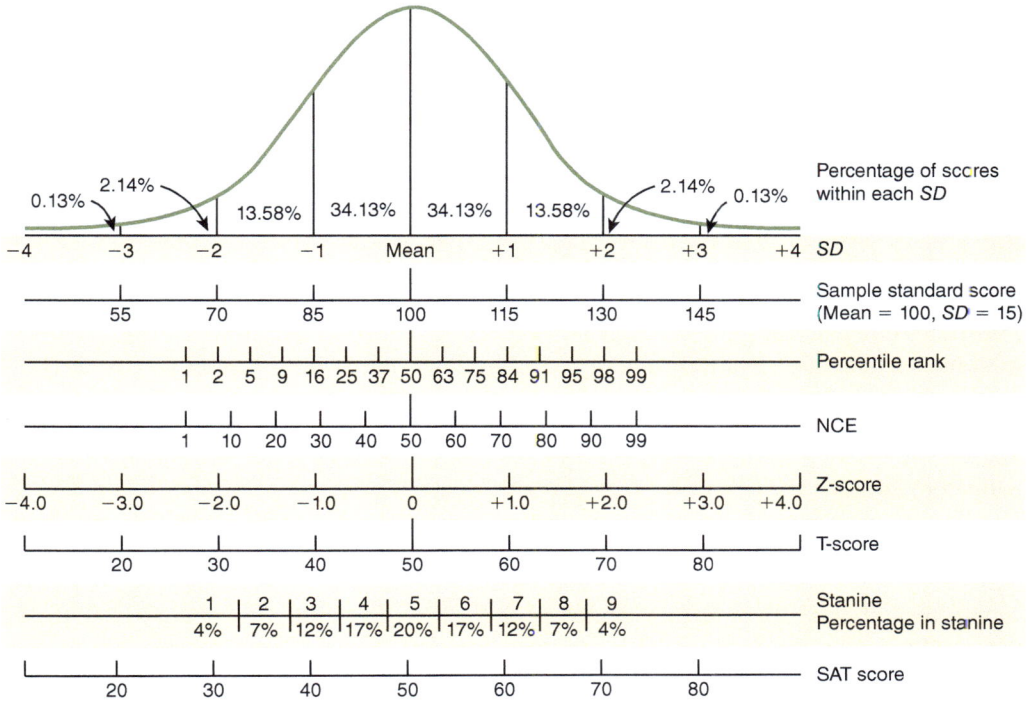

FIGURE 6.6. **Normal curve, percentiles, and select standard scores and conversions.**
NCE, normal curve equivalent; SAT, Scholastic Aptitude Test; SD, standard deviation.

Z-scores tell you how many *SD*s a data point is away from the group mean. If the Z-score is zero, then the data point is exactly the same as the group mean. A positive Z-score would indicate a score above the mean, whereas a negative Z-score would indicate a data point below the mean. To find a Z-score, you must know the individual score (*X*), the mean of the reference group (μ), and the *SD* of the group (σ) and use the following formula: $Z = (X - \mu)/\sigma$.

T-scores also provide information about how many *SD*s a given data point falls from the mean; however, the computation of a T-score includes the size of the reference group, which is important when dealing with smaller sample sizes. To find a T-score, you must know the individual score (*X*), the mean of the reference group (μ), the *SD* of the group (*s*), and the number of individuals in the group (*n*) and use the following formula: $T = (X - \mu)/(s/\sqrt{n})$. Given that smaller samples can produce more variable T-scores, we must be cautious when interpreting test results from smaller reference groups. We might see statistical significance based on T-scores, yet there may be limitations in real-world significance. Both Z-scores and T-scores are utilized in the assessment of psychologic constructs like intelligence, personality, or behavioral functioning.

Stanines, also called "standard nines," are a categorical way of describing scores from a specific group of test takers. They are computed by dividing a range of scores into nine equal intervals with the middle stanine (Stanine 5) representing the group mean. Lower stanines (1–3) indicate scores that fall below the mean, whereas higher stanines (7–9) indicate data points above the mean. Similar to stanines, *sten* ("standard tens") scores describe a range of scores categorically by chunking them into groups of 10. However, where stanine intervals are equal in distribution, sten scores are based on a bell curve, or normal distribution, where a vast majority of the individuals will fall near the mean or average range (sten score 5–7). Very few individuals will receive sten scores of 1 or 10 because this would represent a score extremely below or above average. Both stanines and sten scores are commonly used in educational and achievement assessments as well as psychologic assessments, like the Sixteen Personality Factor Questionnaire (16PF). While not as specific or precise as Z-scores or T-scores, stanines and sten scores provide a simplified comparison of data points that are easy to communicate and understand for educators, individuals, and families who are receiving test results and may not have a strong background in statistics and measurement.

Deviation IQ scores are a specific type of standard score related to intelligence testing. In the early years of intelligence testing, measurement developers calculated the intelligence quotient (IQ) as a ratio of mental age to chronological age. Over time, researchers began to understand the fallacy in this calculation as we learned that mental age does not continue to increase at the same rate as chronological age beyond adolescence. Therefore, intelligence tests, like the Cognitive Abilities Test or Stanford-Binet Intelligence Scale (Roid & Pomplun, 2012), established a deviation IQ of 15 (or 16, in some cases) to describe an *SD* from the mean of 100. Intelligence scores are based on normal distribution, so a score of 115 would indicate one *SD* above the average (100) and a score of 70 would indicate two *SD*s below the average.

Normal curve equivalent (NCE) *scores* assist in measuring student performance in comparison to other students instead of using percentile rank. The NCE score is a standardized score with a mean of 50 and an *SD* of 21.06. An NCE value of 1 corresponds with the 1st percentile, 50 with the 50th percentile, and 99 with the 99th percentile. To calculate NCE scores, you multiply z by the *SD* of the NCE and add the mean score, NCE = z(21.06) + 50.

College entrance exam scores are those scores used to gain entrance into college. The exams measure a student's aptitude in various areas such as verbal, math, analytical, and writing skills. The most common one is the SAT, which is scored on a 200 to 800 scale, respectively.

The mean of the SAT is 500 and the *SD* is 100. To convert to SAT scores, you could use the same formula as the NCE.

NORMATIVE COMPARISONS

Standardized tests, like the ones used in assessment and appraisal, utilize scores that are norm-referenced. This means that raw scores can be converted to a type of standard score, as previously described, and be compared to the distribution of scores represented by the norming sample. A *norming sample* is a large, standardized group that is comprised of individuals who represent the demographic characteristics of the individuals for which the instrument is intended. Standardized norming groups provide information on how an individual's performance compares to a larger group of test takers. Making these comparisons to the normative sample allows counselors to make informed decisions around assessment, intervention, and treatment.

When making norm-referenced comparisons, it is essential to consider how the test taker's demographic characteristics and sociocultural identities are represented in the norming sample. For example, if conducting an assessment of a child's depressive symptoms, it is essential that children of a similar age be represented within the norming group along with similar characteristics like socioeconomic status, geographic location, and racial or ethnic identity. At times, there may be instances where an individual may not align well with the norming group used for a particular instrument either because their cultural identities were not included in the norming sample, or they were not identified and disaggregated in the norming sample.

Developmental Norms

Oftentimes, counselors and educators may want to compare an individual's performance on a test to their expected developmental level. This is achieved through various methods, including norm-referenced assessment tools. In order to make these comparisons, test developers have established age- and grade-equivalent norms.

AGE OR GRADE EQUIVALENT

An *age-equivalent norm* describes an individual's score in terms of the typical age for which that level of performance is expected. For example, an educational assessment might describe a child's vocabulary score as equivalent to what is expected for a 5-year-old. Age-related comparisons are often discussed in terms of physical characteristics in infancy and childhood. A pediatrician may tell a caregiver that their 3-year-old child is in the 95th percentile for height. Compared to other 3-year-olds, this child's height is way above average. However, children almost never develop at a uniform pace, and these age-related comparisons can minimize individual differences in development.

Grade-equivalent norms are similar in that they compare students' scores to those of other students within their grade level. They are often used within educational assessments for their ease of tracking progress and communicating scores with educators and family members who may not have an in-depth understanding of measurement and score calculations. Imagine a student completes a third-grade math calculation test and receives a grade-equivalent score of 3.8, indicating their performance is similar to a student who is in their eighth month of third grade. Based on the school and teacher's expectations, this student is on target for understanding the necessary skills for promotion to the next grade level. Imagine that another third-grade student receives a score of 6.2. Although it may be tempting to associate this score with the math skills of a sixth grader and suggest promotion to more advanced grade levels, it is more accurate to say, "If a sixth grader completed this same third-grade math test, they would score similarly to the third grader who scored a 6.2." A score of 6.2 indicates an above-average performance compared to other third graders, but it may not indicate complete mastery of content that was not assessed on this particular assessment. Both age- and grade-equivalent norms can provide a clear, straightforward way of making meaning out of test scores. However, there are limitations in terms of making assumptions and accounting for individual differences.

MEASURING RELATIONSHIPS

While measures of central tendency and variability are primary ways to examine test scores, we can also use correlational designs to estimate the degree of relationship. When making meaning of scores, we may not only want to compare individuals to groups within a single assessment. In some cases, we may want to see how one person's scores on multiple assessments compare or relate to one another. Measures of relationship describe the degree of relationship, or *correlation*, between two variables, constructs, or scores. Some variables, like age and years of experience, are closely correlated. This means that as individuals continue in their careers, their age will most certainly increase. On the other hand, variables can have low correlation, meaning that there is almost no relationship between the two. For example, if we surveyed 100 people on their eye color and political affiliation, we would expect to see very little to no correlation between the responses as there is no theoretical basis that indicates eye color dictates political affiliation.

Understanding measures of relationships is important for counselors using assessment. For example, we know that anxiety and depression are often highly correlated with one another. If we were to give a client one assessment measuring anxiety symptoms and one assessment measuring depression symptoms, we would not be surprised if we saw a high correlation or relationship between the two. In another example, we might compare a student's performance on an intelligence test with an achievement test. Although these constructs are different, we might expect to see a relationship between the scores. However, if a student with a high intelligence level scores low on an achievement test, we might conclude that additional contextual factors could be contributing to the student's performance level and consider collecting additional data to better understand the circumstances.

To describe the relationship, we use the *correlation coefficient*, a statistical measure that indicates the strength of the correlation as well as the direction. Correlation coefficients can be reported as either positive or negative. A *positive* (+) coefficient indicates that the two variables are changing in the same direction. Therefore, as one variable increases, so does the second variable. Similarly, if one variable decreases, so does the other. On the other hand, a *negative* (-) coefficient indicates that the two variables are changing in different directions. As one variable increases in value, the other variable decreases.

The correlation coefficient also provides information about the strength or magnitude of the relationship. Correlation coefficients range from -1.00 to +1.00 with coefficients closer to +/- 1.00 indicating a stronger relationship than coefficients closer to 0. A correlation coefficient of +1.00 would indicate a perfect positive relationship, meaning that an increase in value of one variable will directly increase the value of another variable. The inverse is true of a -1.00 coefficient, where an increase in value of one variable will directly *decrease* the value of the other variable. A correlation of 0 indicates no relationship or relationship due to chance between the variables. For some practice on understanding correlations, see Box 6.1.

> **BOX 6.1 THINK ABOUT IT**
>
> Would the following sets of variables be positively or negatively correlated, and what directions will each variable go?
>
> 1. The weather and food costs
> 2. Mood and the weather
> 3. Time in therapy and coping skill development
> 4. Hours of screen time and grades
> 5. Hours of exercise and fitness level
> 6. Substance use and quality of life
> 7. Wellness and social support

Often, correlations are depicted using *scatter plots* to visually represent the strength and direction of the relationship (see Figure 6.7). Scatter plots typically consist of large numbers of data points graphed along an X (horizontal) axis and a Y (vertical) axis. The X axis consists of values from one assessment, whereas the Y axis contains the values from the comparing assessment. When graphed, the data points are scattered across the plot to create a graphical representation of the correlation. When the data points are clustered toward a straight line, this indicates a stronger, or more linear, relationship, and we might assume the correlation coefficient is closer to +/- 1.00. A correlation coefficient near 0 would show data points distributed randomly across the scatter plot, indicating no relationship. Depending on the analysis, we might use different types of correlation coefficients to explain the relationship.

The *Pearson product moment correlation* (r), often referred to simply as Pearson's correlation, is used to measure the linear relationship between two continuous variables. Continuous variables can be any value within a specific range of values. Examples of continuous variables are age, height, intelligence, and income. As previously described, Pearson's r provides insights into the strength and direction of two variables' linear relationship. A positive value close to +1.00 indicates a strong positive linear relationship, and a negative value close to -1.00 indicates a strong negative linear relationship. Pearson's correlation is frequently used to describe linear relationships because it is simple and easy to interpret. However, not all variables are continuous and not all relationships are linear. In those cases, Pearson's may not always be the best choice, and we may opt to use a different correlation coefficient.

Spearman's rank correlation coefficient, or Spearman's rho (ρ), is the nonparametric version of Pearson's r, which is used to assess the strength and direction between two rank-ordered variables. Nonparametric means that Spearman's rho does not require that variable relationships be linear. Rank-ordered variables are like the ones we described in scales of measurement that consist of ordered categories. A common example of rank-ordered variables are those that are measured by Likert scales used for agreement, attitude, or perception. For example, the National Institute for Children's Health Quality (NICHQ) Vanderbilt Assessment Scales use rank-ordered scales to understand the frequency of behaviors associated with an attention deficit hyperactivity disorder (ADHD) diagnosis based on reports from teachers and caregivers. The questions use scales with response options like "never," "occasionally," "often," or "very often." We may want to better understand if there is a

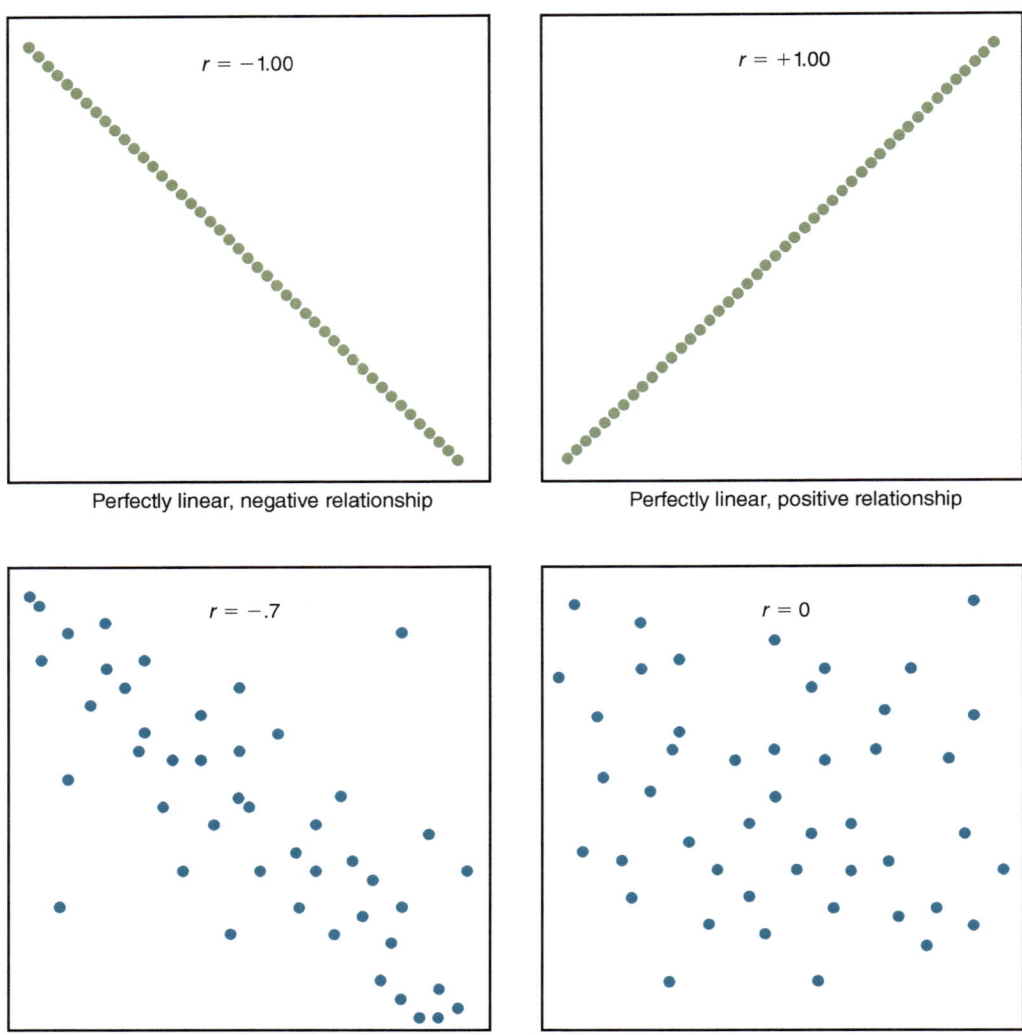

FIGURE 6.7. **Scatter plots.**

relationship between what the parent is reporting and what the teacher is reporting. Since the response options are not continuous variables, we would opt to use Spearman's rho. Unlike Pearson's correlation, which evaluates linear relationships, Spearman's rho focuses on whether, as one variable increases, the other tends to consistently increase or decrease, even if not in a strictly linear fashion. This makes it a valuable tool for data with nonlinear relationships or when the assumption of normality is not met.

The *phi coefficient* (φ) is a measure used to assess the strength and direction of the association between two nominal or categorical variables. Nominal data does not have a numerical value but is better described by categorical distinctions. Sociocultural group affiliation, blood type, and country of origin are all examples of nominal variables. Even variables that are usually thought of as continuous may be grouped in categorical variables for ease of interpretation. For example, we may want to better understand the relationship between college students who are "STEM majors" or "non-STEM majors" and the time it takes to graduate ("4 years," "more than 4 years"). Similar to Pearson's correlation, the phi coefficient quantifies the degree to which the two variables are related but specifically adapted for categorical data. The phi coefficient is used to determine whether there is a meaningful connection between the two categorical variables and the nature of that connection.

In addition to understanding the correlation coefficient, we might also refer to the *coefficient of determination* (R^2), a statistical measure used to assess the proportion of variance shared between two variables. When interpreting assessment scores, it can be a valuable tool to understand how much variance in one variable can be accounted for by another variable or a set of variables. For example, if we want to understand how a particular treatment modality impacts a client's anxiety level, we would examine the relationship between two variables, modality and anxiety. We would likely see a moderately strong negative relationship between participation in counseling and anxiety level. As individuals participate in additional counseling sessions, their anxiety level decreases. However, we could use the coefficient of determination to understand how treatment modality or other factors (e.g., behavioral, environmental) are contributing to variance in anxiety levels.

Regression

Similar to correlations, *regression* is a statistical method for examining the relationship between two or more variables. However, rather than investigating the strength and direction of the relationship, regression describes how changes in one or more variables (independent variables) might predict changes in another variable (dependent variable). Regression methods aim to develop a mathematical equation or model according to the data that represents the relationship between the variables. In counseling assessment, regression analysis plays a significant role in understanding how different factors or variables may influence an individual's performance or outcomes on various forms of measurement. This allows practitioners to uncover patterns, make predictions, and gain insights into the factors that affect counseling and educational outcomes. There are three primary types of regression analysis that we will discuss.

The simplest regression analysis is the *simple linear regression*. This method is used to predict the value of the dependent variable based on the value on the independent variable. More simply, linear regression answers the question, "How do changes in the independent variable affect the dependent variable?" Linear regression answers this question by fitting a linear equation, or straight line, to the data points. This regression line, or *line of best fit*, represents the relationship between the two variables; on a scatter plot, the regression line is plotted straight through the data points where there is minimal deviation of data points from the line. Imagine we wanted to know if participation in a test-taking skills intervention (independent variable) impacts scores on a math test (dependent variable). We would hope to see that those who participate in the intervention would have higher test scores. However, there may be additional factors contributing to the increase in test scores. To better understand the relationship with multiple variables, we would need a different method of regression analysis.

Multiple regression follows the same process of fitting a linear equation to a given set of data points. However, multiple regression allows us to analyze the relationship between multiple independent variables (predictors) on a dependent variable (outcome). Perhaps we want to investigate how gender identity and general anxiety levels, in addition to participation in the test-taking skills intervention, contribute to performance on the math test. Multiple regression will simultaneously include all three predictor variables into the model to consider how they collectively relate to math scores.

Sometimes, we want to know the impact of specific variables on the dependent variable one at a time. *Hierarchical regression* allows us to examine the changes on the dependent variable while controlling for the potential influence of other variables. In hierarchical regression, the predictor variables are considered in a specific order, or hierarchy, which allows us to examine the incremental contribution of each independent variable on the change in the dependent variable. Before we investigate how the intervention predicts test scores, we might first want to see how differences in demographics or baseline data contribute to changes in test scores. For instance, are there gender differences in test scores prior to the intervention? Then, we might introduce general anxiety levels to the model to understand how overall anxiety influences test scores regardless of participation in the intervention. In hierarchical regression, we would enter predictor variables into the model one at a time to understand how they might also be contributing to changes in the dependent variable prior to understanding how participation in the intervention contributes to the outcome.

Error in regression models is called the standard error of estimate. The *standard error of estimate* (SEE) measures the variability or reliability of predictions in regression analysis. Essentially, it indicates how well the regression line (or model) represents the observed data points. SEE is also sometimes referred to as the standard error of the regression with a smaller value indicating a better fit and a larger value indicating a worse fit. It is often represented as σest and is calculated as σest = $\sqrt{\Sigma(y - \hat{y})2/n}$, where y is the observed value, $\hat{y}$ is the predicted value, and n is the total number of observations. SEE is useful for assessing the goodness of fit of a regression model.

In this chapter, we have learned a great deal about the importance of selecting, administering, and scoring assessments. Each of these components are critical in testing and assessment. Scores that come from assessments are able to be applied to measures of central tendency and variance which describe the basic characteristics of a data set or set of scores, while correlations and regression explore the relationships that exist between the variables. Table 6.6, which was referenced a few times in this chapter, contains many of the formulas discussed throughout this chapter. We will continue to put the remaining pieces together in the next chapter and we dive into factors that contribute to test worthiness. Reliability and validity are the foundation of quality measurements and assessments. Together, each of these concepts will contribute to a comprehensive understanding of data in research and assessment contexts.

TABLE 6.6 FORMULA SUMMARY SHEET

Formula Name	Description	Formula
Population Mean	Average of all values in a population	$\mu = \dfrac{\Sigma x}{N}$
Sample Mean	Average value of a sample	$\bar{x} = \dfrac{\Sigma x_1}{n}$
Population Variance	Average of the squared differences from the mean	$\sigma^2 = \dfrac{\Sigma(x_j - \alpha)^2}{N}$
Simple Variance	Average of the squared differences from the mean, for a sample	$s^2 = \dfrac{\Sigma(x_j - \bar{z})^2}{n-1}$
Population SD	Square root of the population variance	$\sigma = \sqrt{\sigma^2}$

(continued)

TABLE 6.6 **FORMULA SUMMARY SHEET** (*continued*)

Formula Name	Description	Formula
Sample SD	Square root of the sample Variance	$s = \sqrt{s^2}$
Raw Score to Z-Score	Number of SDs a raw score is from the mean	$Z = \dfrac{X - \mu}{\sigma}$
Raw Score to T-Score	Standard score that sets the mean to 50 and SD to 10	$T = 10Z + 50$
NCE Score	Standard score with a mean of 50 and SD of 21.06	$NCE = 21.06Z + 50$
Deviation IQ	Standard score with a mean of 100 and SD of 15	$IQ = 15Z + 100$
SAT Score	Standard score with a mean of 500 and SD of 100	$SAT = 100Z + 500$
Sten Score	Standard score that multiplies the Z-score by the SD and adds the mean	$STEN = Z(SD) + M$
Stanine Score	Standard score that ranks the group's results from lowest to highest, then assigns the score based on the percentile they fall in	Based on percentile ranking

IQ, deviation IQ; M, mean; N, total number of values in the population; n, number of values in the sample; NCE, normal curve equivalent; σ, population SD; σ², population variance; s, sample SD; s², sample variance; SAT, Scholastic Aptitude Test score; SD, standard deviation; Stanine, Stanine score; Sten, Sten score; T, T-score; μ, population mean; X̄, sample mean; X, raw score; Z, Z-score.

CHECKING IN WITH JOHN

John is struggling with his mental health and is faced with stress and anxiety over finding a job to help support his family. As a counselor, career assessments would be critical, but consider the following:

1. What considerations and adaptations should be taken into account when selecting and administering psychologic assessments for a veteran like John, who has PTSD and is disabled?

2. How can the assessment process be tailored to ensure a fair and accurate representation of his abilities and mental health status?

3. How might performance-based assessments and authentic assessments be used with John to provide meaningful insights into his abilities, strengths and areas for growth, while also being sensitive to his unique experiences?

4. When John is given an assessment, he is told that he scored a 69. John becomes upset and feels like he is a failure and just can't win in life. He starts to lose hope that he will ever find meaningful employment. What should the counselors have done for John when sharing his raw score?

END-OF-CHAPTER RESOURCES

DISCUSSION QUESTIONS

1. Percentile scores are often used to compare an individual's performance or characteristics to a larger population. What are some advantages and potential limitations of using percentile scores in the assessment process? How might the interpretation of percentile scores differ depending on the specific assessment tool and the population being assessed? Can you provide examples of situations where percentile scores are particularly useful when working with clients and when they might be less informative?

2. In the field of counseling assessment, how can an understanding of distributions, including measures of central tendency and variability, assist counselors and therapists in making informed decisions about their clients? What are the implications of skewed or nonnormal distributions in assessment data? Can you provide examples of how knowledge of distributions has been applied to enhance the counseling process or improve client outcomes?

3. Examine Table 6.1 and look at each of the common ways to access assessment information. Come up with a list of strengths and limitations for each of the methods. Which source is most helpful to you as a future professional counselor and why?

CLASS ACTIVITIES

1. Now that you have learned about what goes into selecting an assessment, let's create your own assessment. Get in small groups and make your own assessment tool to evaluate or rate assessment tool choices when you are in steps 3 and 4 of selecting an assessment tool. What format will you use? What type of scoring? What information would you want to assess and evaluate to make an optimal choice when selecting an assessment tool?

2. Complete the following score transformations.

    a. Z-Score Transformation:

    - Calculate the Z-score for a data point with a value of 85, a mean of 75, and an *SD* of 5.
    - Convert a Z-score of -1.5 to the corresponding raw score given a mean of 60 and an *SD* of 10.

    b. T-Score Transformation:

    - Transform a raw score of 70 into a T-score with a mean of 50 and an *SD* of 10.
    - Given a T-score of 60 with a mean of 55 and an *SD* of 5, calculate the corresponding raw score.

    c. Stanine Transformation:

    - Convert a raw score of 90 into a stanine with a mean of 75 and an *SD* of 10.
    - Determine the raw score corresponding to a stanine of 3 with a mean of 65 and an *SD* of 8.

d. Sten Transformation:

   ○ Calculate the sten score for a data point with a value of 82, a mean of 75, and an *SD* of 6.

   ○ Convert a sten score of 7 to the corresponding raw score given a mean of 60 and an *SD* of 8.

5. A group of clients within an inpatient setting took an anxiety assessment. The raw scores representing anxiety levels reported by the group of clients is as follows: 15, 17, 21, 22, 25, 25, 28, 30, 32, 35, 40, 45, 50, 55, 60, 65, 69, 76.

   a. Calculate the mean, median, and mode for the anxiety scores.

   b. Determine the IQR for the anxiety scores.

   c. Calculate the *SD* for the anxiety scores.

   d. Based on the calculated measures, interpret the central tendency, variability, and distribution of anxiety levels within the group.

   e. Discuss how these measures can inform the assessment and understanding of anxiety levels in counseling practice.

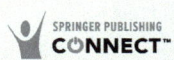

A robust set of instructor resources designed to supplement this text is located at http://connect.springerpub.com/content/book/978-0-8261-8913-4. Qualifying instructors may request access by emailing textbook@springerpub.com.

REFERENCES

American Counseling Association. (2014). *2014 ACA code of ethics*. https://www.counseling.org/docs/default-source/default-document-library/ethics/2014-aca-code-of-ethics.pdf

American Psychiatric Association. (2022). *Diagnostic and statistical manual of mental disorders* (5th ed., text rev.). https://doi.org/10.1176/appi.books.9780890425787

Center for Credentialing & Education. (n.d.). *CPCE: Counselor Preparation Comprehensive Examination: Assessments and exams*. https://www.cce-global.org/assessmentsandexams/cpce

Council for Accreditation of Counseling and Related Educational Programs. (2023). *2024 CACREP standards*. https://www.cacrep.org/wp-content/uploads/2023/06/Combined-version-6.21.23.pdf

Drummond, R. J., & Jones, K. D. (2010). *Assessment procedures for counselors and helping professionals* (7th ed.). Pearson.

Heilbrun, K., DeMatteo, D., Marczyk, G., & Goldstein, A. (2008). Standards of practice and care in forensic mental health assessment: Legal, professional, and principles based consideration. *Psychology, Public Policy, and Law, 14*(1), 1–26. https://doi.org/10.1037/1076-8971.14.1.1

Joint Committee on Testing Practices. (2004). *Code of fair testing practices in education*. https://www.apa.org/science/programs/testing/fair-testing.pdf

Lazowski, L. E., & Geary, B. B. (2019). Validation of the adult Substance Abuse Subtle Screening Inventory-4 (SASSI-4). *European Journal of Psychological Assessment, 35*(1), 86–97. https://doi.org/10.1027/1015-5759/a000359

Oak, E., Viezel, K. D., Dumont, R., & Willis, J. (2019). Wechsler administration and scoring errors made by graduate students and school psychologists. *Journal of Psychoeducational Assessment, 37*(6), 679–691. https://doi.org/10.1177/0734282918787635

Ornstein, A. C. (1993). Norm-referenced and criterion-referenced tests: An overview. *NASSP Bulletin, 77*(555), 28–39. https://doi.org/10.1177/019263659307755505

Palm, T. (2008). Performance assessment and authentic assessment: A conceptual analysis of the literature. *Practical Assessment, Research, and Evaluation, 13*(1), 4. https://doi.org/10.7275/0QPC-WS45

Riccio, C., & Rodriguez, O. (2007). Integration of psychological assessment approaches in school psychology. *Psychology in the Schools, 44*(3), 243–255. https://doi.org/10.1002/pits.20220

Roid, G. H., & Pomplun, M. (2012). *The Stanford-Binet Intelligence Scales*. Guilford Press.

Rudy, H., & Levinson, E. (2008). Best practices in the multidisciplinary assessment of emotional disturbances: A primer for counselors. *Journal of Counseling & Development, 86*(4), 494–504. https://doi.org/10.1002/j.1556-6678.2008.tb00537.x

Whiston, S. C. (2016). *Principles and applications of assessment in counseling*. Cengage Learning.

7

Reliability, Validity, and Test Worthiness

KELLY EMELIANCHIK-KEY, AYSE TORRES, HALEY R. AULT, AND CARMAN S. GILL

2024 CACREP STANDARD
3.G.4. reliability and validity in the use of assessments

I worked with one client for several sessions when I began to wonder just how much impact religious and spiritual issues had on his presenting problem. My colleague recommended a scale that asked questions about faith in God. As I reviewed the questions, I wondered if the assessment actually measured what I needed to know. I wondered, is this assessment applicable and how would I know if the results are accurate?

INTRODUCTION

This chapter is a follow-up to Chapter 6, which focuses on statistical concepts such as measurement scales, measures of central tendency, indices of variability, shapes and types of distributions, and correlations. Aspects of testing reliability and validity are covered in this chapter. Counselors must have a working understanding of these terms and what each concept means, in a practical sense, when selecting or using testing instruments with clients. Both terms have implications for the dependability of test results. For example, *reliability* refers to consistent performance and uniform functioning. The degree to which scores from a testing instrument accurately and consistently measure a construct is referred to as reliability, and statistical methods are used to determine the degree to which psychologic tests are reliable. The Responsibilities of Users of Standardized Tests, Fourth Edition (RUST-4E), statement refers to *test reliability evidence* as "the degree to which scores on a test can be expected to remain consistent across multiple administrations which is influenced by the degree that items are related to one another and sources of error" (Lenz et al., 2022, p. 228). Pertinent methods for determining reliability of testing scores are covered in this chapter.

Validity is just as important to the testing process. This concept refers to how closely the instrument reflects the real-world construct it is intended to measure. The RUST-4E statement also covers validity, noting that *test validity evidence* is "the degree to which formal theory, psychometric evidence, and practical applications support interpretations of test scores with individuals or groups for their intended purpose" (Lenz et al., 2022, p. 228). Because validity is about the use of test scores, counselors should know the intended purpose of the instruments and the impact on validity if the test scores are used for another purpose. Counselors ensure that the tests they use are both reliable and valid. There are many combinations of reliability and validity that can occur within a measurement (see Figure 7.1), but remember we are always aiming for one that hits the bullseye of reliability and validity. Methods for determining the validity and reliability of testing instruments are covered in this chapter, along with developing quality assessment tools.

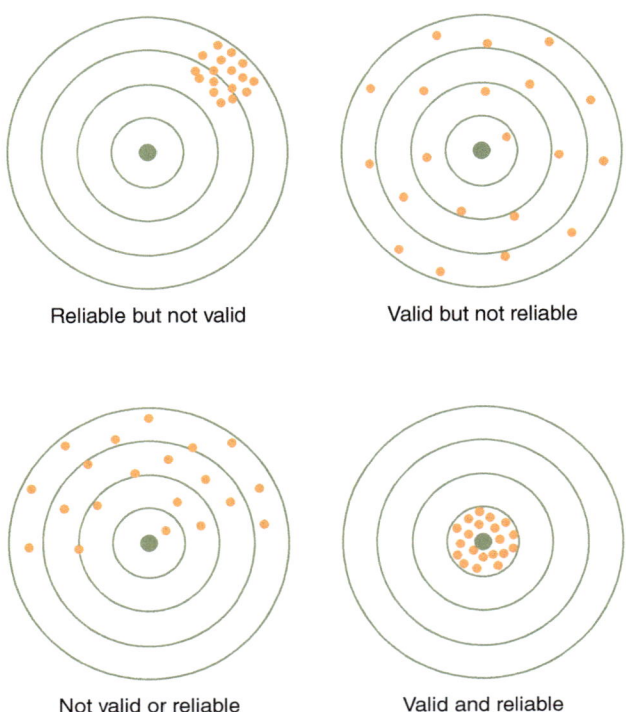

FIGURE 7.1. **Possible combinations of reliability and validity.**
Source: Duran, V., & Topal, S. (2021). *The development of neutrosophic form of the satisfaction with life scale and proposal for a confirmatory analysis based on neutros[o]phic logic.* Research Square. https://doi.org/10.21203/rs.3.rs-188182/v1

RELIABILITY

What makes a test good? In Chapter 2, we covered the history of assessment and testing in counseling. We noted that, historically, some assessments were better than others, and the use of some measures did not continue. Following Galton's passion for using scales and scaling questions, theorists and researchers have made important advancements in determining what makes a good assessment. Reliability is crucial to this, particularly in testing consistency and error measurement. When we think of reliability in our daily lives, we may think of a car that works reliably or a reliable friendship, something or someone that we can count on. Similarly, counting on a testing measure to produce the same or similar results with each use is a sign of a quality instrument. Reliability is an indicator of consistency, which differs from validity or whether the construct intended to be measured is the construct being measured. Reliability is essential to basic components of our lives, such as the performance of our cars to turn on and take us places, the quality and taste of food in a restaurant, and a thermometer that takes our temperature if we are feeling unwell.

The use of a measuring tape is a fairly concrete example of measurement. However, measuring psychologic constructs is not as concrete. *Constructs* are phenomena that we do not directly observe (Balkin & Juhnke, 2018). To measure them, they must first be operationally defined. Researchers have pointed out that most of the constructs counselors evaluate, such as depression, wellness, and spirituality, are not only difficult to define, but they are also difficult to quantify. Further, the process of operationally defining something limits how the construct is measured. For instance, my definition of what it means to be spiritual may be very different from how others define it. This could impact how others might respond to an instrument that I develop toward measuring spirituality and lead to different scores each time a client takes the test. Error is introduced in this and other ways, including poorly worded questions, test-taking anxiety, distractions during the testing process, and inadequate instructions (Neukrug & Fawcett, 2010). The *Standards for Educational and Psychological Testing* document refers to reliability as "the degree to which scores are free of random errors of measurement for a given group" (American Educational Research Association [AERA] et al., 2014, p. 223). Reducing error in tests will increase our ability to obtain reliable, accurate scores. Accurate measurements are always important, but counselors must keep in mind that as the impact of testing outcomes increases, such as with high-stakes testing, so does the need to be accurate. The recognition of error in testing and that error is a random variable, along with the idea that reliability increases as the amount of error variance decreases in a test, underpins classic test theory (CTT). As we cover CTT, keep in mind that reliability refers to accuracy and consistency in test scores, rather than the instruments themselves.

Classic Test Theory

CTT, or true score theory, is assumed to have its foundation in Spearman's work from 1904 (Balkin & Juhnke, 2018; Reynolds et al., 2021), in which he adjusted a correlation coefficient, originally discovered by Galton, to account for weakening in scores due to measurement error. Novick later codified the theory. CTT assumes that measurement results include both the client's response set and the measurement error inherent to any assessment process. An individual's response represents a combination of these factors, rather than "true score."

CTT, and the associated ideas related to reliability, are built upon three specific assumptions. Central to CTT is the assumption that measurement error is random and, as a result, larger data sets or multiple administrations will cancel out errors due to chance. Because random error can sometimes decrease the true score and at other times increase it, the more scores available, the more likely the mean will reflect the true score, resulting in a mean measurement error of zero (Reynolds et al., 2021). Because true score never includes measurement error, there is no relationship between true score and error, so that the correlation is zero. Essentially, your true score for spirituality will never contain measurement error. Further, measurement error on one test administration and subsequent administrations of that test or other testing instruments is unrelated, so that there is no correlation for error among administrations of testing assessments (Reynolds et al., 2021). The principles of CTT provide a basis for understanding reliability and variance, as well as building parameters for the establishment of reliable scores.

Measurement Error

When counselors are interpreting and applying test scores to their clients or students, they must consider hypothetical errors that could arise and contribute to differences within scores. These errors that can cause scores to fluctuate are called *measurement errors*. *True score* refers to the theoretical idea that there is an accurate score in every assessment process. This score is free from measurement error and, as a result, the true score is never known. *Observed scores* always represent the individual's true score with at least some instance of error. *Error* can occur due to the reliability and accuracy of the instrument or fluctuations in the individual's performance or testing conditions. However, if an individual completed the same assessment multiple times over a given time period, we could assume that their observed scores would fall within a similar range or distribution. Measurement error is formally defined as "the difference between an individual's obtained and true score" (Reynolds et al., 2021, p. 136). Because we can never determine the true score, our scores are a function of true score (T) and error (E). Observed (O) score includes error and is the inevitable outcome of testing assessment. Therefore, $O = T + E$, or, in other words, observed score is the result of the true score, and error or observed score minus error will result in the true score. Theoretically, identifying and eliminating error will result in the true score: $T = O - E$.

Reducing error, to the greatest extent possible, will get us closer to the true score. One method by which this occurs is through comparing repeated test measures. For example, if a counselor administers the Beck Depression Inventory (BDI) three times and averages those client scores, the assumption is that they could get much closer to the true score. However, *carryover effects* introduce error in that all clients' scores, except the first administration, are subsequently influenced by seeing the instrument and knowing what questions are asked. The time lapse between administrations of the instrument introduces problems too, as outside events impact responses. For example, if a client takes the BDI and then takes it again in 2 weeks, those scores are influenced by extraneous factors such as getting a new job, losing a pet, starting therapy, and so on. CTT assumes that the true score lies between the results of these administrations. Cohen et al. (2022) hypothesizes that if we could freeze time and have individuals take multiple administrations of the same testing instrument, averaging those scores could result in the true score. Any attempt at measurement includes this and other types of error.

Sources of Error

When we examine the equation $T = O - E$, we note that reducing measurement error gets us closer to the true score. The goal of the perfect test is to completely eliminate error, so that the observed score is the true score; however, this goal is never met. According to CTT, a true score is never accurately known. CTT focuses primarily on random measurement error, understanding the types of error, and methods of reducing error results in a more reliable measure. *Random error* is a type of measurement error that occurs unpredictably, often due to chance, and is not consistent among testing administrations. Disruptions during test administration are considered random errors. Issues with lighting, temperature, sounds, needing to suspend the test for a while, and many other issues frequently impact testing outcomes. These types of errors differ from *systematic error* in that systematic error occurs consistently across administrations. Because they are consistent, this type of error is easier to "fix." For example, if the bathroom scale consistently weighs an individual one pound heavier, subtracting one pound from that weight will obtain your correct weight.

Time sampling error is the type of error that impacts performance and scores related to the testing timing or situation. Because these are chance related and differ from one administration to another, these are random errors. For example, a counseling student who knows the material and is prepared for the National Counselor Examination may not perform as well if they receive bad news, such as the death of a loved one, just prior to taking the examination. This test taker–related scenario reflects the introduction of error into the equation, and true score is not captured as a result. The test taker, test administration, and test environment variables are all influences that can introduce time sampling error. Some examples include time of the day, week, or year; lack of sleep; condition of the testing room; impact of drugs or medications; test taker anxiety; and so on. Time sampling error is common, as tests are never given under identical conditions. However, there are processes for addressing this type of error (Reynolds et al., 2021).

One of the largest and most common sources of error introduced into testing is *item sampling* or *content sampling error*. This concept refers to reducing the content related to a construct down to a few questions within an assessment. Consider the example given earlier in the chapter regarding measuring spirituality. Because I realize my definition of spirituality may not cover all conceptualizations of spirituality, I decided to include all aspects and definitions for this concept. The universe of questions derived from this definition could potentially contain hundreds of questions. Once we begin to reduce the size of this question/item pool, we introduce content sampling error. Content sampling error is the difference between questions or items included on a testing instrument and all potential questions. This type of error is easily estimated, and solutions are available, including examining the relationship among the assessment questions or items, using correlations (Reynolds et al., 2021).

Many modern-day assessment instruments are administered online and scored using computers. For instance, the Graduate Record Examination can now be taken and scored online. However, that is not the case for all assessments. Consider the psychologic evaluations described in Chapter 10. Although you are given step-by-step instructions, variations in how the questions are asked and how you interpret the test taker's responses also introduce error. This type of error is referred to as *interrater error. Interrater* or *interscorer differences* are a common source of error and fluctuate depending upon the assessment process's subjectivity level (Cohen et al., 2022; Reynolds et al., 2021). Observations and projective measures have high levels of subjectivity and can often lead to interrater error. The decreased agreement between those interpreting or scoring the assessment will lead to the differences in the true and observed scores. Proper training and supervision may reduce this type of error. In this chapter, we also discuss interrater reliability to improve the reliability when tests are more subjective.

Other sources of error impacting our quest for true scores and a perfectly reliable assessment measure include administrative or clerical errors, such as leaving out a question or incorrectly calculating scores. Further, the subjective nature of questions can impact the assessment outcome. For example, questions regarding abuse are subject to the test taker's interpretation of what constitutes abuse. For some, corporal punishment, or spanking, does not constitute abuse, whereas for others it does. Additionally, self-report measures frequently used in counseling are subject to *social desirability* and other factors, such as forgetting, fear of disclosure or retribution, and shame. Differing interpretations of subjective constructs can result in overreporting or underreporting (Cohen et al., 2022). Last, as discussed in Chapters 3 and 6, variables within the test taker, such as motivation, fatigue, anxiety, and so on, can all contribute to errors in testing, along with the test administration impacting the test taker's ability to respond appropriately.

Standard Error of Measurement

When counselors interpret and apply test scores for their clients or students, they must consider hypothetical errors contributing to differences in scores. As noted in CTT, a true score is never known. Observed scores always represent the individual's true score with at least some instance of error. Error can occur due to the instrument's reliability and accuracy (which we discuss in depth in this chapter) or fluctuations in the individual's performance or testing conditions. However, if an individual completed the same assessment multiple times over a given time period, we could assume that their observed scores would fall within a similar range or distribution. Given there is a high likelihood of error, the *standard error of measurement* (SEM) describes how an individual's test score fluctuates around their "true score" with hypothetical repetitive administrations of the assessment. It is an absolute estimate of the reliability of a test, meaning it has the units of the test being evaluated and is not sensitive to the between-subjects variability of the data. A high SEM implies a lower reliability in test scores, indicating greater uncertainty in the individual's observed score.

On the other hand, a low SEM indicates greater precision and reliability in the test score. The SEM is directly related to the reliability of a test, with more reliable tests having lower SEMs. It is calculated as: SEM = $SD\sqrt{1-R}$. The R is reliability coefficient of the test, and SD is standard deviation of the test scores. For example, let's say a client takes a test 5 times over the course of a week and attempts to measure overall aptitude on a scale of 0 to 100, and they receive the following scores:

Scores: 88, 90, 91, 94, 86; the sample mean is 89.8, and the sample SD is 3.03.
Provided the test has a known reliability coefficient of 0.85, then we would calculate the SEM as: SEM = $SD\sqrt{1-R}$ = $3.03\sqrt{1-.85}$ = 1.173.

The SEM is used to calculate a *confidence interval* (CI) around the individual's observed score. A *CI* allows counselors and test users to estimate an individual's true score based on their observed score and SEM since we will never know their true score free from error. This helps to determine the confidence or uncertainty one can have in the accuracy of an individual's test score. The CI provides a range of values within which the true score is likely to fall. CIs are commonly reported at the 68%, 95%, or 99% confidence level, meaning there is a 68%, 95%, or 99% chance that the true score falls within the specified range. The formulas for CIs are as follows:

$$68\% \text{ CI} = [x - \text{SEM}, x + \text{SEM}]$$
$$95\% \text{ CI} = [x - 2*\text{SEM}, x + 2*\text{SEM}]$$
$$99\% \text{ CI} = [x - 3*\text{SEM}, x + 3*\text{SEM}]$$

For example, suppose an individual scores a 91 on a certain test that is known to have a SEM of 3. We could calculate a 95% CI as 95% CI = [91 − 2*3; 91 + 2*3] = [85, 97]. This means we are 95% confident that an individual's "true" score on this test is between 87 and 97. If we used the 68% CI, our range would be smaller because we are less confident, [91 − 3; 91 + 3] = [88, 94]. Both SEM and CIs are important concepts in understanding instrument reliability, and they are essential for making informed decisions based on test results.

ESTIMATING RELIABILITY

Using the principles of CTT, we can employ methods for determining the amount of error variance in testing instruments and, thus, the reliability of test scores. Earlier in this chapter, we discussed attempts to obtain true score through multiple administrations of the same testing instrument. True score lies within the range of scores and can be estimated using the mean of multiple administrations. Cohen et al. (2022) states, "If an individual could be tested repeatedly without carryover effects, the long-term average of those estimates is called the true score" (p. 158). For obvious reasons, we are unable to measure repeatedly without carryover effects. However, we can use a variety of methods to estimate error, true score, and the reliability of testing instruments. Understanding measures of variability discussed in Chapter 6 is a crucial component to understanding reliability.

The *reliability coefficient* is a statistical measure used to quantify the degree to which the same results are obtained under reliable conditions over time. Reliability coefficient refers to the quantity of variability in observed scores that is described by the variability of true scores. The reliability coefficient is the ratio of true score variance to observed score variance. This is similar to the correlation coefficient, but the reliability coefficient is specific to the consistency of assessment scores. The larger the reliability coefficient scores, the more variation exists in test scores from differences in the test taker. However, the closer the reliability coefficient is to 0, the more likely the chances are due to random error as opposed to the test taker's ability. Various methods are used to estimate reliability. These methods are test-retest, alternate/parallel form, internal consistency reliability, and interrater reliability.

Test-Retest Coefficient

Test-retest reliability examines the consistency of a testing measure when that measure is taken at one point in time and then taken again at another point in time. This type of reliability reflects the stability of a testing over time, but we must ensure that the results remain stable across multiple repeated test administrations. When a test measure produces consistent results over time, it has high test-retest reliability. Test-retest reliability ensures consistency over time in fields where stable and consistent measurements are essential for tracking changes or assessing progress. The test-retest reliability coefficient is calculated using the Pearson Product Moment Correlation formula (in Chapter 6), where r is the correlation coefficient between the two test scores. For example, suppose the National Counseling Exam (NCE) could be given to a group of students twice, with the second administration occurring a week after the first. In that case, the correlation coefficient may be calculated to indicate the scores' stability between administrations. A high correlation coefficient indicates strong test-retest reliability. Test-retest reliability is particularly useful when tracking changes or stability in a particular construct or attribute over time. Test-retest reliability is influenced by external factors such as memory, practice, and situational variables unable to be accounted for within this method alone. Additionally, this type of reliability may not be satisfactory for measures that are expected to change over time, as it assumes stability of the construct being measured.

Parallel/Alternate Form Reliability

The reliability of a test can be assessed by implementing alternate form reliability, a methodology where two nearly identical versions of the test are created, differing slightly in content, complexity, and other critical parameters (see Figure 7.2). For example, consider an educator constructing two parallel mathematics assessments. Each item on Assessment A has a corresponding item on Assessment B, but with different numerical values or equations. These assessments are given to the same group of students, and then we compare the results. The level of agreement between the results of Assessment A and Assessment B indicates the reliability of the test.

There are two common methods that can be used in this approach. The first method, known as simultaneous alternate form reliability, involves administering both assessments consecutively in the same session. This technique helps to confirm whether the test content consistently measures the intended knowledge or skill. Alternatively, we can administer the second test at a later time. This approach, known as delayed alternate form reliability, evaluates not only the consistency of the test content, but also investigates whether the timing of

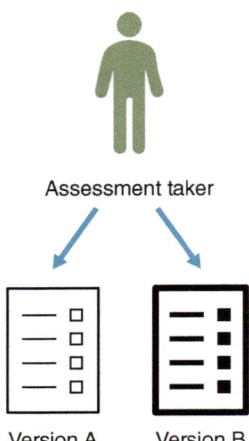

FIGURE 7.2. **Parallel/alternative form.**

the test impacts the results. For instance, students may perform better on the second test due to a heightened familiarity with the question style.

One advantage of using alternative forms is their ability to address the issue of "carry-over effects," where participants remember previous questions and answers. The benefit is that the second test appears different while still measuring the same construct with equally challenging items. However, a potential drawback is that developing a completely new and equivalent test may not be cost-effective. Additionally, establishing reliability becomes challenging when comparing the second test to the first, as ensuring equivalence is a crucial factor to consider. Furthermore, similar to test-retest scenarios, participants may drop out, fall ill, or fail to show up for the subsequent test.

Internal Consistency Reliability

In this chapter, we discussed different ways to assess reliability. Test-retest reliability involves administering the instrument twice to measure consistency. Equivalent forms of reliability require creating a new instrument. Another method to estimate reliability is by examining internal consistency. This type of reliability focuses on content sampling errors and evaluates how well the selected test items represent the intended content. It involves analyzing the relationships between the scores of each item on the instrument. Internal consistency reliability estimates are calculated based on the relationships between items within a single test administration, rather than across multiple tests or occasions. There are various methods to estimate this type of reliability, including the split-half method, Kuder–Richardson Method, and coefficient alpha.

SPLIT-HALF RELIABILITY METHOD

Split-half reliability is a measure of consistency where a test is split in two and the scores for each half of the test are compared with one another (see Figure 7.3). This method is used to examine the consistency of results across items within a test. The main notion is, if the test is consistent it leads to similar results when split in various ways. To calculate split-half reliability, the first step is to divide the test into two halves. Then, administer each half of the test to the same individual; this is then repeated for a large group of individuals. The scores from both halves are then correlated using the standard Pearson correlation.

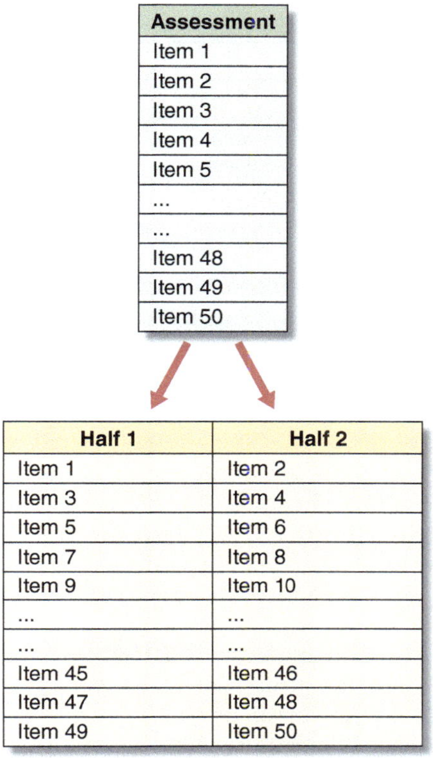

Assessment
Item 1
Item 2
Item 3
Item 4
Item 5
...
...
Item 48
Item 49
Item 50

Half 1	Half 2
Item 1	Item 2
Item 3	Item 4
Item 5	Item 6
Item 7	Item 8
Item 9	Item 10
...	...
...	...
Item 45	Item 46
Item 47	Item 48
Item 49	Item 50

FIGURE 7.3. **Split-half reliability.**

The division of the test into two halves can be achieved through several methods including comparing the first half of the test to the last half, comparing odd-numbered items to even-numbered items, or a random split. A higher correlation between the two halves indicates higher internal consistency of the test or survey, meaning that all parts of the test contribute equally to what is being measured.

One main advantage of split-half reliability is that it is conceptually and computationally simple. It assumes equivalence of the two halves that are created. However, this method does have some disadvantages. Primarily, it evaluates only half a test, which may lead to underestimating the reliability of the full test due to the fewer number of items. This is particularly problematic when a test with many items, like a 100-item test, is split into two 50-item halves. To overcome this, the Spearman-Brown formula is employed. This formula adjusts the correlation to reflect the reliability for the full test, not just the half. Another drawback is the lack of agreement between different splitting methods. This discrepancy, however, usually decreases with larger sample sizes or longer tests.

COEFFICIENT ALPHA

Coefficient alpha, also known as Cronbach's alpha, is a measure of reliability, specifically internal consistency reliability or item interrelatedness, of a scale or test (e.g., questionnaire). It indicates how closely related a set of items are as a group. Internal consistency refers to the extent that all items on a scale or test contribute positively toward measuring the same construct. Coefficient alpha quantifies the level of agreement on a standardized 0 to 1 scale. Higher values indicate higher agreement between items (see Figure 7.4). In other words, a

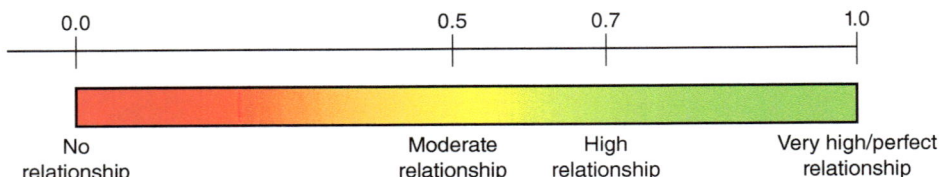

FIGURE 7.4. **Interpreting coefficient alpha.**

coefficient alpha of 1.0 represents perfect consistency in measurement, while an alpha value of 0.0 represents no consistency in measurement.

Coefficient alpha offers multiple benefits for researchers and is used for dichotomous and continuously scored variables. Unlike other reliability estimation strategies that require samples taken at two different points in time (e.g., test-retest reliability or parallel reliability), Coefficient alpha can be calculated using a single sample. A major concern with coefficient alpha is its assessment when there are many scale or test items. Increasing the number of items on a scale, even without changing the intercorrelations, will increase the alpha value. According to research by Cortina (1993), scales with more than 20 items can have a coefficient alpha above 0.70, even when item intercorrelations are very small.

KUDER–RICHARDSON METHOD

The Kuder–Richardson Method, also commonly known as the Kuder–Richardson Formula 20 and abbreviated as KR-20, is a measure of reliability used specifically for tests with dichotomous variables, that is, tests with yes/no or true/false questions. This statistical formula allows us to assess the consistency of results across repeated testing of the same subject, an essential aspect of any reliable measure. The KR-20 is particularly useful in situations where the difficulty of test items varies. For instance, a test may contain a mix of easy and more challenging questions. The reliability score derived from the KR-20 ranges from 0 to 1, with 0 indicating no reliability and 1 signifying perfect reliability. The closer the score is to 1, the more reliable the test.

In contrast, the Kuder–Richardson Formula 21, or KR-21, is used when all test items are assumed to have the same level of difficulty. If your binary test contains equally challenging questions, the KR-21 would be the appropriate measure to use in assessing reliability. KR-20 and KR-21 serve as valuable tools in psychometrics, lending credibility to test results by demonstrating consistency across repeated measurements.

Interrater Reliability

Interrater reliability, also known as interscorer reliability, is a statistical measure used to evaluate the level of agreement between two or more raters when scoring a test or assessment. This measure is particularly important when the scoring of a test is subject to subjective judgment. Essentially, interrater reliability is used to verify the consistency of scores given by different individuals assessing the same performance, thereby ensuring the reliability of the test scores. The interrater reliability in this context is determined by calculating a correlation between the scores the two counselors gave. The higher the correlation, the higher the interrater reliability, indicating a high level of agreement between the two counselors in their scoring. Interrater agreement is estimated by calculating the percentage of times the two counselors assigned the same scores to the client's responses. This approach, referred to as percent agreement, offers another way to measure interrater reliability.

TABLE 7.1 **INTERRATER AGREEMENT (%) = (NUMBER OF AGREEMENTS/TOTAL NUMBER OF ITEMS RATED) X 100**

	Counselor 1	Counselor 2	Agreement
Item 1	1	1	1
Item 2	1	0	0
Item 3	1	1	1
Item 4	1	1	1
Item 5	0	1	0
Item 6	1	1	1
Item 7	0	1	0
Item 8	1	1	1
Item 9	1	1	1
Item 10	1	1	1

The percentage of items the counselors agreed on was (7/10) x 100 = 70%.

For example, let's imagine two counselors are independently conducting and evaluating a behavioral assessment for a client. Both counselors are tasked with observing the client simultaneously and determining the presence or absence of specific behaviors on a scale of 1 (present) to 0 (not present). To calculate the interrater agreement using the percentage agreement method, follow these steps:

1. Start by creating a table with the ratings given by each counselor for each question or item on the assessment (see Table 7.1).
2. For each item, compare the scores given by the two counselors. If the scores are the same, mark it as an agreement (1). If the scores are different, mark it as a disagreement (0).
3. Count the total number of agreements and divide this by the total number of items rated (both agreements and disagreements).
4. Multiply the result by 100 to get the percentage agreement.

VALIDITY

The second important concept in understanding a test's efficacy is testing validity. Broadly, *testing validity* is conceptualized as a test's ability to measure a real-world construct accurately. Imagine a thermometer that consistently reads 10 degrees above the actual temperature regardless of the time of day or weather. Although we could describe the thermometer as reliable, the thermometer's results would be misleading. In instances of telling the weather, this inaccuracy may not be too detrimental. However, in the case of counseling assessment used for diagnosis and treatment, an instrument with low validity could be potentially harmful to clients and students.

When discussing test validity, we do not describe a test as "valid" or "invalid." Rather, we consult multiple sources of validity to understand the degree to which the test's scores most appropriately measure the intended construct. These sources of validity support our interpretations and conclusions from the test scores. According to the *Standards for Educational and Psychological Testing* (AERA et al., 2014), counselors should make judgments regarding an instrument's validity based on their intended use. For instance, an instrument used for screening or selection may require a different degree of validity than instruments used for diagnostic and treatment purposes. Strong sources of validity ensure that the test measures what it claims to measure and allows counselors to make informed decisions around diagnosis and treatment with confidence. Evidence of test validity is established through a variety of sources which are described in the text that follows.

Several factors can act as threats to testing validity. These threats can jeopardize the accuracy and trustworthiness of the results produced by the instrument. Two specific threats to validity are construct underrepresentation and construct irrelevant variance. *Construct underrepresentation* occurs when the test items fail to measure the full range of the intended construct. For example, imagine trying to measure intelligence by providing an instrument that only focuses on mathematical ability. In this assessment, we would miss out on many other aspects of intelligence, which could lead to misinterpretations or biased conclusions. Additionally, *construct irrelevance* describes when the test is influenced by other factors unrelated to the intended construct. Perhaps the test taker is experiencing personal factors, like test anxiety, motivation variances, or social desirability, that lead to an inaccurate depiction of the intended construct. Test users need to consider these threats and implement strategies for minimizing their impact.

Sources of Validity Evidence

An instrument's evidence of validity can be assessed through multiple methods. As previously mentioned, one must consider the assessment's intended use when evaluating the validity evidence's strength. The most common types of validity evidence are content, construct, criterion-related, and treatment validity. Although practitioners do not conduct validity studies themselves, it is important for all test users to be aware of standards for evaluating validity evidence (Lenz et al., 2022).

CONTENT VALIDITY

Content validity refers to the relationship between representativeness of the items, questions, or tasks within an instrument and the instrument's intended construct. This type of validity evaluates whether the instrument covers a balanced representation of all relevant aspects of the target construct. Threats to content validity include items focusing only on specific aspects of the construct, overrepresentation of certain aspects, or neglecting relevant aspects. To establish content validity, test developers will often recruit a panel of content "experts" to evaluate and determine items that appropriately measure an intended construct. Let's take the case of a state that aims to update their school counseling credentialing exam. The first step involves compiling a comprehensive list of test items, drawing from the school counseling curriculum, textbooks, supplementary materials, and items used in previous exams. Then, the test developers would recruit school counseling supervisors, veteran school counselors, and school counselor educators who have demonstrated knowledge and expertise in the foundational concepts that school counselors must master prior to entering the field. The panel of experts would evaluate the sample items to determine their representativeness and importance to professional school counseling. They might identify different domains within the larger construct (e.g., individual counseling, program delivery, consultation) and ensure that the final list of items appropriately corresponds to each domain without over- and underrepresentation of any core aspect. Ideally, the expert reviewers would reach a level of agreement or consensus to provide additional trustworthiness to the content selected for the final instrument.

Face validity is often described as a type of content validity. This term indicates that an assessment "looks like" it measures the content at "face value." Quizzes and tests found on the internet may demonstrate face validity because they ask questions that generally describe the focus of the quiz. Face validity may be useful in the preliminary stages of item development or in gaining client buy-in for participating in an assessment. However, face validity is not a trustworthy source of test validity because there is no statistical or theoretical basis for deeming an assessment as face valid. Test users should be wary if an instrument's only source of validity is face validity.

CONSTRUCT VALIDITY

Another type of validity evidence is *construct validity*. Construct validity differs from content validity in that it assesses whether the instrument actually measures what it claims to measure. As you know, assessments in counseling tend to examine constructs that are not easily observed or measured, like anxiety, depression, or self-esteem. We call these *latent constructs* because they represent underlying processes, abilities, or characteristics that explain observed characteristics. For example, we can observe physiological symptoms, self-reported worry or fear, and avoidance behaviors in the real world. Observation of these characteristics may lead a clinician to infer that an individual is experiencing the latent construct of "anxiety." To establish evidence of construct validity, test developers want to ensure that the observable variables or items on the test accurately measure the latent construct it intends to measure.

There are two main types of construct validity: convergent and discriminant validity. *Convergent validity* assesses the degree to which a test correlates with other measures of the same construct. Alternatively, *discriminant validity* assesses the level to which a test does not correlate with measures of different constructs. To assess for either type of construct validity, we would provide multiple instruments to an individual or group and compute the correlation of scores between the tests. We would hypothesize that scores on two different instruments measuring depression would be highly correlated, an indication of high convergent validity. On the other hand, we would expect scores on a depression inventory to not correlate significantly with tests measuring happiness or life satisfaction. The lack of correlation between dissimilar constructs is an indication of discriminant validity.

In addition to ensuring the test measures the intended construct, we want to ensure the test measures the intended construct across groups of individuals. *Measurement invariance* indicates that a test score holds true regardless of the test taker's social and cultural identities or the time the test is administered. It is important to be aware of measurement invariance when selecting an instrument for a given individual. Counselors must be aware of the norming sample and consider whether the norm group contains social and cultural identities that reflect their client. Instrument developers should provide information for consumers regarding the measurement invariance to reduce bias and erroneous conclusions for diverse populations.

Factor analysis is a common statistical method for measuring construct validity as it is used to explain the relationship between multiple variables. However, factor analysis is not used for prediction purposes but rather to explain the underlying structure or patterns in a data set with numerous variables. In psychometrics and assessment, factor analysis helps researchers condense a large set of variables into a smaller number of meaningful dimensions, or factors, for easier interpretation of the latent variable. There are two types of factor analysis: exploratory factor analysis (EFA) and confirmatory factor analysis (CFA).

EFA explores the underlying factor structure of a set of variables or items and explains the relationship between them. Test developers use EFA to explore a new or novel concept when little is known about the underlying makeup of the construct. In contrast, CFA is used to test a previously hypothesized theoretical model and the relationship between the individual variables and the overall construct. The CFA is most frequently used to confirm the findings of EFA. Each type of factor analysis will produce the sets of models that group items together in the best fit structures, as discussed briefly in Chapter 6 on measuring relationships and correlations.

Omega coefficient (ω), similar to coefficient alpha, is often used in the context of factor analysis. Omega describes the relationship between a set of observed variables and an underlying latent construct. A latent construct is something that is not directly observable or easily measured. Many counseling and psychology constructs are latent, like empathy, wellness, intelligence, and motivation. However, assessment researchers have worked to develop instruments to measure these constructs using more observable indicators. The omega coefficient provides information about the strength of the relationship between those individual indicators and the overall latent construct (Kalkbrenner, 2023). A stronger relationship may indicate a more accurate assessment. Omega coefficient is often used as an alternative to coefficient alpha. More accurate reliability estimates are said to be found in omega as compared to alpha when assessment items are measured on ordinal scales (McNeish, 2018).

Both types of factor analysis (EFA and CFA) are often used in test development and scale validation (we discuss this a bit more in the text that follows). For example, the Counselor Burnout Inventory (Lee et al., 2007) consists of 20 items for assessing the level of burnout counselors experience, specifically due to their work environment. Rather than examining how each of the 20 individual items contribute to change in overall counselor burnout, the test creators conducted a factor analysis to identify five dimensions that describe the underlying factors of counselor burnout: (1) exhaustion, (2) negative work environment, (3) devaluing client, (4) incompetence, and (5) deterioration of personal life. By doing this, we have simplified 20 items into 5, which allows us to reduce the complexity of the data set and make interpretations of the data easier. Factor analysis is a much more complex procedure than we have described here. However, it is important to note that you will likely come across studies about factor analysis while learning about different counseling assessments. Although practitioners will not need to conduct a factor analysis, factor analysis allows counseling researchers to uncover the latent constructs within complex data sets, facilitating a deeper understanding of psychologic phenomena and enhancing the development and refinement of assessment tools and interventions.

CRITERION-RELATED VALIDITY

The next type of validity source is *criterion-related validity*, which describes the extent to which a test score relates to performance on a specific criterion measure. Criteria include a variety of attributes that are observable in the real world but may be discrete from the specific construct measured by the instrument. For example, we might reference a student's grade point average to determine their potential for future academic success. Additionally, we might anticipate the same student to be similarly ranked when considering their performance on a college aptitude test like the American College Testing (ACT). Each of these measures (i.e., grade point average [GPA], ACT) provides some criterion-related validity to the construct of academic achievement.

There are two main types of criterion-related validity. *Concurrent validity* examines the relationship between test scores and a criterion measure observed simultaneously. Perhaps a researcher wants to develop a new anxiety questionnaire. To establish concurrent validity, they might ask participants to complete the new questionnaire alongside a well-established anxiety questionnaire, such as the Beck Anxiety Inventory. The researcher would correlate the results of both measures and hope for a high positive correlation to indicate concurrent validity. Evidence of concurrent validity can help counselors choose appropriate assessments for their clients, particularly when considering the accessibility of a specific instrument (i.e., cost, language).

Alternatively, *predictive validity* examines the relationship between test scores and a criterion measure observed in the future. As in the previous example, a college admissions board may reference a high school student's ACT score as a predictor of their future college success. At the end of the student's freshman year, the college may assess their GPA and expect to see a high correlation between the two measurements. Suppose there is not a high correlation between the ACT score and first-year GPA. In that case, it may indicate that ACT scores do not predict college success or other variables may impact students' college success (e.g., motivation, study habits, extracurricular activities). An instrument with strong predictive validity may be helpful for counselors selecting appropriate interventions for specific clients or providing evidence for the efficacy of new treatment programs.

TREATMENT VALIDITY

The last type of validity evidence to discuss is *treatment*, or *experimental validity*. Broadly, treatment validity assesses the extent to which a particular intervention or treatment is responsible for observed changes in an observed outcome. Within counseling assessment, participation in the assessment process through administration or interpretation can contribute to changes in outcomes, providing evidence of treatment validity. For example, individuals who receive personalized interpretation of their career interest assessments tend to make more significant progress on their career planning (Randahl et al., 1993). As we know, assessment and appraisal are key components of counseling practice, and high-quality assessment practices can provide additional benefits for those receiving counseling treatment.

Test Worthiness as a Cornerstone of Assessment Practice

Test worthiness is paramount in counseling to ensure the effectiveness, as well as the ethical and quality use, of assessments. *Test worthiness* refers to the credibility, integrity, and dependability of assessments utilized in counseling to make insightful clinical determinations about a client's mental health, character traits, or behaviors. The appropriateness of these tests in counseling encompasses various elements such as validity, reliability, practicality, and cultural awareness.

All types of formal and informal assessments will have their strengths and weaknesses. The process for test selection is discussed in depth in Chapter 6; however, counselors should select tests based on principles of test worthiness that align with the assessment's specific goals, context, and intended use. Using a combination of both formal and informal assessments allows for a comprehensive understanding of the client's issues and will provide a well-rounded foundation for evidence-based treatment. Formal assessments are commonly designed with specific purposes, are carefully validated, provide consistent or reliable results over time, have clear scoring criteria and guidelines, and are typically standardized. Additionally, test worthy tests show cross-cultural fairness and are practical with regard to administration and scoring, as discussed in Chapters 3 and 6. These qualities result in a test worthy formal assessment. Informal assessment can be test worthy and demonstrate the four principles of trustworthiness as well. An example of an informal counseling assessment that can have trustworthiness is an observational rating scale for children's behaviors or emotional well-being. Counselors can use these scales to gain valuable data, have structured and consistent rating scales, obtain accurate and holistic understanding, and work with diverse groups in context. The adaptable and flexible nature allows a counselor to capture a wide range of skills and behaviors quickly, reflecting real-world and authentic situations, and it is often less intimidating, which could produce more accurate results. However, the same level of rigor may not be present as with formal assessments. Trustworthiness is also a term often associated with qualitative research to ensure the reliability of the findings.

ESTABLISHING TRUSTWORTHINESS IN QUALITATIVE ASSESSMENT

Often, qualitative assessments provide rich data that other methods may not capture. Qualitative assessment methods are commonly more informal, allowing for flexibility, and counselors can ask additional questions that go beyond the preset items. Qualitative assessments often do not require statistical knowledge and the ability to calculate scores or norm scores. Clients can participate actively with counselors and build a better rapport, leaving opportunities for self-awareness and growth experiences during the assessment process. Additionally, these assessments are not restricted to preset scales or required scales and scores that place clients into categories, allowing for a more open-ended, divergent, and holistic interpretation, which is helpful with diverse groups of clients. With this flexibility, we also need to consider the critical nature of trustworthiness. While we cannot statistically evaluate reliability and validity as we do with standardized tests, we can maintain trustworthiness via concepts coined by Lincoln and Guba (1985), including *credibility, transferability, dependability*, and *confirmability*. *Credibility* is similar to internal validity and reflects the degree of accuracy in results. The concept relies heavily on individuals administering the assessment and whether their process and scoring procedures are accurate. There are methods to assist in maintaining credibility, which include: (a) triangulation, which includes collecting multiple sources of data; (b) prolonged engagement that requires meeting with the client enough times to assess accurately; (c) persistent observation and ensuring the assessor is watching the phenomenon being assessed (e.g., anxiety symptoms) over a long period of time; (d) negative case analysis where the counselor or assessor solicits information on times the phenomenon being assessed did not happen; and (e) member checks where the counselor checks in with the client on findings and interpretations for each session to ensure that the information is synthesized accurately during assessment of the client (Kline, 2008). *Transferability* in qualitative assessment is similar to external validity and relates to whether the assessment results can be extended to other contexts and settings. To establish and maintain transferability, counselors use methods such as providing thorough descriptions of the assessment results to aid in formulating case conceptualizations, to help select methods for treatment plans, and to create comprehensive assessment reports. *Dependability* in qualitative assessment is most aligned with reliability and is related to the consistency of the findings over time and in various conditions or settings. Peer debriefing, a process that is used to enhance dependability, involves consulting with a supervisor or colleague about the assessment results and interpretations that were found. *Confirmability* refers to whether findings can be substantiated and are accurate, as reported by the client. The researchers confirm that participant narratives shape and influence the results rather than researcher bias or misinterpretations. Detailed audit trails of the assessment process, which contain notes and quotations from the client that provide examples of the findings, help to enhance confirmability.

REDUCING BIAS IN QUALITATIVE ASSESSMENT

Bias resulting from the evaluator's personal perspective and life experiences is a source of error in qualitative research and assessment. In qualitative research, reflexivity refers to the practice of researchers openly discussing their own experiences and beliefs to mitigate bias. This involves a continuous and collaborative process where researchers self-reflectively evaluate and disclose their potential biases throughout the research endeavor. Reflexivity is crucial in enhancing the transparency, credibility, and rigor of qualitative research and assessment practices. It is essential for maintaining ethical standards and ensuring the integrity of qualitative practices.

In counseling, we are trained to monitor self-disclosure with our clients. A critical component of our ethics is to ensure we are using self-disclosures in an ethical way that does not create a dual relationship or change the relationship dynamics, and which keeps client growth and needs in mind. Given this, employing reflexivity in assessment seemingly contradicts our ethical mandates and can be confusing. However, when completing qualitative assessments, reflexivity involves the counselor or assessment provider critically examining their own beliefs, practices, and judgments related to the assessment process, subject, and client prior to engaging in the assessment process or interpretation with the client. Counselors should consider how their background and perspectives could influence how they provide or interpret the results of an assessment. Additional strategies counselors can complete inside or outside the session to promote reflexivity while providing assessments include taking notes about client statements that may trigger personal thoughts during assessments, processing with a supervisor regarding personal thoughts that could impact your work, and peer debriefing with a colleague or supervisor after a session.

DEVELOPING QUALITY ASSESSMENTS

Establishing content-oriented assessments is a complex process in order to ensure that psychometric rigor and validity is established. Lambie et al. (2017) outline the steps for establishing content-oriented evidence in counseling assessments. Content is critical in assessment and assists in establishing reliability and content validity. Lambie et al. (2017) note that content-oriented validity is difficult to establish in counseling because constructs such as personal qualities, attributes, and values can be challenging to capture and quantify. A very brief overview of the steps for establishing content-oriented evidence follows:

1. *Defining the concept measured by the counseling assessment.* A clear definition of the construct or criterion should be established from relevant theories, literature, and other measures. Additionally, a case for the need or necessity of the new instrument should be established through a thorough search of the literature and other established existing assessments that measure the same or similar constructs. What will this new assessment do for counselors and researchers?

2. *Setting the structural framework.* This process involves establishing the assessment criteria, which define the areas to be evaluated or assessed within a theoretical framework that links items to the performance domain and includes subscales. A theory-based model is recommended.

3. *Developing assessment items.* It is crucial to craft the language and structure of assessment items carefully. Those developing assessments should follow precise guidelines when creating effective scale items, such as ensuring each item focuses on a single central idea, using concise and accurate wording, staying away from double-barreled items where two concepts are measured in one item (e.g., Do you ever feel

sad or tired?), and avoiding unnecessary details. It is always recommended to review established assessments, acquaint yourself with the items, and assess their quality by asking targeted questions regarding specificity and readability.

4. *Surveying experts in the field.* After you develop your assessment, a panel of qualified experts in the field should be identified to review the scale. These can include people who are experts in the topic being assessed, experts in test development, and even clinicians in the field who might be interested in using this assessment with clients. Prompts to ask the reviewers include (a) Do the items fit the specified content domains? (b) Do the items match the specified skill? (c) Are the items technically correct? (d) Are the items clear? (e) Do the items adhere to the specified item format (Schmeiser & Welch, 2006, as cited in Lambie et al., 2017)? Clear guidelines and instructions for providing feedback are important. Asking reviewers questions about clarity, readability, flow, or relevance is helpful. A modification section with suggested edits also can be useful. Additionally, having a rating scale or yes/no if an item should be retained is helpful. With this, interrater reliability determines if an item accurately measures a construct. For example, if the established criterion for retaining an item is interrater reliability of 75 and 8/10 experts endorse the item as good, the interrater reliability is 80 for that item. After this step, the scale may be revised based on feedback, potentially soliciting one more round of feedback from those expert reviewers after changes are made.

5. *Pretesting items.* Pretesting the scale once all revisions are made is the last step. Finding a small sample from the identified population that the new scale seeks to assess is needed. Ask them to take the scale and give detailed feedback while also collecting the data to examine psychometric features.

6. *Exploratory factor analysis.* A data sample is collected. This sample typically includes five participants for every one item (Costello & Osborne, 2005). Then an EFA (as previously described) is completed to identify the underlying relationships between measured variables and to reduce data to a smaller set of summary variables. The best-fit structure determines what items should be kept and eliminated for your scale.

7. *Confirmatory factor analysis.* The scale is adjusted based on the EFA, and a new sample is gathered. Then the CFA (as described earlier) is conducted. This allows researchers to test whether the measures of a construct are consistent with their understanding and if the factor structure holds true. After this step, the resulting scale is the final product.

Additional Steps to Designing Quality Assessments

Quality test items are imperative for the reliability and validity of a testing instrument. As test developers continue to review item performance and refine and improve the quality of items on a test, the test quality (i.e., reliability and validity) will increase. This systemic and ongoing review of items is called *item analysis*. The scores' accuracy depends on the quality of items on the test, which makes item analysis critical to test development. Item discrimination and item difficulty are vital elements in evaluating the effectiveness of test items. *Item discrimination* assesses how well an item can distinguish between test takers who have varying levels related to what the test measures. In contrast, *item difficulty* refers to the proportion of individuals who answer the item correctly. The item difficulty level (p) is calculated with the following formula:

$$P = \frac{\text{Number of Examinees Correctly Answering the Item}}{\text{Number of Examinees}}$$

For example, in a counseling class of 20 students, if 15 students get the answer correct on a test of theories, the item difficulty index is 0.75. While the item difficulty index indicates the percentage of individuals who answer a specific item correctly, the *discrimination index* measures how items perform to distinguish between those test takers who possess the knowledge being assessed and those who do not. The extreme group method is one of the more common ways to measure the item discrimination index. The method compares the number of people with high test scores who answered an item correctly to those people with low scores who answered the same item correctly. The item discrimination index is then computed by subtracting the proportion of those in the lower group from those in the upper group; scores range from +1.0 to –1.0. Negative scores are highly challenging to assessment developers. Item analysis is a critical process in evaluating the quality of individual test items and scales, as well as the relationship of each item to other items.

Item Response Theory

Item response theory (IRT) is a complex yet flexible approach to test development and validation compared to CTT. It allows assessments tailored to the test takers' specific abilities to be developed, while providing more accurate and detailed information about an individual's abilities. IRT has similar goals of CTT, but uses a robust statistical approach for evaluating the accuracy of measurement scales, building further upon item analysis. IRT supports assessment development, evaluation, and scoring by focusing on the connection between an individual's ability or trait and their likelihood of correctly responding to a specific test item. This theory centers on representing how individuals' positions on an unobservable continuum relate to their responses to particular test items in order to establish insights into performance, strengths, and areas needing improvement (Whittaker & Worthington, 2016).

IRT operates under the two assumptions of unidimensionality and local independence. Unidimensionality assumes each test item is constructed so it can only measure one ability or latent trait (or underlying unobservable characteristic). This can be challenging because there are often other factors that can outperform the ability of the test to measure latent traits, such as test anxiety (Strout, 1990). The second assumption of local independence is that the response to each item is independent of their response to other items. The answer on one item should not impact the answer on another item. Biased parameter estimates can affect the validity of the inferences drawn from the IRT model and stem from violations of local independence (Strout, 1990). IRT has broad applications across psychometrics, health sciences, and educational psychology. It provides insights into the performance of individual test items and their ability to differentiate between individuals with varying levels of a latent trait through a process of modeling the relationship between item responses and latent traits. The process can be helpful in identifying and addressing possible sources of bias in test items, such as differential item functioning across different demographic groups (discussed in Chapter 3). Additionally, it aids in pinpointing individual abilities and difficulties with specific sets of items while enabling comparisons across different populations. IRT is instrumental in ensuring assessment instruments' reliability, validity, and efficiency, ultimately enhancing the quality and accuracy of the data collected in counseling assessments and further advancing the field.

CHECKING IN WITH ARTURO

As Arturo struggles with his faith, depression, and sense of fulfillment in life, there are many assessments that his counselor wants to use. But the counselor also knows, from Chapter 3, that they must be sensitive to cultural factors.

1. How might Arturo's cultural background and religious beliefs influence the reliability and validity of a counseling assessment? Consider the potential impact of cultural factors on the interpretation of assessment results and the choice of assessment tools.

2. What impact would Arturo's emotional state have on the reliability and validity of counseling assessments? How could the counselor ensure that assessment results are reliable and valid, and how does trustworthiness play a role?

3. How might the therapist address limitations of reliability and validity for Arturo? Discuss the importance of understanding the limitations of assessment tools and different approaches.

END-OF-CHAPTER RESOURCES

DISCUSSION QUESTIONS

1. How does reliability affect the validity of a test? Can a test with low reliability still be valid?

2. How does the internal consistency reliability differ from test-retest and equivalent forms reliability?

3. Describe the coefficient alpha. How does it measure internal consistency and what are some of its potential limitations?

4. What is the importance of interrater reliability and how can it be determined? Provide an example of a scenario where it might be used.

CLASS ACTIVITIES

1. **Parallel/Alternate Form Reliability:** Students will create two similar tests, Test A and Test B. Each test should be based on the same material but should feature different questions or problems. Students should ensure that the complexity and content of both tests are similar. After creating the tests, students will take both tests. The scores from both tests will then be compared to determine the level of agreement, indicating the reliability of the tests.

2. Given a set of test scores (e.g., 85, 90, 88, 92, 87), calculate the SEM and the 95% CIs if the reliability coefficient is 95 around the observed scores. Discuss the implications of these CIs in interpreting the precision and accuracy of the test scores in the context of psychologic assessment.

PERSPECTIVE FROM THE FIELD

The goal of this chapter is to provide further insight into the importance of reliability and validity regarding counseling assessment, appraisal, and research. Listen to Dr. Tiffany Vastardis to learn more about concepts related to the validity and reliability of psychometric instruments. Dr. Vastardis is a counselor educator and alumnus of Florida Atlantic University, whose research specialties include instrument design, psychosocial trauma, psychologic intimate partner violence (P-IPV), and neuropsychology. Dr. Vastardis serves as an adjunct professor across several  universities and has taught most courses within the Council for Accreditation of Counseling and Related Educational Programs (CACREP) curriculum. Dr. Vastardis is a licensed mental health counselor and has developed numerous National Board for Certified Counselors (NBCC)-accredited credentialing courses for practitioners across the United States. Dr. Vastardis was named Emerging Leader for 2018–2020 by the Southern Association of Counselor Education and Supervision (SACES). She was also awarded Dissertation of the Year in 2020 by the Florida Atlantic University Department of Education for her development of the Covert Traumatic Experience Scale (CoTES).

Access podcasts via the QR code or http://connect.springerpub.com/content/book/978-0-8261-8913-4/chapter/ch00.

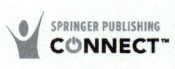 A robust set of instructor resources designed to supplement this text is located at http://connect.springerpub.com/content/book/978-0-8261-8913-4. Qualifying instructors may request access by emailing textbook@springerpub.com.

REFERENCES

American Educational Research Association, American Psychological Association, & National Council of Measurement in Education. (2014). *Standards for educational and psychological testing*. https://www.testingstandards.net/uploads/7/6/6/4/76643089/standards_2014edition.pdf

Balkin, R. S., & Juhnke, G. A. (2018). *Assessment in counseling: Practice and application*. Oxford University Press.

Cohen, R. J., Scheider, W. J., & Tobin, R. M. (2022). *Psychological testing and assessment: An introduction to tests and measurement* (10th ed.). McGraw-Hill Education.

Costello, A. B., & Osborne, J. (2005). Best practices in exploratory factor analysis: Four recommendations for getting the most from your analysis. *Practical Assessment, Research, and Evaluation, 10*(7), Article No. 7. https://doi.org/10.7275/jyj1-4868

Council for Accreditation of Counseling and Related Educational Programs. (2023). *2024 CACREP standards*. https://www.cacrep.org/wp-content/uploads/2023/06/Combined-version-6.21.23.pdf

Cortina, J. M. (1993). What is coefficient alpha? An examination of theory and applications. *Journal of Applied Psychology, 78*(1), 98–104. https://doi.org/10.1037/0021-9010.78.1.98

Kalkbrenner, M. T. (2023). Alpha, omega, and H internal consistency reliability estimates: Reviewing these options and when to use them. *Counseling Outcome Research and Evaluation, 14*(1), 77–88. https://doi.org/10.1080/21501378.2021.1940118

Kline, W. B. (2008). Developing and submitting credible qualitative manuscripts. *Counselor Education and Supervision, 47*(4), 210–217. https://doi.org/10.1002/j.1556-6978.2008.tb00052.x

Lambie, G. W., Blount, A. J., & Mullen, P. R. (2017). Establishing content-oriented evidence for psychological assessments. *Measurement and Evaluation in Counseling and Development, 50*(4), 210–216. https://doi.org/10.1080/07481756.2017.1336930

Lenz, A. S., Ault, H., Balkin, R. S., Minton, C. B., Erford, B. T., Hays, D. G., Kim, B. S. K., & Li, C. (2022). Responsibilities of Users of Standardized Tests (RUST-4E): Prepared for the Association for Assessment and Research in Counseling. *Measurement and Evaluation in Counseling and Development, 55*(4), 227–235. https://doi.org/10.1080/07481756.2022.2052321

Lincoln, Y., & Guba, E. (1985). *Naturalistic inquiry.* Sage.

McNeish, D. (2018). Thanks coefficient alpha, we'll take it from here. *Psychological Methods, 23*(3), 412–433. https://doi.org/10.1037/met0000144

Neukrug, E. S., & Fawcett, R. C. (2010). *Essentials of testing & assessment: A practical guide for counselors, social workers, and psychologists* (2nd ed.). Brooks/Cole Cengage Learning.

Reynolds, C. R., Altmann, R. A., & Allen, D. N. (2021). *Mastering modern psychological testing: Theory and methods* (2nd ed.). Springer Publishing Company.

Schmeiser, C. B., & Welch, C. J. (2006). Test development. In R. L. Brennan (Ed.), *Educational measurement* (4th ed., pp. 307–353). Praeger.

Strout, W. F. (1990). A new item response theory modeling approach with applications to unidimensionality assessment and ability estimation. *Psychometrika, 55*(2), 293–325. https://doi.org/10.1007/BF02295289

Whittaker, T. A., & Worthington, R. L. (2016). Item response theory in scale development research: A critical analysis. *The Counseling Psychologist, 44*(2), 216–225. https://doi.org/10.1177/0011000015626273

Assessment Types

8

Assessment of Intelligence, Aptitude, Ability, and Achievement

NADIYA BOYCE-ROSEN, AYSE TORRES, AND CARMAN S. GILL

2024 CACREP STANDARD

3.G.8. use of assessments in academic/educational, career, personal, and social development

During my sophomore year at university, I had the opportunity to serve as a peer counselor for first-year students. It was during this period that I encountered the significance and complexity of intelligence assessments. I remember a fellow peer counselor, who happened to be an international student, expressing his frustration about the culturally biased questions on certain standardized tests, such as the SAT. This sparked a series of discussions among our team, leading us to explore the various theories of intelligence testing, their historical evolution, and their cultural implications. It was a transformative experience that highlighted the immense responsibility borne by test administrators and the ethical considerations they must adhere to.

INTRODUCTION

Section III of this book shifts us from the fundamentals of assessment and understanding psychometrics of testing to examining assessment designed for specific settings and purposes. In this chapter, we begin with history and the basics of intelligence theory and assessment, and move to assessments of ability, achievement, and aptitude. Resources are provided for counselors in school and other academic settings. For any construct or assessment within this chapter, counselors will apply the principles of ethics and cultural competencies as covered in Chapters 2 and 3.

ASSESSING ABILITY, APTITUDE, AND INTELLIGENCE

Throughout history, the evaluation of cognitive abilities, aptitude, and existing knowledge has been employed to categorize individual capacities and differentiate between participants. When considering the measurement of abilities, instruments can be broadly categorized into two divisions: (1) tests of general abilities and (2) tests of specific abilities (Strauser et al., 2020). Tests of general ability attempt to measure a construct that represents overall intelligence and are associated with the capacity to understand, integrate, and utilize information, as well as identify, analyze, and solve problems. Tests of specific abilities, often known as aptitude tests, provide an assessment of particular strengths in specific domains. Achievement testing, on the other hand, refers to measuring knowledge or proficiency gained through learning or training. This measure often reflects the degree of learning attained after a period of instruction.

Intelligence tests, achievement tests, and aptitude tests may seem to measure a similar construct, but they each serve distinct purposes. Intelligence tests evaluate general cognitive ability and are used for distinct reasons. These include: (a) assessing intellectual disabilities, (b) identifying specific types of learning disabilities, (c) identifying exceptionally talented individuals, (d) evaluating intellectual ability after a disabling injury or the onset of a cognitive condition (e.g., dementia), and (e) serving as a component of a personality assessment to gain a comprehensive understanding of an individual. Achievement tests determine the level of knowledge or skills acquired. Similar to intelligence tests, achievement tests are valuable in identifying both learning disabilities and individuals with exceptional academic abilities. Aptitude tests are employed to assess cognitive abilities. These assessments are frequently utilized to determine one's suitability for higher education or vocational pursuits.

Intelligence

As noted in Chapter 2, the fascination with human intelligence has a long history dating back over a century (Boeck et al., 2020). You will remember that Sir Francis Galton (1822–1911), a key figure in the field of differential psychology, conducted some of the earliest scholarly works exploring the nature of intelligence. Galton proposed that intelligence is inherited and can be assessed through sensorimotor tasks (Jastrzębski et al., 2021). Regarded as one of the fathers of modern-day intelligence research, Galton pioneered psychometric and statistical methods. Alfred Binet (1857–1911), a French psychologist, was fascinated by Galton's efforts to measure cognitive functions. Binet devised a set of questions with the purpose of identifying children who might require additional support due to learning disabilities. Binet, along with his colleague Theodore Simon, created the initial test that resembled a modern intelligence test. The Binet-Simon Intelligence Scale, also known as the Simon-Binet Scale, laid the foundation for modern intelligence assessments.

The concept of IQ was introduced by the German psychologist William Stern (1871–1938). He proposed a formula for determining mental age, which could be evaluated through a test like the one developed by Binet. This formula involved dividing the mental age by the chronological age and then multiplying the result by 100. Lewis Madison Terman (1877–1956), who was a cognitive psychology professor at Stanford University, brought standardization to the original test created by Binet. He did this by testing a group of participants in the United States. The first publication of the Stanford-Binet test was in 1916 (Terman, 1916). Terman's adaptation of Binet's intelligence test, known as the Stanford-Binet Intelligence Scales, has become the widely recognized standard in assessing cognitive abilities (Becker, 2003). The Stanford-Binet intelligence test has undergone several revisions and remains a widely utilized assessment tool in present times.

In the 1930s, David Wechsler (1896–1981), an American psychologist, expanded on the idea of assessing adult intelligence through written exams. Similar to Alfred Binet's belief, Wechsler recognized that intelligence encompasses various cognitive abilities; however, he had concerns about the limitations of the Stanford-Binet test. To address this, he introduced his own intelligence test in 1955, known as the Wechsler Adult Intelligence Scale (WAIS). Additionally, he developed two separate tests for children: the Wechsler Intelligence Scale for Children (WISC-V) and the Wechsler Preschool and Primary Scale of Intelligence (WPPSI). The adult version of the test has undergone revisions since its initial release and is now referred to as the WAIS-IV.

Definitions and Theories of Intelligence Testing

Despite more than a century of historical exploration, a clear consensus on the definition and measurement of intelligence has yet to be reached. The various interpretations arise from the complex nature of intelligence, which combines both genetic factors and socially learned aspects. Scholars and researchers have engaged in heated debates about the attributes that make up intelligence. Intelligence is a concept that can be defined in various ways, depending on the underlying theory. However, it is commonly seen as the expression of abilities that arise from the complex interaction of cognitive and emotional faculties, which are shaped by the environment.

Throughout history, various definitions of intelligence have been proposed by renowned scholars. Charles Spearman (1904) posited that intelligent behavior is generated by a single, unitary quality within the human mind. In the early 1990s, Alfred Binet conceptualized intelligence as the ability to judge, reason, and adapt. Lewis M. Terman (1921) defined it as the capacity for abstract thinking, while Louis Thurstone (1925) described it as the ability to abstract. David Wechsler (1945) defined intelligence as the overall capacity of an individual to act purposefully, think rationally, and effectively navigate their environment. Howard Gardner (1983/2011) viewed intelligence as the ability to solve problems or create valued products within cultural contexts. Robert Sternberg (2003) interpreted intelligence as the capacity for lifelong adaptation to one's environment.

Spearman's "g" Factor

In 1904, Charles Edward Spearman introduced his groundbreaking two-factor theory of intelligence. Spearman was the first to propose the concept of a general factor of intelligence, known as the "g" factor. He was also a pioneer in the field of statistics, particularly in the development of factor analysis, and is renowned for his work on Spearman's rank correlation coefficient. Spearman observed that individuals consistently performed similarly across different mental tests. Those who excelled in one aptitude test tended to excel in others, whereas those who struggled in one test faced similar challenges in other tests. This suggested the presence of a common factor that influenced all intellectual and cognitive abilities.

Through factor analysis, a technique that reduces multiple correlated variables to a smaller number of factors, Spearman examined cognitive tests and determined that intelligence-related factors could be measured and quantified. He postulated that these measures of intelligence converged on a unitary factor known as the general factor, or "g." According to Spearman, various mental traits were not independent of each other; instead, they shared a common factor across all cognitive abilities, which he referred to as the general factor or "g" (Gregory, 2014).

Spearman's theory proposed that intelligence comprises two factors: the general factor ("g"), which influences overall mental ability, and the specific factor ("s"), which accounts for specific intellectual abilities. It is worth noting that while the theory is called "two-factor," there are multiple specific subfactors within the "s" factor, depending on the specific abilities assessed in each test (Wasserman, 2003). Spearman's theory proposes that the "g" factor measures an individual's ability to solve complex problems, learn from past experiences, and adapt to new situations. According to Spearman, this factor is primarily influenced by genetics and is not affected by environmental factors like education or socioeconomic status. On the other hand, the "s" factor assesses specific abilities. Spearman suggests that each mental activity has unique characteristics or a certain level of distinctiveness, which can be attributed to a specific factor. These specific factors have three important properties: they can change, their magnitude can vary within an individual over time, and they are influenced by learning.

In the field of IQ testing, most assessments today are based on factor models inspired by Spearman's work on general intelligence ("g"). One example is the well-known Stanford-Binet test, designed to evaluate different aspects of cognitive performance that contribute to overall intelligence. These include working memory, which involves retaining and manipulating information, and visual-spatial reasoning, which relates to mentally visualizing and manipulating objects in space. By incorporating these measures, the Stanford-Binet test provides a comprehensive evaluation of cognitive abilities and potential for intellectual achievement.

Thurstone's Multifactor Theory

In 1938, Louis Leon Thurstone proposed his multiple-factor theory of intelligence, challenging the prevailing notion at the time of the "g" factor put forth by Charles Spearman. Thurstone introduced the concept of multiple factors contributing to human intelligence, as opposed to a single factor. According to Thurstone, individuals possess varying levels of seven primary mental abilities: verbal comprehension, word fluency, numerical ability, spatial visualization, perceptual speed, memory, and inductive reasoning (Sternberg, 2003; see Table 8.1). According to Thurstone, each person has varying levels of these seven factors. These levels are independent of each other, and each ability can be assessed individually. He recommended placing more emphasis on a person's scores in different mental abilities rather than solely focusing on their IQ. Thurstone's theory laid the groundwork for future research exploring different forms of intelligence.

TABLE 8.1 **THURSTONE'S MULTIFACTOR THEORY: PRIMARY MENTAL ABILITIES**

Mental Ability	Description
Verbal comprehension	This factor involves a person's ability to understand verbal material. It is measured by tests such as vocabulary and reading comprehension.
Word fluency	This ability is involved in rapidly producing words, sentences, and other verbal material. It is measured by tests such as one that requires the examinee to produce as many words as possible beginning with a particular letter in a short amount of time.
Numerical ability	This ability is involved in rapid arithmetic computation and in solving simple arithmetic word problems.
Spatial visualization	This ability is involved in visualizing shapes, rotations of objects, and how pieces of a puzzle fit together. An example of a test would be the presentation of a geometric form followed by several other geometric forms. Each of the forms that follows the first is either the same rotated by some rigid transformation or the mirror image of the first form in rotation. The examinee has to indicate which of the forms at the right is a rotated version of the form at the left, rather than a mirror image.
Perceptual speed	This ability is involved in proofreading and in rapid recognition of letters and numbers. It is measured by tests such as those requiring the crossing out of A's in a long string of letters or in tests requiring recognition of which of several pictures at the right is identical to the picture at the left.
Memory	Ability to remember details or data such as lists or words, mathematical formulas, and definitions.
Inductive reasoning	This ability requires generalization—reasoning from the specific to the general. It is measured by tests, such as letter series, number series, and word classifications, in which the examinee must indicate which of several words does not belong with the others.

Source: Sternberg, R. J. (2003). Contemporary theories of intelligence. In I. B. Weiner, W. M. Reynolds, & G. E. Miller (Eds.), *Handbook of psychology: Vol. 7. Educational psychology* (pp. 23–45). John Wiley & Sons.

Vernon's Hierarchical Model of Intelligence

In 1950, Philip E. Vernon proposed a hierarchical model of intelligence that organizes abilities into four distinct levels. Vernon's hierarchical model has gained widespread adoption as one of the most prominent models of intelligence. According to Vernon, intelligence can be understood as a cumulative "g" factor score, with subcomponents of intelligence added in a hierarchical fashion. The model consists of four levels, with factors from each lower level contributing to the next level in the hierarchy.

At the first level of the hierarchy is Spearman's general factor ("g") of intelligence. The second level encompasses two broad abilities: verbal-educational ability and practical-mechanical spatial ability. Each broad ability is further subdivided into specific abilities at the third level. Verbal-educational ability includes verbal fluency and numerical ability, whereas practical-mechanical spatial ability includes mechanical ability, psychomotor ability, and spatial relations. The fourth level comprises specific factors that are unique to the abilities within each domain at the third level (see Figure 8.1).

Vernon's model not only accounts for the higher-order "g" factor but also includes specific factors associated with each domain. It served as a bridge between Spearman's two-factor theory and Thurstone's multiple factor theory, providing a comprehensive framework for understanding intelligence.

Cattell-Horn-Carroll Theory of Cognitive Ability

The Cattell-Horn-Carroll theory of cognitive abilities (CHC theory) is a significant framework in the study of human intelligence. It is based on the combined work of three influential psychologists: Raymond B. Cattell, John L. Horn, and John B. Carroll. The theory integrates two established models: Cattell's theory of fluid and crystallized intelligence (Gf-Gc) and Carroll's three-stratum theory (see Figure 8.2).

In 1963, psychologist Raymond Cattell introduced the concepts of fluid intelligence (g_f) and crystallized intelligence (g_c). According to Cattell's psychometric theory, general intelligence (g) can be further divided into g_f and g_c. Fluid intelligence refers to the ability to adapt and think flexibly when faced with new problems, regardless of prior knowledge. It represents our capacity to learn. On the other hand, crystallized intelligence involves problem-solving and decision-making based on acquired knowledge, experiences, and verbal conceptualizations. It encompasses the application of secondary relational abstractions.

Carroll's three-stratum theory, developed using the psychometric approach, focuses on objectively measuring individual differences in abilities and utilizing factor analysis to reveal underlying relationships. This theory presents a hierarchical model of intelligence, consisting of three levels of cognitive abilities (Horn & Noll, 1997). At the highest level, stratum III represents general ability, "g." Moving down to stratum II, there are nine broad cognitive abilities:

- Crystallized Intelligence (Gc): This includes the breadth and depth of a person's acquired knowledge, the ability to communicate one's knowledge, and the ability to reason using previously learned experiences or procedures.

- Fluid Intelligence (Gf): This includes the broad ability to reason, form concepts, and solve problems using unfamiliar information or novel procedures.

- Quantitative Reasoning (Gq): This is the ability to comprehend quantitative concepts and relationships and to manipulate numerical symbols.

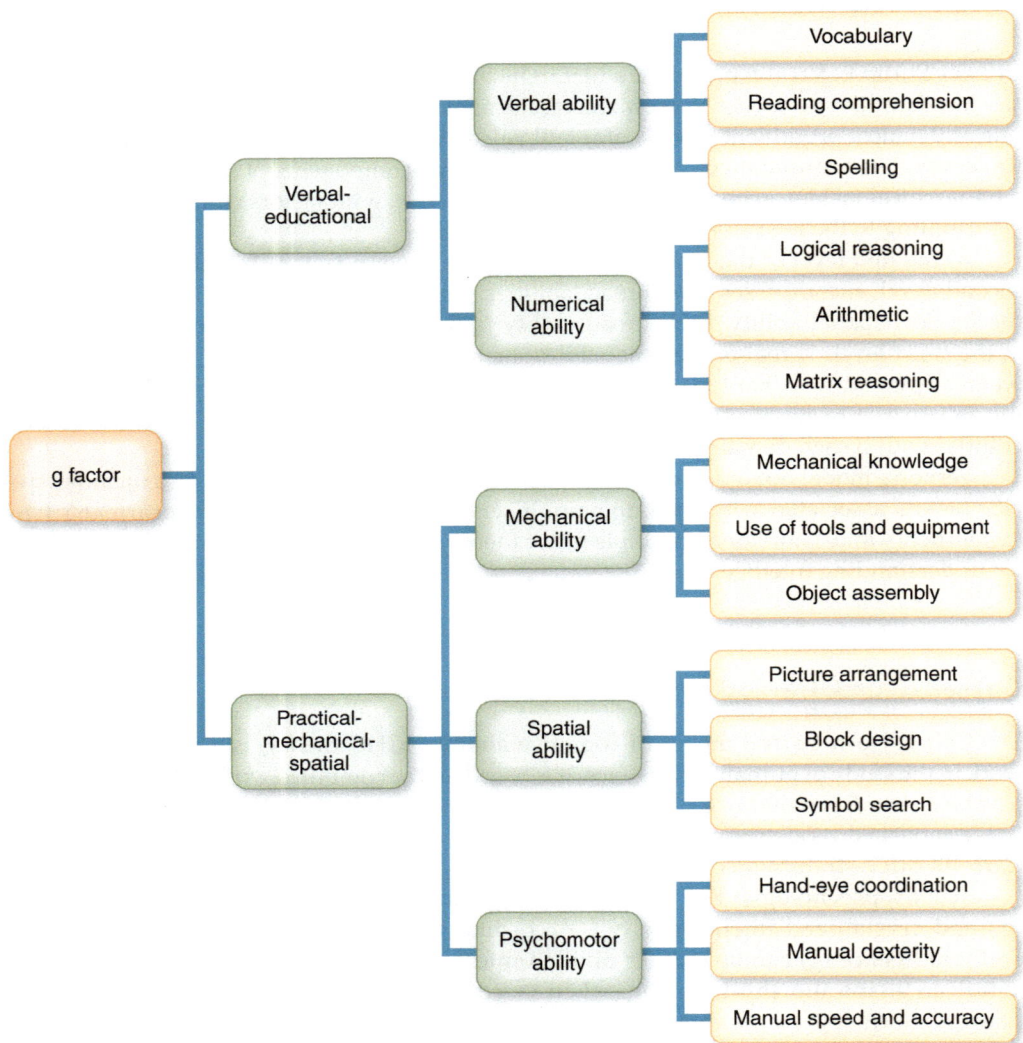

FIGURE 8.1. **Vernon's hierarchical model of intelligence.**

- Reading and Writing Ability (Grw): This includes basic reading and writing skills.

- Short-Term Memory (Gsm): This is the ability to apprehend and hold information in immediate awareness and then use it within a few seconds.

- Long-Term Storage and Retrieval (Glr): This is the ability to store information and fluently retrieve it later in the process of thinking.

- Visual Processing (Gv): This is the ability to perceive, analyze, synthesize, and think with visual patterns, including the ability to store and recall visual representations.

- Auditory Processing (Ga): This is the ability to analyze, synthesize, and discriminate auditory stimuli, including the ability to process and discriminate speech sounds that may be presented under distorted conditions.

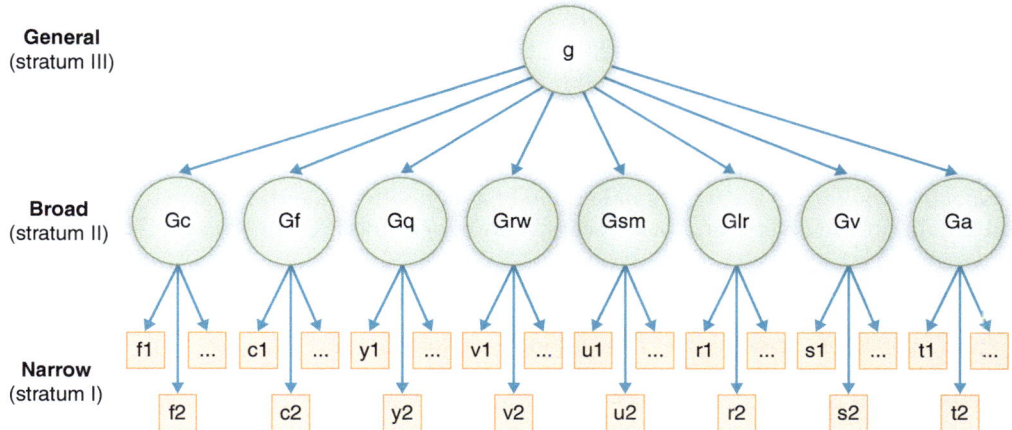

FIGURE 8.2. **The Cattell-Horn-Carroll model of intelligence: Overview of cognitive abilities.**
Ga, auditory processing; Gc, crystallized intelligence; Gf, fluid intelligence; Glr, long-term storage and retrieval; Gq, quantitative reasoning; Grw, reading and writing ability; Gsm, short-term memory; Gv, visual processing.
Source: Tansey, T. N., Brinck, E. A., Wu, J.-R., Estala-Gutierrez, V. Y., & Espino, M. L. (2020). Tests of ability. In D. R. Strauser, T. N. Tansey, & F. Chan (Eds.), *Assessment in rehabilitation and mental health counseling* (pp. 67–82). Springer Publishing Company.

- Processing Speed (Gs): This is the ability to perform automatic cognitive tasks, particularly when measured under pressure to maintain focused attention. The CHC model has undergone numerous revisions and updates over time. Notably, the latest version by Schneider and McGrew, released in 2018, includes the Gs ability (Schneider & McGrew, 2018). As a result, Figure 8.2, which features the original CHC model of intelligence with 8 abilities, does not account for this addition.

A tenth ability, Decision/Reaction Time/Speed (Gt), is considered part of the theory, but is not currently assessed by any major intellectual ability test, although it can be assessed with a supplemental measure such as a continuous performance test (Flanagan et al., 2000). Finally, at stratum I, there are at least 69 narrow abilities (Flanagan et al., 2000). Carroll's three-stratum theory provides a comprehensive framework for understanding and assessing intelligence, offering valuable insights into the diverse range of cognitive capabilities.

Based on the Gf-Gc theory, Carroll developed the CHC theory in 1990, which has been continuously refined since then. By analyzing extensive research spanning several decades, this theory explores the essence, recognition, and organization of human cognitive abilities using factor analysis. Compared to other theories, the CHC theory stands out as the most comprehensive and empirically supported framework for understanding the structure of cognitive and academic abilities.

Gardner's Theory of Multiple Intelligences

Howard Gardner, a psychologist and professor at Harvard University, introduced the theory of multiple intelligences in his 1983 book *Frames of Mind* (Gardner, 1983/2011). In this influential work, Gardner expanded the conventional definition of intelligence and identified several distinct types of intellectual competencies. He challenged the narrow scope of traditional psychometric assessments, which focus solely on cognitive abilities, by proposing that intelligence encompasses a much broader range of aptitudes and talents (Gardner, 1993). Gardner defines intelligence as a "biopsychological potential to process information that can be activated in a cultural setting to solve problems or create products that are of value in a culture" (Gardner, 1983/2011, p. 28).

Gardner has identified eight intelligences, with the possibility of expanding this taxonomy to include additional categories such as "existentialist intelligence." This innovative perspective challenges the traditional notion of a monolithic, one-dimensional intelligence, and highlights the diverse and multifaceted nature of human cognitive capabilities.

1. Visual-Spatial Intelligence: Visual and spatial judgment

2. Linguistic-Verbal Intelligence: Words, language, and writing

3. Logical-Mathematical Intelligence: Analyzing problems and mathematical operations

4. Bodily-Kinesthetic Intelligence: Physical movement and motor control

5. Musical Intelligence: Rhythm and music

6. Interpersonal Intelligence: Understanding and relating to other people

7. Intrapersonal Intelligence: Introspection and self-reflection

8. Naturalistic Intelligence: Finding patterns and relationships to nature

COMMON INTELLIGENCE MEASURES

Stanford-Binet

Since 1916, the Stanford-Binet Intelligence Scales-Fifth Edition (SB5) have held a prominent position as the gold standard for measuring intelligence. Its reputation for accuracy and reliability has made it widely recognized in the field. The SB5 is the latest version of the intelligence test originally created by Alfred Binet. The SB5 measures both verbal and nonverbal intelligence and has a new, simplified format for administering and scoring. It assesses cognitive abilities across five factors: Knowledge, Quantitative Reasoning, Visual-Spatial Processing, Working Memory, and Fluid Reasoning, in both verbal and nonverbal domains. The SB5 is suitable for individuals aged 2 to 85+ years and is widely used in psychologic assessment to identify intellectual disabilities, giftedness, and cognitive impairments. It takes approximately 45 to 75 minutes to administer individually.

The battery provides a Full-Scale Intelligence Quotient (FSIQ) score, as well as Nonverbal and Verbal IQ scores, along with five factor index scores: Fluid Reasoning, Knowledge, Quantitative Reasoning, Visual-Spatial Processing, and Working Memory. Verbal tests assess age-appropriate English reading and speaking abilities, whereas nonverbal tests require fine-motor coordination for manipulating and pointing to objects.

The reliability of SP5 scores has been extensively studied using three different methods: internal consistency, test-retest reliability, and interscorer agreement. The internal consistency coefficients for the IQ scores ranged from 0.95 to 0.98, and from 0.90 to 0.92 for each of the factor index scores. The reliabilities of the 10th subtests ranged from 0.76 to 0.91. Test-retest reliability coefficients were reported to be between 0.89 and 0.95 for the IQ scores, and between 0.83 and 0.95 for the factor index scores. The agreement among different scorers was also found to be high, with a median correlation of 0.90. The standard errors of measurement were determined to be 2.30 for FSIQ, 3.26 for Nonverbal IQ, and 3.05 for Verbal IQ. Furthermore, the SB5 demonstrated strong convergent validity through its high correlations with other cognitive tests, including the Wechsler scales and previous editions of the Stanford-Binet (Bain & Allin, 2005). A confirmatory factor analysis of the subtests provided evidence in support of the five-factor solution. The construction of the SB5 was based on a hierarchical model of intelligence, with FSIQ representing the highest level and five factors representing the intermediate level, which further branched into third-level subtests. The SB5 can be scored manually, or counselors can receive assistance from a computer program that generates an extended score.

Wechsler Adult Intelligence Scale, Fourth Edition

The WAIS is an IQ test specifically designed to assess intelligence and cognitive abilities in adults and older adolescents. Developed by David Wechsler and first published in February 1955, the WAIS has undergone multiple revisions. The WAIS-IV, released by Pearson in 2008, is widely regarded as the most commonly used IQ test worldwide for adults and older adolescents.

The WAIS-IV consists of 15 subtests that are further grouped into four index scales: Verbal Comprehension, Perceptual Reasoning, Working Memory, and Processing Speed. Each subtest is tailored to evaluate specific cognitive abilities, providing a comprehensive profile of an individual's intellectual capabilities.

The Verbal Comprehension Index includes subtests such as "Similarities," "Vocabulary," and "Information," which assess an individual's ability to understand, apply, and articulate verbal information. The Perceptual Reasoning Index measures nonverbal and fluid reasoning through subtests like "Block Design," "Matrix Reasoning," and "Visual Puzzles." The Working Memory Index, comprising of "Digit Span" and "Arithmetic," evaluates an individual's capacity to retain information in immediate awareness while performing mental operations. Lastly, the Processing Speed Index, which includes the "Symbol Search" and "Coding" subtests, appraises the speed of mental and graphomotor processing.

Scoring in the WAIS-IV employs a point system, where each correct response earns a specific number of points. The raw scores from each subtest are then converted into scaled scores, with a mean of 10 and a standard deviation of 3. These scaled scores are subsequently combined to generate index scores, with a mean of 100 and a standard deviation of 15. The sum of these index scores yields the Full-Scale IQ score, which represents an individual's overall cognitive ability.

The WAIS-IV demonstrates strong psychometric properties, making it valuable in both clinical and research settings. Test-retest reliabilities, conducted over a period of 2 to 12 weeks, ranged from 0.70 to 0.90 across the subscales. Inter-scorer coefficients were consistently high, surpassing 0.90. The test manual highlights three target areas for the instrument's application: psychoeducational disability, neuropsychiatric and organic dysfunction, and giftedness. The WAIS also exhibits a high correlation (0.88) with the Stanford-Binet IQ test and demonstrates significant concordance with various measures, including memory, language, dexterity, motor speed, attention, and cognitive ability.

The Wechsler Intelligence Scale for Children (WISC-V; Wechsler & Kodama, 1949) is a common instrument used to measure a child's cognitive abilities and IQ. Children aged 6 years old to 17 years old are able to take this assessment. School counselors and school psychologists can use the results from the assessment to determine if a student qualifies for gifted services, measure the severity of brain injuries on cognitive processing, and diagnose other intellectual and learning disabilities. The overall test can take around 60 minutes to complete and can be done digitally or using paper and pencil.

Woodcock–Johnson Tests of Cognitive Abilities

The Woodcock–Johnson Tests of Cognitive Abilities were developed in 1977 by Richard Woodcock and Mary E. Bonner Johnson. Since then, there have been several revisions. The latest version, the Woodcock–Johnson IV Tests of Cognitive Abilities-Fourth Edition (WJ-IV; Schrank et al., 2014), aligns with contemporary CHC theory. It measures general intellectual ability (GIA; g) and specific cognitive abilities across a wide age range from 2 to 90+ years old.

The WJ-IV is composed of 18 different tests, each designed to assess various aspects of cognitive functioning. These tests are divided into a Standard Battery and an Extended Battery. The Standard Battery includes 10 tests that evaluate GIA and other cognitive capabilities. Specific tests in this battery assess cognitive abilities like comprehension, fluid reasoning, working memory, and processing speed. The WJ-IV includes an Extended Battery with eight additional tests. These tests explore cognitive functioning in more detail, offering specialized assessments of areas like auditory processing, long-term retrieval, and visual processing.

Together, the tests in both batteries allow for the generation of composite scores, offering a broader understanding of a person's cognitive abilities. Some of these composite scores include the GIA score and the CHC Factors, which encompass abilities like comprehension-knowledge (Gc), fluid reasoning (Gf), short-term working memory (Gwm), and more. Finally, the WJ-IV is designed to work in conjunction with other tests, such as the WJ-IV Tests of Achievement (WJ-IV ACH), described later in this chapter, and the WJ-IV Tests of Oral Language (WJ-IV OL), to offer a comprehensive assessment of a person's cognitive abilities.

Cultural and Ethical Considerations in the Administration of Intelligence Tests

The concept of intelligence and its measurement through testing is a deeply debated topic with a multitude of theories and models, but no universally accepted definition or standard. There is ongoing dispute whether intelligence is a single entity or an amalgamation of various abilities, with varying terminologies adding to the confusion. Additionally, the role of heredity in intelligence is a subject of debate. It is often misunderstood that IQ is solely determined by genes, which can downplay the significance of education. The diverse theories proposing different definitions and metrics lead to inconsistent findings from intelligence tests, raising concerns about their breadth and applicability. IQ tests are often criticized for being biased toward certain cultures due to their grounding in specific cultural contexts, leading to questions about their standardization, scope, and overreliance. Historical, social, scientific, and methodological factors have further fueled concerns about the validity of intelligence testing, including issues of bias, privacy, and cultural appropriateness.

Critics argue that many IQ tests are biased, particularly against individuals who deviate from mainstream Western society. For instance, tribal communities possess a rich repository of indigenous knowledge, which may not be reflected in mainstream IQ tests. Recognizing the prevalent bias in intelligence tests, many of which were developed by Western psychologists without considering cultural and ethical factors, there have been significant efforts in the latter half of the 20th century to revise test protocols and address these biases.

IQ tests have the potential to inaccurately measure an individual's intelligence and cause problems including low confidence, unrealistic expectations, and just a generally flawed understanding of a person's potential. Additionally, IQ tests are unable to measure variable aspects of intelligence like emotional and social intelligence. Both of these are crucial factors in assessing an individual's potential for success. In conclusion, it is worth noting that, while IQ tests can be useful for identifying certain strengths and weaknesses, they do not capture the full breadth of a person's intelligence. As such, it is crucial to look beyond IQ scores when assessing an individual's learning needs and potential for success.

ACHIEVEMENT, READINESS, AND APTITUDE ASSESSMENTS IN EDUCATIONAL SETTINGS

In educational settings, there are generally three types of tests: achievement, readiness, and aptitude tests. An easy way to remember what separates aptitude, ability, and readiness from each other is *achievement* represents what the student already knows or has learned in the *past*, *readiness* suggests the student's *present* potential or knowledge, and *aptitude* can assess the student's *future* behavior. Zyromski and Mariani (2016) provide a comprehensive list of assessments that measure academic, career, and social/emotional growth; we cover a few here.

Assessments of Achievement

The Measures of Academic Progress (MAP) Standardized Assessments (Burns & Young, 2019) are growth assessments that measure reading, language usage, math, and science achievement in children grades K through 12. It generally takes 45 to 60 minutes to complete and provides Lexile scores. Lexile scores allow educators to quantify a student's reading and math abilities by grade level. The data received from MAP assessments and Lexile scores assist school counselors with identifying academic self-efficacy small group participants and can help inform whether a child is suited for placement in special education or gifted services. MAP assessments are offered in English and Spanish, and text to speech, screen readers, and visual aids can be provided for those needing accommodations.

The Woodcock–Johnson Tests of Achievement (WJ-IV; Ding & Alfonso, 2016) can measure a student's reading, mathematics, and written language skill. The achievement, cognitive abilities, and oral language components have all been co-normed so that each battery can be administered all together or separately. There is a general and extended form to measure levels of fluency in all three areas. These tests can be given to individuals between the ages of 2 and 90 years old and generally take about 5 minutes to complete per subtest. This exam also allows for progress monitoring to be completed 2 to 3 times a year. Professional school counselors (PSCs) can use the results from the WJ-IV to screen, diagnose, and monitor progress toward academic achievement areas. Though this assessment is often administered by psychologists or outside mental health professionals, school counselors can use the data from this resource to determine if a student is appropriately placed in a course, advocate for special education services, and identify if a student needs additional resources and support like one-on-one academic coaching.

The Kaufman Test of Educational Achievement (KTEA-3; Frame et al., 2016) is an achievement test that measures a broad range of skills in reading, math, written language, and oral language. The KTEA-3 can be used for progress monitoring and diagnosing learning disabilities. Logical processing, letter and word recognition, and math fluency are also included as subtests on the exam. School counselors can use this assessment to assist with determining appropriate classes and special education services for students.

Assessments of Readiness

Many school districts elect to implement kindergarten readiness screeners to determine the level of instructional support needed for incoming kindergartners and first graders. Kindergarten readiness assessments can be used throughout the year as a progress monitoring tool and assess a child's knowledge of English language arts, math, science, social studies, and personal/social development. School counselors can use the data from kindergarten readiness assessments to identify students for behavioral small groups, individual counseling, and to provide feedback to caregivers when making decisions related to class placement in special education services.

The Bracken School Readiness Assessment, Fourth Edition (BSRA-4; Panter & Bracken, 2009), is an example of a kindergarten readiness assessment. The BSRA-4 features six subtests designed to measure a child's cognitive skills, language skills, and early academic achievement.

The ACCESS for ELLs (WIDA Consortium, 2007), based out of the Wisconsin Center for Education Research at the University of Wisconsin–Madison School of Education, has designed assessments to gauge English language proficiency for early language learners. ACCESS for ELLs assessments can be administered to children in kindergarten through 12th grade in both paper and digital formats. ACCESS tests are used as a summative measure of a student's listening, reading, speaking, and writing proficiency. Student scores range from level one (entering) to level six (reaching). School counselors can use the data received from ACCESS testing to decide whether or not a student should remain in English language support services, to determine appropriate placement in classroom instruction, and to demonstrate progress within a subject area.

Assessments of Aptitude

Gifted and talented tests like the CogAT (Cognitive Abilities Test; Lohman, 2011) and IA (Iowa Assessments, formerly the Iowa Tests of Basic Skills; Lindquist & Hieronymus, 1955; University of Iowa College of Education, n.d.) may be administered as a screener for all students at the elementary and middle school levels to identify students who would benefit from placement in accelerated and gifted programs and services. These tests provide schools with screening data in the multistep process of screening, eligibility testing, and placement in gifted services. The CogAT and IA measure a student's reasoning abilities, reading and mathematical abilities, and intellectual curiosity and motivation.

Despite having the word *abilities* in its name, the CogAT test is an aptitude test designed for grades K through 12 and measures analysis, problem-solving skills, and intellectual ability. This test has three sections (verbal, quantitative, and nonverbal) with three subtests in each section and can take 2 to 3 hours to complete. The CogAT is usually administered as a group exam, delivered digitally or on a paper form, and can be administered over the course of 2 to 3 days. The CogAT is a timed test. Note: Educators and caregivers of students receiving 504 or Individualized Education Program (IEP) accommodations such as extended time should discuss the implications regarding eligibility for gifted student services.

The IA assessment often accompanies the CogAT assessment and is actually an achievement test used to determine if a student is eligible for accelerated, gifted, and talented services. The IA measures what a student has already learned and works in conjunction with the CogAT to demonstrate a child's cognitive and academic achievement abilities.

Scholastic Aptitude Test and American College Testing

The Scholastic Aptitude Test (SAT) and American College Testing (ACT) are intended to measure a student's future performance at the college or university level (ACT, n.d.; College Board, n.d.). Students often take the SAT and ACT as a component of their application to attend a 2-year or 4-year college or university. The SAT is composed of reading, writing, language, and math tests and can take up to 3 hours to complete. Generally speaking, students in ninth through 12th grade take the SAT (usually during 11th or 12th grade) or Preliminary Scholastic Aptitude Test (PSAT; ninth or 10th grade), which is a precursor to the SAT. The questions on the SAT are mostly multiple choice. The ACT is similar to the SAT, and covers English, mathematics, reading, and scientific reasoning skill areas. The ACT takes just under 3 hours to administer, and per ACT, Inc., students of all ages are eligible to take the ACT, including those in sixth through ninth grades and high school graduates.

After a student has received results from their test, their school counselor can work with them to identify postsecondary education options. College entrance exams like the SAT and ACT are meant to accompany a comprehensive application that includes a letter of recommendation from the student's teacher, counselor, or mentor; the student's academic record; the student's extracurricular activities; and the student's interest and goal statement. The school counselor can help the student with crafting an application that will encourage acceptance to their ideal educational setting.

Special consideration should be made for dual language students and English as a second language students when conducting aptitude, readiness, and ability assessments. Using assessments that have been adapted to multiple languages can make the difference between a student being placed in gifted or disability services. For example, a student who speaks Mandarin may perform well on the Chinese (Mandarin/Cantonese) version of the CogAT, but struggle to understand the directives in an English-language version of the same assessment.

Graduate Record Examination

The Graduate Record Examination (GRE) general test is intended to measure an individual's ability to succeed in a graduate level program (Educational Testing Services [ETS], 2016). The GRE is generally accepted across a range of disciplines including counseling, psychology, business, law, public health, nursing, and so on. The GRE general test includes three scored sections that measure analytical writing, verbal reasoning, and quantitative reasoning. There are two additional sections that are unscored or used for research that do not count toward an individual's overall GRE score. The exam consists of both multiple choice and written responses and takes around 3 hours and 45 minutes to complete. Individuals can also take a GRE subject test within the mathematics, physics, and psychology disciplines.

Though the GRE is usually taken by those who have completed or are in the process of completing an undergraduate degree, school counselors can develop a student's understanding of the type of assessments they will encounter when they complete their postsecondary schooling. Also, there are academic school programs that give students the opportunity to complete the first 2 years of college while enrolled in high school. Given this accelerated pace, a high school student might consider applying for graduate level programs shortly after enrolling in a 4-year undergraduate program. Having an awareness of the components of the GRE and the expectations of graduate-level standardized testing can help a student confidently navigate their postsecondary education opportunities.

Social/Emotional Domain Assessments

From a social/emotional standpoint, databases such as the RAND Education Assessment Finder and the Collaborative for Academic, Social, and Emotional Learning (CASEL) provide helpful information about interventions and assessments that gauge a student's social/emotional growth, strengths, and weaknesses. A wide range of psychometrically defensible inventories are available that can be used across all age groups. When deciding on which assessment to choose, it may be helpful to look for assessments that have qualities that align with the CASEL 5 (self-awareness, self-management, responsible decision-making, relationship skills, and social awareness). School counselors can use the assessments that follow to measure students' current strengths and areas of need, to measure growth after participation in a school counselor-led intervention, or to serve as progress monitoring tools.

Additionally, skills like Emotional Intelligence (EQ) can be transformative for the social/emotional growth of students across all grade levels. EQ can be described as the process of having awareness and management of your emotions and an understanding of how they affect others. Bradberry et al. (2009) suggest there are two EQ competencies—personal competence and social competence—and within each of these competencies there are two skills. Self-awareness and self-management fall within personal competence, and social awareness and relationship management fall within social competence. EQ can grow and improve over time, but it is important to note that level of growth may look different for those who are neurodivergent.

EXAMPLES OF SOCIAL/EMOTIONAL ASSESSMENTS

The Bar-On Emotional Quotient Inventory: Youth Version (Bar-OnEQ-i:YV; Bar-On, 2000) is designed to measure a student's EQ and can be used for children and adolescents aged 7 to 18 years old. The assessment is a student self-report and provides an overall score as well as subscores for skills such as adaptability, interpersonal and intrapersonal skills, and stress management. The Bar-OnEQ-i:YV can take up to 30 minutes.

The Behavior Assessment System for Children (BASC-3PRS; Reynolds, 2010) measures the behavioral and emotional functioning of children and adolescents between the ages of 2 and 21 years old. The assessment takes up to 20 minutes to complete and includes three major scales—externalizing problems, internalizing problems, and adaptive skills. This assessment includes writing skills for parents/caregivers and teachers, as well as student observation and student self-report.

The Behavior Intervention Monitoring Assessment System (BIMAS-2; McDougal et al., 2011) is an assessment for children and adolescents ages 5 to 18 years old and is widely known as a progress monitoring assessment and universal screener. The BIMAS-2 provides subscores for conduct, negative affect, and cognitive/attention scales, as well as adaptive scales for social and academic functioning. There is a teacher form, parent/caregiver form, and student form available, and the assessment can be completed within 5 to 10 minutes.

The Delaware Social-Emotional Competency Scale (DSECS–S; Mantz et al., 2018) uses the CASEL framework to assess students' social emotional competencies. It can be used as a progress monitoring assessment for children and adolescents in the third to 12th grades. The DSECS–S is a student self-report assessment and provides an overall score as well as subscores for responsible decision-making, relationship skills, self-management, and social awareness.

The Devereaux Student Strengths Assessment (DESSA; LeBuffe et al., 2018) is a widely used and extremely comprehensive assessment that can be used in school, community, and mental health counseling settings as a progress monitoring and outcomes evaluation tool. This assessment can be completed by parents/guardians, teachers, or school staff in under 10 minutes. The DESSA provides an overall score as well as subscores for self-awareness, social-awareness, self-management, goal-directed behavior, relationship skills, personal responsibility, decision-making, and optimistic thinking.

The Mayer–Salovey–Caruso Emotional Intelligence Test (MSCEIT; Mayer et al., 2003) is an EQ self-report measure designed to provide an overall EQ score, as well as subscores for experiential and strategic EQ. This test can take up to 45 minutes to complete and can be used for individuals age 17 and older.

School Climate Assessments

In addition to individual assessment, psychometrically defensible universal screeners provide school counselors with valuable data they can use to inform their Comprehensive School Counseling Programs (CSCPs). Screeners like My Class Inventory (MCI); the Strengths and Difficulties Questionnaire (SDQ); and the Social, Academic, and Emotional Behavior Risk Screener (SAEBRS) are commonly used due to their reliability and concurrent validity (Reinbergs & Fefer, 2018). These screeners can measure prosocial behaviors, peer relationship behaviors, emotional behavior, and academic behavior concerns.

The MCI (Sink & Spencer, 2005) measures are a set of instruments for use with students in fourth through sixth grade. Teachers, parents/caregivers, and students can complete this instrument. The MCI provides the school counselor with a snapshot of how students and other educational partners perceive their school and classroom environment. School counselors can use this information to further hone existing programs, introduce new school-wide programs, and identify a need for more intensive or small group programs.

The SDQ (Goodman, 1997) can be used with children ages 2 to 17 years old and measures emotional symptoms, conduct problems, hyperactivity/inattention, peer relationships, problems, and prosocial behaviors. The SDQ is primarily an informant measure, but there is a version available for self-report for adolescents aged 11 to 17 years old.

The SAEBRS (Kilgus et al., 2013) is a teacher-respondent assessment for understanding student risk for social, academic, and emotional behavior problems. Students can complete this assessment in 3 minutes, and it is a useful resource as a universal screener to understand the needs of students within their school, classroom, and individual settings.

Model for School Counselors and Assessment

Assessing students, particularly at an early age, has important implications across the life span, making the purposeful, accurate, and ethical use of these types of assessments particularly important. For example, PSCs use achievement, readiness or ability, and aptitude assessments to determine what classroom settings and courses to recommend for student placement, to assist students and families with developing postsecondary academic and career plans, and to determine what supports and services students will need to ensure they receive an appropriate level of education or Free Appropriate Public Education (FAPE; American School Counselor Association [ASCA], 2019; U.S. Department of Education, 2023). Whereas ethics in assessment is covered in Chapter 2, in this section we cover the ASCA model for appropriate assessment in school settings.

Assessment within school counseling is weaved throughout the services that PSCs provide to their school communities. PSCs assess schoolwide and individual data to identify student aptitude, ability, and readiness for academic and postsecondary opportunities and determine the necessary academic, social-emotional, and career-based programs needed within the collective school community. The ASCA National Model is the cornerstone of a PSC's program and comprises four central components: *Define, Manage, Deliver,* and *Assess* (ASCA, 2019). The goal of the ASCA National Model is to help PSCs develop CSCPs that are evidence-based, data-driven, and "results-oriented in design and developmental in nature" (ASCA, 2023, p. 12; Zyromski & Mariani, 2016). CSCPs address achievement and opportunity gaps and improve student outcomes through data-informed decision-making and program planning and delivery of postsecondary readiness and success. Each component of the ASCA National Model is developed to consider the needs of the school community. *Define* includes standards for both PSCs and their students. *Manage* incorporates program focus and program planning. Program focus centers on program beliefs, vision, and mission statements. Program planning refers to using school data summaries to develop annual student outcome goals, action plans, lesson plans, and so on. *Deliver* includes direct services (student appraisal and advisement, instruction, and counseling) and indirect services (consultation, collaboration, and referrals). *Assess* involves evaluation of the professional school counseling program to identify equity gaps, highlight gains related to the PSC's programmatic efforts, and investigate areas of potential growth in a PSC's mindset and behaviors (ASCA, 2019). Data and assessment play integral roles throughout the National Model as they inform the opportunities and services that students receive and the types of service that PSCs provide.

Of the four areas in the ASCA National Model, the deliver component most explicitly highlights the application of student assessment and appraisal in school counseling. As recommended by ASCA, 80% of a PSC's time should be focused on the delivery of direct and indirect services (ASCA, 2019). PSCs use ability, readiness, and aptitude assessments to help students understand their social and emotional needs and personal and professional interests. With the knowledge gleaned from assessments, PSCs, students, and their community work collaboratively to identify a plan to achieve the goals related to the student's needs and interests. PSCs can reference the ASCA Student Standards: Mindsets & Behaviors for Student Success to conceptualize how they might approach appraisal and advisement with their students and the desired outcomes related to appraisal and advisement (ASCA, 2021).

Though there are many resources on the internet that assist PSCs with finding assessments, it is useful to use databases and resources that critically evaluate the psychometric properties and other elements of test fairness mentioned in Chapter 3.

Resources: RAND Education Assessment Finder

The RAND Education Assessment Finder is a comprehensive database that allows users to search for assessment instruments that measure K through 12 social/emotional, academic, and career growth (RAND Corporation, 2018). You can use the RAND database to decide which assessments are the best fit for your school community and their goals. This database allows you to filter assessments by competency (cognitive, intrapersonal, interpersonal) and by grade level, responded type, method of administration, administration time, format, and cost. Many of the assessments found on the RAND website align with the ASCA National Model, and the assessments in the RAND provide a thorough resource for school counselors to implement evidence-based interventions using reliable, psychometrically sound measures.

Resources: The Collaborative for Academic, Social, and Emotional Learning

The CASEL (n.d.) provides tools and resources to support growth in social and emotional learning of children, adolescents, and adults. CASEL, which began in 1994, is a collaborative that incorporates data and feedback from a multidisciplinary network of educators, practitioners, researchers, and child advocates. These partners in education have developed a database of interventions and assessments that measure five social/emotional learning competencies (CASEL 5: self-awareness, self-management, responsible decision-making, relationship skills, and social awareness). Each assessment and intervention undergoes a thorough review process to gauge their rigor in regards to reliability, construct, grade and developmental level, and content.

Resources: National Center on Safe Supportive Learning Environments

The National Center on Safe Supportive Learning Environments (NCSSLE; n.d.) offers a compendium of school climate survey assessments and batteries that are verified for validity and reliability in measuring students', educators', administrators', and parents/caregivers' perceptions of school communities. The compendium was developed in partnership with the U.S. Department of Education and can be used by states, school districts, and schools to measure a wide range of constructs, such as bullying and cyberbullying, school connectedness, student support, substance abuse, and so on. PSCs can use the data from school climate surveys to identify schoolwide initiatives that address student engagement, suicide prevention, and student mental health.

The ED School Climate Surveys (EDSCLS), American Institutes for Research Conditions for Learning Survey, and the Academic Optimism of School Surveys are also examples of school climate surveys that provide school counselors with a snapshot of how students, teachers, and caregivers perceive the school's ability to support the academic, career, and social/emotional needs of students.

Student Voice in Assessment

As Zyromski and Mariani (2016) note, students' perspectives on what they consider to be barriers or challenges in education may differ from the perspectives of the adults in their lives. Hatch and Hartline (2021) recommend PSCs use the "ASK" approach to gauging student growth in relation to counseling interventions. ASK is an acronym for Attitudes,

Skills, and Knowledge. Though different from the achievement, readiness, and aptitude assessments mentioned in this chapter, needs assessments and school climate surveys give students an opportunity to share their thoughts regarding their experiences within the educational environment. Student voice is an emerging topic within the school counseling field and PSCs can serve as advocates for students and their voice, needs, and personal agency (Lemberger-Truelove & Bowers, 2018). When developing schoolwide or individual needs assessments, consider how you can include your students' perspectives and collaborate with educational partners (teachers, staff, administration, and caregivers) to develop a comprehensive needs assessment. There are many needs assessments available online; these should ideally be distributed via digital means using tools like Google Forms, Microsoft Forms, SurveyMonkey, and so on.

In this chapter, we discussed the background and history of intelligence and cognitive ability testing and assessment. We also covered a wide range of assessments that can be completed within the school system and utilized by school counselors. It is important to note that ability, aptitude, readiness, and intelligence are individually defined, meaning someone scoring high on an ability or intelligence assessment may not be ready for accelerated coursework or a good fit for a specific career type. You may find that a student qualifies for your school's gifted program based on their CogAT or IA scores but may need additional behavioral or emotional support before they are ready for the demands of a gifted program. Intelligence and aptitude assessments make up one part of the "assessment puzzle." Maturity, motivation, and mental health can significantly impact a student's success, even if they score high on an exam like the CogAT, SAT, or WAIS. Alternatively, a student might not meet the threshold for more advanced coursework based on their performance on the PSAT or SAT, but may demonstrate the maturity and readiness needed to be successful in an advanced or gifted program. The best way to identify appropriate placement for a student is to connect and build relationships with the student and the adults in their life. Learning more about the student and their interests can be instrumental in determining appropriate supports and opportunities for them. Additionally, developing relationships with the student's caretakers and teachers can help with developing a more comprehensive view of what the student can benefit from within their educational experience. As you develop your knowledge and comfort with implementing assessments in your settings, remember that having a holistic understanding of the student and their needs is integral to their success.

CHECKING IN WITH SARAH

Sarah has a number of concerning behaviors and changes—lack of interest in school and drop in grades, emotionally withdrawn and distant, decreased interaction with friends, reduced appetite and weight loss, and suspected self-injury behaviors.

1. How do Sarah's concerns impact her development within the academic, career, and social/emotional domains?

2. Let's say you've applied the ethical considerations recommended in Chapter 2. What are your next steps to help Sarah?

3. In addition to providing referrals for long-term counseling, what assessments and services can you provide as a school counselor to better assess Sarah's needs while at school?

END-OF-CHAPTER RESOURCES

DISCUSSION QUESTIONS

1. Think back to when you were a K through 12 student. What assessments do you recall taking?

2. What assessments within the academic, career, and social/emotional domains would have been helpful to guide your personal and professional decisions when you were a student?

3. As a counseling professional, what academic, career, and behavioral or social/emotional assessments would you use to assess the students or clients that you work with?

CLASS ACTIVITIES

1. **Group Work:** Break out into small groups (3–4 people). With your partners, identify how to approach the following scenarios:

   The students at your school recently completed the CogAT and IA, as well as a universal screener made up of questions from the DESSA and the SDQ. You notice the following:
   The second- and third-grade students who qualify for gifted services are 60% White, 30% African American, and 10% Hispanic/Latinx. Among the qualifying students, 80% identify as female, 19% identify as male, and 1% identify as transgender. The total second- and third-grade level population is 55% African American, 30% Hispanic/Latinx, and 15% White. Of this total population, 63% identify as female, 35% identify as male, and 2% identify as transgender.

   - What do you notice about the race and gender differences of students who qualify for gifted services compared to your second- and third-grade population?

   - How would you address equity concerns and who would you discuss these concerns with within your school community?

2. **Group Work:** With a partner, develop a plan to administer and implement a schoolwide universal screener to identify students' needs within the academic, career, and social/emotional domains. Select one grade level of focus (elementary, middle, or high school).

   - Consider how the universal assessment may differ between each grade level, and what assessments would provide a comprehensive picture of the student's abilities and their outlook on their educational experience.

   - Describe the assessments you would use and why they are necessary in measuring academic career or social-emotional supports.

   - Identify how you would disseminate the universal assessment to your school community, including who you would work with within your school and the consents needed to assess your students.

   - Reflect on how you would address disparities in equity and educational access using the data received from your schoolwide universal screener.

III: ASSESSMENT TYPES

PERSPECTIVE FROM THE FIELD

The goal of this chapter was to provide you with an overview of the assessments and measures of intelligence, aptitude, ability, and achievement. Throughout the chapter, we emphasize the importance of using assessment to understand the needs of the individuals and the population you work with. Collaboration with key partners within your organization, like other mental health professionals, medical professionals, caregivers, educators, and wraparound services, like community organizations, is integral to the success of an appropriate assessment plan. It is also important to clarify what you are attempting to assess. For example, an intelligence assessment may not be appropriate in circumstances when you are aiming to assess an individual's interest or aptitude for a specific career path. As you consider how these instruments are applied by professionals like school counselors, we invite you to listen to our conversation with Dr. Sandra Logan-McKibben. In our conversation, we discuss her experience with implementing assessments while working in a high needs community, using data and assessments for professional advocacy, and collaborating with school-level professionals.

Dr. Logan-McKibben is a leader in the school counseling profession, having served in practice and as a school counselor educator for more than 15 years. She boasts more than 100 professional presentations at scholarly and community conferences; consults with schools, districts, and county offices of education from across the nation; and has coauthored the first-of-its-kind book focusing on comprehensively understanding assessment, data collection, and data-driven school counseling, *The Ultimate School Counselor's Guide to Assessment and Data Collection*.

Access podcasts via the QR code or http://connect.springerpub.com/content/book/978-0-8261-8913-4/chapter/ch00.

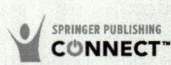 A robust set of instructor resources designed to supplement this text is located at http://connect.springerpub.com/content/book/978-0-8261-8913-4. Qualifying instructors may request access by emailing textbook@springerpub.com.

REFERENCES

ACT (n.d.). *Assessment solutions for schools and districts*. https://www.act.org/content/act/en/products-and-services.html#solutions

American School Counselor Association. (2019). *ASCA National Model: A framework for school counseling programs* (4th ed.). Author.

American School Counselor Association. (2021). *ASCA student standards: Mindsets & behaviors for student success*. https://www.schoolcounselor.org/Standards-Positions/Standards/ASCA-Mindsets-Behaviors-for-Student-Success

American School Counselor Association. (2023). *The school counselor and school counseling programs*. https://www.schoolcounselor.org/Standards-Positions/Position-Statements/ASCA-Position-Statements/The-School-Counselor-and-School-Counseling-Program

Bain, S. K., & Allin, J. D. (2005). Book review: *Stanford-Binet Intelligence Scales*, fifth edition. *Journal of Psychoeducational Assessment, 23*(1), 87–95. https://doi.org/10.1177/073428290502300108

Bar-On, R. (2000). *Bar-On Emotional Quotient Inventory. Youth Version (Bar-On eq-i:Yv): Technical manual*. MHS.

Becker, K. A. (2003). *History of the Stanford-Binet Intelligence Scales: Content and psychometrics* (Stanford-Binet Intelligence Scales, Fifth Edition Assessment Service Bulletin No. 1). Riverside Publishing.

Boeck, P., Gore, L., González, T., & Martín, E. (2020). An alternative view on the measurement of intelligence and its history. In R. Sternberg (Ed.), *The Cambridge handbook of intelligence* (Cambridge Handbooks in Psychology, pp. 47–74). Cambridge University Press. https://doi.org/10.1017/9781108770422.005

Bradberry, T., Greaves, J., & Lencioni, P. (2009). *Emotional intelligence 2.0*. TalentSmart.

Burns, M. K., & Young, H. (2019). Test review: Measures of academic progress skills. *Journal of Psychoeducational Assessment, 37*(5), 665–668. https://doi.org/10.1177/0734282918783509

Collaborative for Academic, Social and Emotional Learning. (n.d.). *CASEL program guide*. https://pg.casel.org/review-programs

College Board. (n.d.). *What's on the SAT?* https://satsuite.collegeboard.org/sat/whats-on-the-test

Council for Accreditation of Counseling and Related Educational Programs. (2023). *2024 CACREP standards*. https://www.cacrep.org/wp-content/uploads/2023/06/Combined-version-6.21.23.pdf

Ding, Y., & Alfonso, V. (2016). Overview of the Woodcock–Johnson IV. In D. P. Flanagan & V. C. Alfonso (Eds.), *WJ IV clinical use and interpretation* (pp. 1–30). Elsevier. https://doi.org/10.1016/B978-0-12-802076-0.00001-3

Educational Testing Services. (2016). *The GRE® tests*. https://www.ets.org/gre.html

Flanagan, D. P., McGrew, K. S., & Ortiz, S. O. (2000). *The Wechsler Intelligence Scales and Gf-Gc theory: A contemporary approach to interpretation*. Allyn & Bacon.

Frame, L. B., Vidrine, S. M., & Hinojosa, R. (2016). Test review: Kaufman, A. S., & Kaufman, N. L. (2014). Kaufman Test of Educational Achievement, third edition. *Journal of Psychoeducational Assessment, 34*(8), 811–818. https://doi.org/10.1177/0734282916632392

Gardner, H. (1993). *Multiple intelligences: The theory in practice*. Basic Books/Hachette Book Group.

Gardner, H. (2011). *Frames of mind: The theory of multiple intelligences*. Basic Books. (Original work published 1983)

Gardner, R. C. (1983). Learning another language: A true social psychological experiment. *Journal of Language and Social Psychology, 2*(2-3-4), 219–239. https://doi.org/10.1177/0261927X8300200209

Goodman, R. (1997). The strengths and difficulties questionnaire: A research note. *Journal of Child Psychology and Psychiatry, 38*(5), 581–586. https://doi.org/10.1111/j.1469-7610.1997.tb01545.x

Gregory, R. J. (2014). *Psychological testing: History, principles, and applications* (7th ed.). Pearson.

Hatch, T., & Hartline, J. (2021). *The use of data in school counseling: Hatching results (and so much more) for students, programs, and the profession*. Sage Publications.

Horn, J. L., & Noll, J. (1997). Human cognitive capabilities: Gf-Gc theory. In D. Flanagan, J. Genshaft, & P. Harrsion (Eds.), *Contemporary intellectual assessment: Theories, tests, and issues* (pp. 53–91). Guilford Press.

Jastrzębski, J., Kroczek, B., & Chuderski, A. (2021). Galton and Spearman revisited: Can single general discrimination ability drive performance on diverse sensorimotor tasks and explain intelligence? *Journal of Experimental Psychology: General, 150*(7), 1279–1302. https://doi.org/10.1037/xge0001005

Kilgus, S. P., Chafouleas, S. M., & Riley-Tillman, T. C. (2013). Development and initial validation of the social and academic behavior risk screener for elementary grades. *School Psychology Quarterly, 28*(3), 210–226. https://doi.org/10.1037/spq0000024

LeBuffe, P. A., Shapiro, V. B., & Robitaille, J. L. (2018). The Devereux Student Strengths Assessment (DESSA) comprehensive system: Screening, assessing, planning, and monitoring. *Journal of Applied Developmental Psychology, 55*, 62–70. https://doi.org/10.1016/j.appdev.2017.05.002

Lemberger-Truelove, M. E., & Bowers, H. (2018). An advocating student-within-environment approach to school counseling. In C. T. Dollarhide & M. E. Lemberger-Truelove (Eds.), *Theories of school counseling for the 21st century*. Oxford University Press. https://books.google.com/books?id=jlByDwAAQBAJ

Lindquist, E. F., & Hieronymus, A. N. (1955). *Iowa tests of basic skills*. Houghton Mifflin Co.

Lohman, D. F. (2011). *Cognitive abilities test (Form 7)*. Riverside.

Mantz, L., Bear, G., Yang, C., & Harris, A. (2018). The Delaware Social-Emotional Competency Scale (DSECS-S): Evidence of validity and reliability. *Child Indicators Research, 11*, 137–157. https://doi.org/10.1007/s12187-016-9427-6

Mayer, J. D., Salovey, P., Caruso, D. R., & Sitarenios, G. (2003). Measuring emotional intelligence with the MSCEIT v2.0. *Emotion, 3*(1), 97–105. https://doi.org/10.1037/1528-3542.3.1.97

McDougal, J. L., Bardos, A., & Meier, S. T. (2011). *Behavior Intervention Monitoring Assessment System: Technical manual*. Multi-Health Systems Incorporated.

National Center on Safe Supportive Learning Environments. (n.d.). *School climate survey compendium*. https://safesupportivelearning.ed.gov/topic-research/school-climate-measurement/school-climate-survey-compendium

Panter, J., & Bracken, B. (2009). Validity of the Bracken School Readiness Assessment for predicting first grade readiness. *Psychology in the Schools, 46*, 397–409. https://doi.org/10.1002/pits.20385

RAND Corporation. (2018). *Choosing and using SEL competency assessments: What schools and districts need to know*. https://measuringsel.casel.org/pdf/Choosing-and-Using-SEL-Competency-Assessments_What-Schools-and-Districts-Need-to-Know.pdf

Reinbergs, E. J., & Fefer, S. A. (2018). Addressing trauma in schools: Multitiered service delivery options for practitioners. *Psychology in the Schools, 55*(3), 250–263. https://doi.org/10.1002/pits.22105

Reynolds, C. R. (2010). Behavior assessment system for children. In I. B. Weiner & W. Edward Craighead (Eds.), *The Corsini encyclopedia of psychology* (pp. 1–2). Wiley. https://doi.org/10.1002/9780470479216.corpsy0114

Schrank, F. A., McGrew, K. S., Mather, N., & Woodcock, R. W. (2014). *Woodcock–Johnson IV*. Riverside Publishing.

Schneider, W. J., & McGrew, K. S. (2018). The Cattell–Horn–Carroll theory of cognitive abilities. In D. P. Flanagan & E. M. McDonough (Eds.), *Contemporary intellectual assessment: Theories, tests, and issues* (4th ed., pp. 73–163). The Guilford Press.

Sink, C. A., & Spencer, L. R. (2005). My Class Inventory-Short Form as an accountability tool for elementary school counselors to measure classroom climate. *Professional School Counseling, 9*(1), 37–48. http://www.jstor.org/stable/42732642

Spearman, C. (1904). "General intelligence," objectively determined and measured. *The American Journal of Psychology, 15*(2), 201–292. https://doi.org/10.2307/1412107

Sternberg, R. J. (2003). Contemporary theories of intelligence. In I. B. Weiner, W. M. Reynolds, & G. E. Miller (Eds.), *Handbook of psychology: Vol. 7. Educational psychology* (pp. 23–45). John Wiley & Sons.

Strauser, D. R., Tansey, T. N., & Chan, F. (2020). *Assessment in rehabilitation and mental health counseling*. Springer Publishing Company.

Terman, L. M. (1916). *The measurement of intelligence: An explanation of and a complete guide for the use of the Stanford revision and extension of the Binet-Simon Intelligence Scale*. Houghton, Mifflin and Company.

Terman, L. M. (1921). Intelligence and its measurement: A symposium—II. *Journal of Educational Psychology, 12*(3), 127–133. https://doi.org/10.1037/h0064940

Thurstone, L. L. (1925). *The fundamentals of statistics* (Vol. 4). Macmillan.

University of Iowa College of Education. (n.d.). *Iowa testing programs*. https://education.uiowa.edu/research/research-centers-and-research-initiatives/iowa-testing-programs

U.S. Department of Education, Office for Civil Rights. (2023). *Free appropriate public education for students with disabilities: Requirements under Section 504 of the Rehabilitation Act of 1973 (1999, 2010, 2023)*. U.S. Department of Education. https://www2.ed.gov/about/offices/list/ocr/docs/edlite-FAPE504.html

Wasserman, J. D. (2003). Assessment of intellectual functioning. In I. B. Weiner, J. R. Graham, & J. A. Naglieri (Eds.), *Handbook of psychology: Vol. 10. Assessment psychology* (pp. 417–442.). John Wiley & Sons.

Wechsler, D. (1945). A standardized memory scale for clinical use. *The Journal of Psychology, 19*(1), 87–95. https://doi.org/10.1080/00223980.1945.9917223

Wechsler, D., & Kodama, H. (1949). *Wechsler Intelligence Scale for Children* (Vol. 1). Psychological Corporation.

WIDA Consortium. (2007). *WIDA English language proficiency standards and resource guide: Prekindergarten-grade 12*. WIDA Consortium.

Zyromski, B., & Mariani, M. A. (2016). *Facilitating evidence-based, data-driven school counseling: A manual for practice*. Sage Publications.

9

Career and Occupational Assessments and Interest Inventories

AYSE TORRES

2024 CACREP STANDARDS

3.G.8 use of assessments in academic/educational, career, personal, and social development

Rehabilitation Counseling

5.G.8. career- and work-related assessments, including job analysis, worksite modification, transferable skills analysis, job readiness, and work hardening

5.G.9. evaluation and application of assistive technology with an emphasis on individualized assessment and planning

During my time as a graduate student in a counseling program, I had the opportunity to work with individuals with disabilities as a practicum student. I distinctly remember my first client, who was at a crossroads in her professional journey. Having recently completed her university education with a degree in liberal arts, she found herself unsure about the different career paths available to her. This uncertainty brought about feelings of anxiety and helplessness. To assist her, I recommended a comprehensive career exploration process that involved various assessments. Although she initially had some reservations, she made the decision to move forward. The assessments helped identify her strengths and shed light on different roles that matched her desired lifestyle. They also provided valuable insights into supportive work environments. With this newfound clarity, she chose a role in a not-for-profit organization that emphasized inclusivity and offered the flexibility and support she needed. Being able to provide guidance and support during such a crucial phase in her life was an absolute privilege. Witnessing her transformation and subsequent success has been incredibly rewarding. This serves as a reminder of how counseling can profoundly and positively impact the lives of those we serve.

CAREER ASSESSMENTS

Work is a significant part of adult life, providing financial security, personal fulfillment, and social connections. It is a vital aspect of well-being, gives us purpose, and contributes to overall life satisfaction. Beyond economic benefits, work cultivates skills, builds confidence, and fosters relationships. It is an opportunity for growth and achievement. When we engage in work that aligns with our interests, values, and abilities, we experience higher job satisfaction, improved mental health, and greater well-being. Career assessments play a pivotal role in promoting well-being by helping individuals find meaningful, satisfying, and enriching work.

Career assessments are tools designed to evaluate individuals' interests, values, abilities, and personality traits to assist them in making informed career choices and planning their professional development. These assessments employ a systematic approach to gather information about an individual's vocational preferences and capabilities, providing valuable insights for career exploration, planning, and development (Savickas & Porfeli, 2012). Career assessments aim to align individual attributes with suitable occupational fields, thereby enhancing the likelihood of career satisfaction and success. These assessments not only reveal the desired destination but also shed light on the journey, empowering individuals to fully grasp and leverage their potential in the professional realm. Career assessments have diverse applications in various contexts, including education, career counseling, vocational rehabilitation, and human resources. Employing a range of techniques, such as self-report questionnaires, inventories, interviews, tests, and online platforms, these assessments gather data and provide valuable insights, enabling a deeper understanding of an individual's career preferences and potential.

Career assessment revolves around key traits such as personality, interests, values, and abilities. It is a collaborative process between counselors and clients. Counselors guide clients in exploring and understanding these traits, creating a comprehensive framework that integrates an individual's unique attributes. This framework offers a holistic view of a client's career identity and serves as the foundation for effective career counseling. By leveraging this framework, counselors can help clients discover career paths that align with their traits, enhancing their career satisfaction and success.

The following are the most commonly used types of career assessments.

- *Interest Inventories*: One commonly used type of career assessment is interest inventories. These inventories measure an individual's preferences for specific activities, industries, tasks, and work environments and can help individuals identify potential career options that align with their interests. The Strong Interest Inventory (SII), for instance, assesses an individual's interests across six broad occupational themes and provides information about corresponding job titles and work environments (Donnay et al., 2004). Interest inventories are reliable predictors of career satisfaction and occupational choice (Su et al., 2019).

- *Aptitude Tests*: Aptitudes are innate abilities that result from inheritance and early development. Aptitude tests provide quantitative estimates of a person's potential for learning the knowledge and skills needed for school, training, or career success (Krane & Tirre, 2005). Occupational aptitude assessments are commonly used to evaluate an individual's capacity to quickly acquire the necessary skills for competent performance in various occupations. The underlying principle behind these assessments is that individuals can make more informed and thoughtful decisions about their educational and career paths when they have a better understanding of their inherent strengths and areas that may require additional effort. By recognizing what comes naturally to them and what may pose challenges, individuals can make more informed choices for a successful future (Feller et al., 2014).

- *Personality Assessments*: Personality assessments play a vital role in career evaluation, providing valuable insights into an individual's character traits. These tests shed light on how individuals interact with others, their preferred work styles, and problem-solving approaches. This understanding guides individuals toward career paths that align with their personality types, enhancing job satisfaction and long-term career success. For example, extroverts thrive in team-oriented and public-speaking roles, whereas introverts excel in individualized positions. By incorporating personality tests into career assessment, individuals can pursue careers that align not only with their skills and interests but also with their innate personality traits. The Big Five Inventory (BFI) is an assessment tool that measures personality dimensions, including extraversion, conscientiousness, openness, agreeableness, and emotional stability.

- *Values Assessments*: Values assessments play a crucial role in career evaluation by exploring an individual's personal values, beliefs, and preferences. By aligning career choices with core principles, individuals gain a deeper understanding of how their beliefs and priorities intersect with different career paths. These assessments shed light on various aspects, such as the importance of financial security, work–life balance, and contributing to society. Identifying and understanding these values allows individuals to pursue careers that meet their needs, resulting in increased job satisfaction and performance. For instance, those who value community service may find fulfillment in nonprofit or social work careers. Therefore, values assessments are essential for making informed career decisions that ensure harmony between personal values and professional pursuits. Tools such as the Work Values Inventory (WVI) help individuals identify work environments and job characteristics that align with their core values.

CAREER ASSESSMENTS IN ONLINE PLATFORMS

The emergence of technology has sparked a revolution in the field of career assessments. Online career assessments have emerged as a convenient and flexible option, offering self-report questionnaires and interactive tools that aid individuals in exploring various aspects of themselves—their interests, personality traits, values, and skills. Accessible through websites or mobile applications, these assessments have transformed the way people make informed decisions about their careers. One such example is the Occupational Information Network (O*NET) Interest Profiler (IP), which provides personalized career recommendations based on users' interests and work values. These assessments not only help individuals explore diverse career options but also foster self-awareness and facilitate decision-making. However, it is imperative to recognize and comprehend the advantages and limitations of online platforms when guiding individuals toward well-informed career choices. The text that follows highlights some key strengths and weaknesses associated with the use of online career assessments, which aim to provide individuals with comprehensive and accurate guidance in their decision-making process.

Strengths of Online Career Assessments

- *Awareness*: Career assessments help individuals gain self-awareness by reflecting on their interests, values, and strengths. This process helps individuals gain a deeper understanding of themselves and their unique qualities, enabling them to make informed decisions about their career paths. By encouraging individuals to explore different career options and consider a wider range of possibilities, career assessments can provide valuable insights and open up new avenues for personal and professional growth. This is especially helpful for those who are unsure of their career goals or those who have not had a chance to extensively explore different career options.

- *Accessibility*: Online platforms have revolutionized the way career assessments are conducted, offering individuals the convenience of completing them at their own pace and convenience. Accessibility eliminates geographical barriers, empowering individuals worldwide to participate in the assessment process with ease, requiring only a simple internet connection.

- *Practicality*: Online platforms provide a wide array of career assessments, ranging from interest inventories to personality assessments. This diverse range of options empowers individuals to explore various aspects of themselves and acquire a comprehensive understanding of their career preferences. Furthermore, online career assessments are often available at no cost or at a minimal expense, making them easily accessible to all.

- *Individualized Feedback*: Numerous career assessments employ sophisticated algorithms and artificial intelligence (AI) techniques to analyze extensive data sets. They then deliver customized career recommendations based on individual responses and profiles. These personalized feedback reports and resources provide invaluable insights into individual strengths, weaknesses, and potential career matches. They empower individuals to make informed decisions.

Weaknesses of Online Career Assessments

- *Validity and Reliability Issues*: Some online career assessments may not have undergone thorough validation and reliability studies, which can make it difficult to determine their accuracy and effectiveness in predicting career success or satisfaction. A lack of professional supervision during the assessment process may undermine the accuracy of the results.

- *Constraints of Self-Reporting*: Online career assessments predominantly depend on self-reported measures, which can be influenced by biases, self-perception, and social desirability. Relying solely on subjective responses could compromise the accuracy and validity of the assessment results.

- *Limited Personalization*: Online career assessments often overlook the unique personal and contextual factors that shape an individual's trajectory. Although AI has made significant strides, it still falls short in capturing the complex tapestry of human experiences and the nuances of individual differences. Algorithms may inadvertently introduce biases or oversimplify career decision-making. Hence, the involvement of human career professionals in interpreting assessment results and offering guidance based on their expertise is vital.

CULTURAL CONSIDERATIONS IN CAREER ASSESSMENTS

Considering cultural factors in career assessments is crucial for ensuring fairness, accuracy, and inclusivity in evaluating individuals' career choices and potentials. Tailoring career assessments to diverse cultural contexts is key to maximizing their effectiveness, and thereby ensuring their validity and reliability across different populations. In today's globally interconnected world, a one-size-fits-all approach falls short as it overlooks the unique cultural elements that shape individuals' values, beliefs, and career aspirations. Factors such as collectivism versus individualism can significantly impact career-related decisions. Thus, adapting career assessment tools to account for these cultural nuances is of utmost importance. This adaptation will result in more accurate, valid, and culturally sensitive assessments that effectively guide individuals on their career paths (Blustein & Ellis, 2000).

Cultural considerations in career assessments involve recognizing and addressing the influence of cultural factors on individuals' career development, aspirations, and decision-making processes. These factors encompass, but are not limited to, race, ethnicity, socioeconomic status, language, religion, and gender. Neglecting cultural considerations can lead to biased assessments, inaccurate predictions, and limited opportunities for individuals from diverse backgrounds. Taking cultural considerations into account in career assessments means acknowledging cultural norms, values, and expectations related to career choices and pathways. Understanding these variations is crucial for accurately evaluating individuals' satisfaction and compatibility with their careers in diverse cultural settings. Language and communication also play a significant role in cultural considerations. Providing career assessments in multiple languages and adapting assessment methods ensures accurate and meaningful results for diverse populations.

VOCATIONAL INTEREST

Vocational interests are defined as trait-like preferences for activities, environments, and outcomes that motivate goal achievement through specific behaviors and attitudes (Rounds, 1995; Su et al., 2009, 2018, 2019). Measuring vocational interests typically involves using vocational interest inventories or assessments. These assessments consist of a series of questions or statements to which individuals respond, indicating their level of interest or preference for different work-related activities, environments, or job characteristics. The responses are then analyzed to generate a profile or score that reflects the individual's vocational interests.

Assessing individual differences in vocational interests is a common practice in various practical settings. Every year, millions of individuals complete interest inventories to understand how their interests align with different job roles and work environments. For instance, the IP on the O*NET receives an average of one million visits per month (Rounds et al., 2008; U.S. Department of Labor, 2018). Similarly, the SII, another popular assessment, is used by millions of career seekers annually (Hoff et al., 2020).

The use of vocational interests to predict job satisfaction has been a topic of study since the 1940s. Interest assessments were introduced as a tool to help individuals find fulfilling work. In popular career guidance literature, aligning one's interests with their job is crucial for job satisfaction. However, despite this assumption, several meta-analyses conducted on the subject did not find a significant relationship between interest fit and job satisfaction (Assouline & Meir, 1987; Tranberg et al., 1993; Tsabari et al., 2005). Based on a recent meta-analysis by Hoff et al. (2020), researchers suggest the following key points to inform decision-making in career guidance when using vocational interest inventories:

1. Combine interest inventories with other career assessments (e.g., abilities, values, personality) that predict work outcomes.

2. Discuss interest fit as a predictor of multiple career-related outcomes (e.g., job satisfaction, job performance, and career success).

3. Encourage individuals to retake interest inventories at various stages throughout their career, especially after significant educational or work transitions. Additionally, inquire about the importance individuals place on being interested in their work compared with other factors such as pay, relationships, and autonomy.

WIDELY USED CAREER ASSESSMENT TOOLS

For more than a century, the assessment of career and vocational interests has been a cornerstone of scholarly research. This rich tradition traces back to Parsons's (1909) theoretical framework for aligning individuals with suitable careers, as well as E. K. Strong's (1927a) empirical approach using contrasting groups. Through this enduring legacy, we have gained valuable insights into the intricate dynamics between individuals and their professional paths. The use of interest inventories in career counseling can be traced back to the emergence of career guidance programs in the 1930s, which aimed to address the high unemployment rates during the Great Depression. These programs provided individuals with valuable guidance and support in navigating their career paths. Furthermore, World War II played a significant role in the development of career counseling programs. Specifically, through initiatives such as the Veterans Administration, efforts were made to assist returning veterans in taking advantage of the educational opportunities provided by the G.I. Bill. These programs not only helped veterans transition into civilian life but also enabled them to explore new occupational avenues and make informed career choices.

Strong Interest Inventory

The SII has a rich and esteemed history, beginning with the pioneering work of E. K. Strong Jr. and the release of his initial formal assessment inventory in 1927. The SII holds the distinction of being the longest-standing psychologic test in current use. Not only is it widely regarded as the most commonly used interest inventory, but it also ranks among the most frequently employed psychologic instruments overall (Donnay, 1997).

Strong's vocational interest inventory, now called the SII, was previously known as the Strong Vocational Interest Blank (E. K. Strong, 1927b) and later as the Strong-Campbell Interest Inventory (Campbell, 1974). Throughout its history, it has undergone six revisions and expansions to keep pace with advancements in the field. The current SII contains 291 items and takes an average of 35 to 40 minutes to complete. Respondents are asked to rate themselves using a five-point Likert scale from strongly like to strongly dislike in six broad areas (occupations, subject areas, activities, leisure activities, people, and characteristics). The Strong assessment is suitable for individuals with a 9th-grade reading level or higher (Donnay et al., 2005). It is appropriate for high school students, college students, and adults aged 15 years and above. One advantage of SII is that it suits the needs of clients with different levels of career maturity.

The SII measures interests in four main categories of scales: General Occupational Themes (GOTs), Basic Interest Scales (BISs), Personal Style Scales (PSSs), and Occupational Scales (OSs). The following section provides an overview of each scale. The SII has received significant research that provides compelling evidence for its reliability and validity. The reliability reported for the GOTs' internal consistency ranged from 0.90 to 0.95, and test-retest reliability ranged from 0.83 to 0.91; the BISs' internal consistency ranged from 0.80 to 0.92, and its test-retest reliability ranged from 0.78 to 0.89; and the OSs' test-retest reliability ranged from 0.71 to 0.93 (Donnay et al., 2004).

GENERAL OCCUPATIONAL THEMES

The six GOTs form the most comprehensive layer of SII. These themes are based on the model proposed by John L. Holland (1959, 1997), which is widely regarded as the most extensively researched theory on vocational interests. It serves as a framework for categorizing careers and occupational interests. According to Holland, individuals can be classified into six broad personality types based on their interests, preferences, and abilities: Realistic (R),

Investigative (I), Artistic (A), Social (S), Enterprising (E), and Conventional (C), collectively referred to as RIASEC. This classification system, known as the RIASEC model or the Holland Occupational Codes, is represented by a hexagonal structure (Figure 9.1). Let's take a closer look at each of the six RIASEC personality types.

- Realistic (R): Realistic individuals are practical, hands-on, and enjoy working with tools, machinery, and physical tasks. They typically prefer occupations such as carpentry, engineering, farming, or athletics.

- Investigative (I): Investigative individuals are analytical, curious, and enjoy intellectual pursuits. They have a strong interest in scientific and mathematical activities, research, and problem-solving. Careers in fields such as science, technology, medicine, or academia often attract them.

- Artistic (A): Artistic individuals are creative, expressive, and enjoy activities involving art, design, and self-expression. They often have a passion for music, painting, writing, or acting. They may pursue careers in fields such as graphic design, writing, photography, or performing arts.

- Social (S): Social individuals are people-oriented, compassionate, and enjoy helping others. They have excellent interpersonal skills and often gravitate toward careers that involve working with people, such as counseling, social work, teaching, or healthcare.

- Enterprising (E): Enterprising individuals are ambitious, persuasive, and enjoy leadership roles. They have strong entrepreneurial skills and a desire to influence and persuade others. They are often drawn to careers in sales, marketing, business management, or politics.

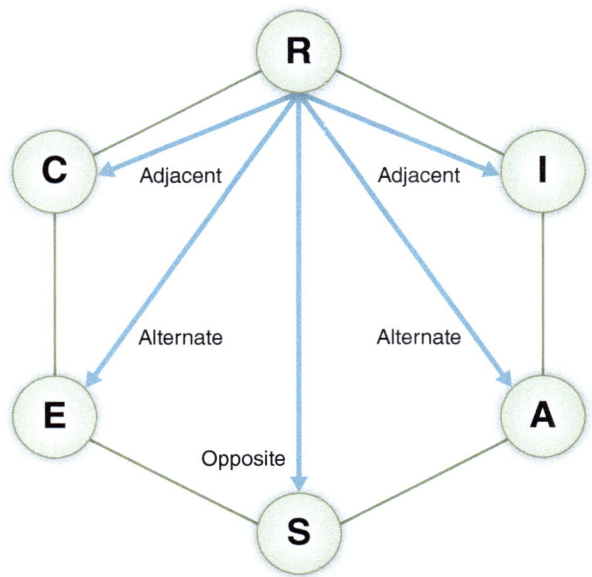

FIGURE 9.1. **RIASEC model.**
RIASEC, realistic, investigative, artistic, social, enterprising, conventional.
Source: Nye, C. D., Su, R., Rounds, J., & Drasgow, F. (2012). Vocational interests and performance: A quantitative summary of over 60 years of research. *Perspectives on Psychological Science, 7*(4), 384–403. https://doi.org/10.1177/1745691612449021

- Conventional (C): Conventional individuals are organized, detail-oriented, and enjoy working with data, numbers, and systems. They prefer structured and orderly environments and may excel in administrative, financial, or technical roles. Careers such as accounting, banking, office management, or computer programing may appeal to them.

The RIASEC model suggests that individuals are more likely to be satisfied and successful in careers that align with their dominant personality types. It's important to note that while the RIASEC model can be a useful framework, it's not definitive or exhaustive. Many individuals may have interests and abilities that span multiple categories, and personal factors such as values, skills, and life circumstances also play a significant role in career decision-making.

BASIC INTEREST SCALES

BISs provide a deeper layer of understanding, moving beyond personality traits to explore specific fields of interest. These scales allow the client to align their interests with potential career fields. They include scales such as:

- mechanics and construction,
- medical science,
- visual arts and design,
- counseling and helping,
- entrepreneurship, and
- office management.

Individuals with high scores on the mechanics and construction scale may find satisfaction in roles such as engineers or contractors. Those with a high score in medical science might thrive in health-related careers, perhaps as doctors or biomedical researchers. Visual arts and design enthusiasts might excel in graphic design or interior decorating, while individuals scoring high on the counseling and helping scale might be ideally suited to roles in social work, therapy, or education. The entrepreneurship scale suits those who are inventive, resourceful, and prefer to chart their own course, with potential careers in startup ventures or business development. Lastly, those who score high on the office management scale might thrive in roles that require meticulousness organization, such as administrative management or secretarial roles. BISs bridge the gap between personal attributes and practical career paths, allowing individuals to map their future with greater clarity and confidence.

OCCUPATIONAL SCALES

The OSs directly compare the interests of the respondents to those of people happily employed in similar occupations. The profile comprises 130 occupations, fostering a detailed and nuanced understanding of career preferences. Approximately 25% of these scales represent occupations that are typically accessible without a college degree, such as carpentry, cosmetology, floristry, opticians, or respiratory therapist. The remaining scales mirror occupations of a more professional nature, including but not limited to architect, registered nurse, psychologist, social science teacher, and executive. OSs fortify the bridge between personal interests and practical career paths, promoting an informed and confident approach toward career planning.

PERSONAL STYLE SCALES

The PSS consists of five distinct scales that offer valuable insights into an individual's preferred learning style, perspective on achieving a work–life balance, risk-taking tendencies, leadership approach, and teamwork inclination.

1. *The Learning Environment (LE) Scale* offers a profound insight into an individual's affinity for academic pursuits. Those who score highly on this scale typically exhibit a deep-rooted curiosity and passion for learning, often pursuing advanced degrees to quench their intellectual thirst. Individuals with average scores on the LE scale tend to align with those who had completed undergraduate college degrees, showcasing a moderate interest in academic endeavors. Conversely, individuals who score lower on the LE Scale are often comparable to those who do not pursue college degrees, favoring practical or vocational paths over academic ones. Therefore, this scale serves as a significant tool for navigating and predicting an individual's academic inclinations and potential.

2. *The Work Style (WS) Scale* offers a unique perspective on an individual's inclination toward social interaction versus solitary activities. Those who score high on this scale, such as event planners, flight attendants, and sales agents, demonstrate a strong preference for roles that involve frequent engagement with people. They thrive in environments that prioritize interpersonal skills, empathy, and emotional intelligence. Conversely, those who score low on the WS Scale, such as graphic designers, computer programmers, and writers, gravitate toward activities centered around ideas, data, and objects. These individuals excel in roles that demand analytical thinking, problem-solving, and independent work. Therefore, the WS Scale serves as a valuable tool for predicting an individual's suitability for either people-oriented or task-oriented work environments.

3. *The Risk-Taking (RT) Scale* offers valuable insights into an individual's propensity for RT and their openness to novel experiences. High scorers on the RT Scale, such as fire fighters and drivers, exhibit a willingness to undertake social, financial, and physical risks. In contrast, individuals who score low on the RT Scale, including accountants and librarians, tend to prefer predictability and stability in their roles. They are more comfortable with familiar routines and are less likely to put themselves in risky situations. The RT Scale is a critical instrument for predicting an individual's inclination toward RT and their comfort with unpredictability in their work and personal environments.

4. *The Leadership Style (LS) Scale* primarily correlates with introversion–extroversion personality traits. Individuals scoring high on the LS Scale, such as CEOs, supervisors, and team leaders, exhibit a strong interest in leading and managing others. These high scorers are typically extroverted with inherent qualities such as assertiveness, social dominance, and persuasiveness. Conversely, low scorers on the LS Scale, such as technical experts, often reflect the interests of those who prefer to work alone. These individuals are usually introverted and find fulfillment in solitary tasks that allow them to focus on detail and independence. Hence, the LS Scale is a pivotal instrument for predicting an individual's likelihood of leadership or autonomous roles based on personality tendencies.

5. *The Team Orientation (TO) Scale* highlights an individual's preference for how they approach tasks, either independently or collectively within a group setting. Those scoring high on this scale, such as project managers or social workers, exhibit a strong inclination toward teamwork and collaboration. They thrive in environments where collective effort and interdependence are valued and tasks are accomplished through shared responsibility. Conversely, individuals with low TO scores, such as park rangers or data entry clerks, usually exhibit an affinity for independent work. They are inclined toward roles in which they can control their work pace and the process, preferring solitary tasks that allow for self-reliance. The TO Scale is an essential tool for predicting an individual's preference for teamwork or independent roles based on personality tendencies.

TIPS FOR COUNSELORS

Professionals who use SII in their counseling sessions have access to various strategies to optimize outcomes. Employing these strategies can enhance the effectiveness of the SII and ultimately provide improved career guidance to its clients.

- Get acquainted with the instrument. Ensure that you have a solid grasp of SII and its functioning. Engage in the manual, guidelines, and supplementary materials provided by the publisher to comprehend the theoretical framework and its application in your practice.

- To effectively administer and interpret SII, it is crucial to obtain proper certification or training. Many organizations mandate counselors to be certified before using the assessment with clients. This ensures that you are adequately equipped to accurately administer and interpret the results with precision.

- Building rapport with clients is crucial when introducing SII. Before administering the assessment, ensure that your clients understand its purpose, format, and structure. Address any questions or concerns they may have and emphasize that the SII is not a definitive answer, but rather a valuable tool for generating ideas and gaining insights. By clarifying these points, you can create a more effective and collaborative assessment process.

- To effectively administer SII, adhere to the administration guidelines provided by the publisher. It is crucial to maintain consistency and accuracy throughout the process. Be sure to allocate sufficient time for your clients to complete the assessment and ensure they understand the instructions clearly. While offering assistance, when necessary, encourage them to answer the questions independently.

- Engage in collaborative interpretation of the results. After the results are accessible, arrange a session with your clients to comprehensively discuss and interpret the findings. Use the SII report as a foundation for initiating a dialog about their interests, preferences, and potential career trajectories. Foster active involvement and invite clients to openly express their thoughts, emotions, and reflections.

- Assist clients in career exploration. Use the SII results as a launching pad to explore diverse career possibilities. Engage in discussions about potential occupations that align with their interests, values, and skills. Offer valuable resources, such as occupational handbooks, websites, and professional networks, to facilitate exploration.

- It is crucial to consider the unique characteristics of each client, including personality traits, abilities, values, and life circumstances, when interpreting the results. In addition, it is essential to consider the broader context in which clients plan to pursue their career goals, such as market demands, job availability, and educational requirements. By considering these individual factors and the overall context, a more comprehensive understanding can be gained to effectively guide clients.

- Foster a collaborative approach with your clients to craft action plans aligned with their SII results. Aid them in setting attainable and practical goals, breaking down the necessary steps to achieve those goals, and identifying valuable resources or support systems to facilitate their career development.

- Progress monitoring and ongoing support: Consistently track the progress of your clients and offer continuous support as they navigate and pursue their career paths. Ensuring their satisfaction, proactively addressing any challenges they may face, and offering guidance as needed are of utmost importance.

Occupational Information Network Interest Profiler

The O*NET IP is a vocational interest inventory designed for use in educational planning, career exploration, and career guidance. The IP is one of several O*NET career exploration tools publicly available through O*NET websites. The IP assesses career interests according to Holland's (1997) RIASEC types. Clients are asked to identify their likes and dislikes for different career tasks using a questionnaire. Results are aggregated into scales based on Holland's RIASEC types, which together form an interest profile. A client's interest profile is then linked to the interest profiles of different careers based on the Standard Occupational Classification system (Rounds et al., 2021).

The O*NET IP has three forms: the IP Long-Form, the IP Short-Form, and the Mini-IP. The IP Short-Form, a web-based version, is currently delivered through My Next Move (www.mynextmove.org). In addition to the English version delivered through My Next Move, a Spanish version of the instrument is available on the Mi Proximo Paso website (www.miproximopaso.org). My Next Move sites average over one million visits per month (U.S. Department of Labor, 2018).

IP is a useful tool for helping students, teachers, counselors, and parents align educational planning and workforce preparation with personalized interests. By completing the IP, individuals gain access to a wealth of information linked to the O*NET OnLine website, which catalogs over 900 occupations through the lens of interests (RIASEC coded), requisite education, experience, and training. This direct connection allows users to explore the prerequisites required for careers that pique their curiosity. Furthermore, O*NET OnLine provides comprehensive data on technology skills, knowledge, and abilities pertinent to various professions.

TIPS FOR COUNSELORS

To effectively utilize IP for their clients, counselors can employ various strategies to achieve the best outcomes.

- Invest time in gaining a comprehensive understanding of the O*NET IP and its functionality. Familiarize yourself with the assessment questions, scoring process, and significance of the interest domains (RIASEC). This will empower you to articulate the assessment effectively to your clients and address any inquiries they may have with confidence.

- When introducing the O*NET IP to your clients, it is important to explain its purpose and the benefits they can gain from using it. Emphasize that this assessment is designed to provide valuable insights into their interests, enabling them to explore potential career paths and make informed decisions about their future. Highlight the tool's capability to generate a comprehensive list of related occupations, accompanied by detailed information about each one.

- To ensure accurate completion of the assessment, it is crucial to provide clear instructions to your clients. Clearly explain the instructions and provide examples if needed. Motivate individuals to respond to questions honestly, reflecting their genuine preferences, rather than feeling compelled to select a specific option. By doing so, you can optimize the accuracy and reliability of the assessment results.

- After your clients finish the O*NET IP, support them in understanding the implications of their scores. Review their interest profile together and explore how their interests align with various work environments. Discuss the potential impact on their career choices.

- Engage in conversations about occupational matches. Delve into a comprehensive array of professions that resonate with your clients' interests. Assist them in comprehending the essence of each occupation, encompassing job responsibilities, essential skills and qualifications, salary insights, and future prospects. Motivate them to conduct further research and gather additional information on specific occupations that captivate their curiosity.

- To create a holistic understanding of your clients' career preferences, strengths, and potential areas of growth, it is important to integrate the IP with other assessment tools. Consider incorporating personality assessments and skill inventories. By doing so, you will assemble a comprehensive career assessment puzzle that provides valuable insights for your clients.

- As a counselor, it is important to offer comprehensive guidance and unwavering support to individuals throughout their career exploration journey. This entails helping clients navigate the vast array of information about various occupations, providing valuable insights into industry trends, and assisting them in crafting actionable plans to pursue their desired career paths. By doing so, you play a vital role in empowering individuals to make informed decisions and achieve their professional aspirations.

Vocational Evaluation

Vocational evaluation (VE) is a systematic assessment that provides reliable and valid data on an individual's current work abilities, limitations, and need for training or services in specific and general skills required for successful employment (Rubin & Roessler, 2008). VE combines standardized psychometric tests, structured interviews, and work samples or simulated tasks to gather information on the client's educational, psychologic, physiological, social, cultural, and economic functioning, all of which are relevant to their vocational pursuits. VE plays a crucial role in the field of vocational rehabilitation, helping to determine suitable employment goals for individuals with disabilities, as well as in the field of forensic rehabilitation.

During the vocational rehabilitation process, VE helps individuals with disabilities understand their vocational readiness and work skills. It incorporates various assessments to identify work-related soft skills and assist individuals in gaining a better understanding of themselves in the workplace. This comprehensive process includes a battery of work, aptitude, and interest tests, as well as clinical interviews and situational assessments. The key objectives of VE include identifying jobs that the client can perform with or without additional vocational services and determining potentially feasible job options that may require further vocational support. VE also provides recommendations for enhancing vocational potential or achieving specific job goals, such as through training, education, job coaching, or additional services and supports (Roessler et al., 1998; Rubin & Roessler, 2008). By considering aspects such as the individual's previous work history, academic achievements, personal interests, physical capacities, and psychologic makeup, VE paves the way for creating a personalized rehabilitation plan. This plan is instrumental in enhancing an individual's employability, thereby fostering their independence and improving their overall quality of life.

In the context of forensic rehabilitation, VE often relates to determining an individual's employability and earning capacity following an injury or disability resulting from an incident or accident. This form of VE is critical in legal proceedings where compensation or damages might need to be awarded. The evaluator must conduct a meticulous analysis, including an examination of the individual's functional abilities, transferable skills, residual capacities, and demands of the labor market. This process can greatly assist in determining the extent of vocational disability or impairment and thus influence the amount of compensation to be awarded. The clear and precise report produced after the evaluation not only provides the courts with a comprehensive understanding of the individual's vocational potential but also serves as a robust platform for planning future vocational rehabilitation interventions (Strauser, 2021).

Vocational evaluators must possess a thorough comprehension of both the intricacies of the labor market and the effects of disability on work and human behavior (Chan et al., 1997). The specific skills required in VE include reviewing files, conducting diagnostic interviews, administering psychometric tests, making clinical observations, interpreting data, and providing career counseling (Farnsworth et al., 2005). After completing the VE, the evaluator is responsible for creating a comprehensive report that covers all the findings and establishes clear conclusions. This report needs to be well-crafted, with no ambiguity, and serve as a clear roadmap for the individual's career development plan (Rubin & Roessler, 2008).

Situational Evaluation

Situational evaluation (SE) plays a crucial role in career assessments as it offers a comprehensive understanding of an individual's vocational potential and capabilities. This process involves assessing an individual's skills, abilities, and work behavior in either a real or simulated work environment. By observing and evaluating individuals in an authentic or work-like setting, SE provides a realistic and holistic picture of their performance in a real-life work situation. It not only evaluates an individual's ability to perform specific tasks but also considers interpersonal skills, problem-solving abilities, work habits, and stress tolerance. While SE offers numerous advantages, there are also some associated disadvantages. For instance, it relies heavily on the observer's subjectivity, which may introduce bias. Furthermore, performance in a simulated environment may not always accurately reflect an individual's potential in a real work situation. The pressure of being observed can influence behaviors and performance, and the artificial setting may not fully capture the complexities and challenges of a genuine work environment. Lastly, setting up and conducting SE can be resource-intensive, especially when simulating complex work environments.

Various professionals and organizations widely use SE. This includes vocational rehabilitation counselors, career development professionals, occupational therapists, and human resources managers. Additionally, educational institutions often employ SE in programs focused on career readiness and occupational training. Moreover, businesses may incorporate it into their recruitment and training processes to assess potential employees' skill sets and adaptability to real-world work scenarios. In the public sector, government agencies may use SE to evaluate candidates for roles that require strong decision-making abilities under pressure, such as emergency response or law enforcement.

CAREER ASSESSMENT FOR YOUTH WITH DISABILITIES TRANSITIONING FROM SCHOOL TO ADULTHOOD

Promoting workforce readiness has long been a central goal of ongoing legislative and policy endeavors aimed at equipping individuals, regardless of disabilities, for successful employment. The importance of career development and vocational experiences is particularly crucial for youth with disabilities. Individuals with disabilities who are of working age are more than two times less likely to be employed when compared to their peers without disabilities (Oertle & O'Leary, 2017). The adverse effects of unemployment on health, such as depression and anxiety, alcohol abuse, and poor physical well-being, have been well documented (Langi et al., 2017; McKee-Ryan et al., 2005). The effects vary by subgroup of individuals, with youth being particularly vulnerable.

To assist students with disabilities to achieve their postschool and career goals, Congress enacted two key statutes that address the provision of transition services: The Individuals with Disabilities Education Act (IDEA, 2004) and the Rehabilitation Act of 1973, as amended by Title IV of the Workforce Innovation and Opportunity Act (WIOA). IDEA mandates schools to provide a coordinated set of transition activities that facilitates the student's movement from school to postschool activities, including postsecondary education, vocational education, integrated employment, continuing and adult education, adult services, independent living, or community participation (IDEA, 2004). Transition-age youth with disabilities, under the IDEA, who have turned 22 or graduated from high school with the regular diploma no longer have the legal right to appropriate transition services, such as age-appropriate life skills training, vocational training, individual and family counseling, and transportation assistance. Nevertheless, these services play a crucial role in facilitating a successful transition to adulthood for young adults with disabilities. The WIOA aims to address these needs and provide assistance accordingly. This legislation represents a renewed commitment to the workforce development system and is designed to strengthen our nation's workforce to address the needs of current employees, job seekers, and employers. The purpose of WIOA is to provide workforce activities to assist job seekers in accessing employment, education, training, and related supports; integrate and improve service delivery to assist workers in achieving a family-sustaining wage; and ensure that the workforce meets the skill requirements of employers to compete in the global economy. The focus of Title IV of the WIOA legislation is specifically transition-related regulations for youth and students with disabilities.

Both the IDEA and WIOA make clear that transition services require a coordinated set of activities for students with disabilities within an outcome-oriented process. The term *transition* can be used at different transitional points in the public education system. In this section, transition refers to the movement from school to postschool activities. Transition students often experience significant academic, social, emotional, physical, or developmental changes that may adversely affect their lives. Students with disabilities, in particular, face additional challenges in managing their disability while they are getting ready for a new chapter in their lives. The transition should be coordinated as a systematic, individualized process based on the individual student's needs, strengths, preferences, and interests.

Career assessments play a crucial role in students with disabilities during transition for several reasons. First, these assessments help identify the unique abilities and strengths of each student, providing a solid foundation for them to excel in areas where they naturally thrive. Second, they assist in charting a career path that aligns with students' preferences and interests, fueling their motivation to achieve success. These assessments also foster self-confidence by emphasizing strengths rather than limitations, enabling individuals to overcome potential challenges on their career journey and empowering them to reach their full potential. Lastly, career assessments offer invaluable guidance in making informed decisions, enabling students with disabilities to choose fulfilling and prosperous career paths.

Counselors working with youth with disabilities should ensure that the assessment measures are accessible and inclusive, avoiding any bias or discrimination. The primary objective should be to identify suitable assessments that empower young individuals with disabilities to gain a deeper understanding of their strengths, skills, and needs. It is vital to provide clear feedback and guidance pre- and postassessment. This allows students to make informed decisions about the assessment process and later their career paths. In addition, counselors should maintain open communication with the students' support system, parents, teachers, and mentors to ensure a comprehensive approach to career planning. This inclusive approach can empower youth with disabilities to carve their own path in the professional world.

CAREER ASSESSMENT FOR VETERANS

The challenges of unemployment, underemployment, and work instability lead to hardships in daily living and significantly affect mental well-being. Conversely, mental health issues can impede individuals' ability to secure and sustain employment (J. Strong et al., 2014; Zalaquett, 2010). This correlation holds particular significance for active duty servicemembers and veterans, given their distinct military culture and transition from the military to civilian life (Coll et al., 2011).

Veterans represent a population distinctly different from the larger society in the United States, which maintains a strict hierarchy. Their shared experiences in the military (i.e., training, reporting structure, exposure to harm, adherence to personal codes of conduct) often result in a deeply ingrained sense of camaraderie, mutual understanding, and shared identity. These factors often shape their worldview and influence their relationships and interactions within the community. Upon entering the military, service members are systematically trained to develop a new sense of self-confidence, creating a military identity that supplants civilian orientations (Kintzle et al., 2018). Ultimately, the development of a "strong and stable identity" appears to be the prime goal of military training (Grojean & Thomas, 2006, p. 52).

Military culture has its own values, customs, ethos, selfless duty, codes of conduct, and implicit patterns of communication (Burke, 2004). The collectivist approach encourages interdependency, group orientation, and group cohesion (Hoge et al., 2006). Joining the military offers a profound sense of purpose, providing individuals with structure, support, and the ability to thrive. It instills a sense of direction and empowers its members to fulfill their potential (Petrovich, 2012). This distinct culture allows service personnel to cope with the isolation, ambiguity, danger, powerlessness, boredom, and intense workload that characterize military operations (Bartone, 2006). For some individuals, separating from the military can result in an "identity crisis" (Higate, 2003, p. 102; Hunniecutt, 2022), or a culture shock in which individuals unable to resocialize appear to equate their discharge with being powerless (Higate, 2003). While transitioning to civilian life, veterans also face several issues such as home-front stressors (e.g., family, occupational problems; Elnitsky et al., 2017; Haselden et al., 2019), redefined roles within the family and community (McCormack & Ell, 2017), moral injury (Pyne et al., 2019) due to postcombat deployments, adjustment to service-related disabilities, and chronic physical and psychologic pain (Flynn et al., 2019; Phillips et al., 2016; U.S. Department of Veterans Affairs [VA], 2015).

For many transitioning service members, employment is a critical component of their reintegration into civilian society. Employment can serve as a form of rehabilitation for service members returning home with psychologic wounds (Ainspan, 2011; Wehman et al., 2005). However, in addition to the myriad challenges of transitioning to civilian life, veterans may face difficulties in finding suitable employment. This can exacerbate symptoms related to anxiety, depression, and posttraumatic stress disorder. These mental health challenges impede job search efforts and workplace performance, creating a complex cycle. Comprehensive support systems that address both career and mental health needs are essential for transitioning veterans (Zalaquett & Chatters, 2016). One frequently overlooked challenge during the recruitment and selection process for veterans is effectively communicating their military skills, experience, and qualifications on their resumes in a manner that civilian employers can understand and appreciate (Sargent, 2014). Veterans often need assistance in translating their military jargon into a language that can be easily understood and valued by civilian employers (Sargent, 2014; Troutman & Gagnon, 2014). This is critical, particularly for veterans who are prospective employees (Hunter-Johnson et al., 2020).

Counselors must be mindful of two essential steps to meet the career development needs of veterans. First, military competence is crucial when providing service to veterans (Hayden & Buzzetta, 2014). Counselors often perceive cultural diversity based on geographical, ethnic, religious, or national differences. While all these cultural values are valid, it is important not to overlook the military population as a distinct culture. The military encompasses language, a code of conduct, behavioral norms, belief systems, attire, and rituals. In fact, military culture is more defined than many other cultures, and its principles are established by law. Given the unique challenges veterans face when transitioning from military to civilian life, counselors would greatly benefit from an understanding of military culture to avoid any therapeutic barriers (Buzzetta & Rowe, 2012). Approaching a new therapeutic relationship with a basic knowledge of military culture helps foster a stronger therapeutic alliance, which is a significant factor in determining the success of mental health treatment. Second, it is essential to consider the readiness of the veterans with whom they work. Career development is typically viewed as an active and ongoing journey that involves exploration and achievement. However, veterans may face obstacles that limit their ability to fully engage in these activities, such as mental health challenges, personal circumstances, or limited resources. These factors can introduce varying levels of complexity in addressing career-related issues and making informed decisions. Therefore, before implementing interventions, it is crucial to assess an individual's readiness for career decision-making (Sampson et al., 2004).

Career assessment plays a vital role in veterans transitioning to civilian employment. It helps translate military skills and experiences into job skills, identifies new career opportunities, and highlights additional training needed. It fosters self-awareness and recognizes veterans' values in the job market. When working with veterans, there are various career assessments that can be used. Here are a few notable ones that stand out (Hayden & Buzzetta, 2014).

- *The Career Thoughts Inventory (CTI)*: The CTI is a theory-based assessment and intervention designed to help individuals identify, challenge, and alter negative career thoughts that interfere with effective career decision-making. The CTI yields a total score and scores on three construct scales: Decision-Making Confusion, Commitment Anxiety, and External Conflict. Furthermore, the CTI provides a comprehensive workbook as a valuable learning tool. This resource contains informative content and practical exercises aimed at assisting individuals in recognizing and transforming negative career thoughts. By challenging and modifying these thoughts, individuals can take proactive steps toward making informed career decisions. This self-administered inventory consists of 48 items and can typically be completed by most clients within a time frame of 7 to 15 minutes.

- *The Self-Directed Search (SDS)*: The SDS, founded on Holland's RIASEC theory, is designed to assist individuals in identifying occupations and fields of study that align with their interests and abilities. The SDS operates on the premise that individuals who find a close match between their personality, interests, and work environment tend to experience greater satisfaction and success in their chosen careers. It is a self-administered, self-scored, and self-interpreted tool. Completing the assessment typically takes just around 20 minutes.

- *The Veterans and Military Occupations Finder (VMOF)*: The VMOF is an adjunctive resource for the SDS (Messer et al., 2013). It was developed using Holland's typology and designed to bridge military and civilian employment by conceptualizing military occupations in accordance with the Holland Occupational Codes (Gottfredson & Holland, 1975). This allows exploration of civilian employment options associated with veterans' interests.

- *Transferable Skills Analysis (TSA)*: TSA is a long-standing procedure used by vocational rehabilitation professionals to assist the job search process and serve as a forensic tool for calculating loss of employment potential or earnings. Understanding how military skills translate into workforce skills can be challenging. However, the TSA offers a highly effective approach to bridge this gap by translating military skills and training into civilian work fields. TSA relies solely on individuals' past records, thus adding validity to the results. Vocational rehabilitation professionals often rely on computerized software programs to generate a TSA, which allows them to enter background information on a veteran and obtain a TSA within a few minutes. Additionally, self-administered versions can be found on the internet, such as at www.careeronestop.org/Veterans/ExploreCivilianCareers/YourSkillsAndInterests/transferable-skills.aspx.

CHECKING IN WITH JOHN

Thinking back to the case of John, he has been struggling in various aspects of his life. John is seeking guidance in developing a new career path. He is confident in his abilities to find his own way but believes that a little assistance from you would be beneficial to share his career decision-making.

1. As you have not worked with a veteran before, how would you initially approach working with John?

2. John is curious about your perspective on the use of career assessment tools, and which one would be appropriate for him. How would you address his inquiry?

3. What guidance and insights can you offer regarding self-administered career assessment tools?

END-OF-CHAPTER RESOURCES

DISCUSSION QUESTIONS

1. Considering the historical trajectory and the role of career assessment tools in guiding individuals toward suitable careers, what are some of the most effective contemporary assessment tools being utilized in career counseling today?

2. Given the outlined strategies for counselors to effectively utilize the O*NET IP for their clients, discuss how you can incorporate these tactics into your counseling sessions. Specifically, how would you introduce the O*NET IP to your clients and ensure they understand its purpose and benefits?

3. How can the implementation of career assessments be improved to better serve youth with disabilities transitioning from school to adulthood, given the current legislative and policy framework such as the IDEA (2004) and the Rehabilitation Act of 1973, as amended by Title IV of the WIOA?

4. Considering the effectiveness of career assessment tools such as interest inventories, aptitude tests, and personality assessments in identifying an individual's career direction, how can they be further enhanced to cater to the diverse needs of individuals? Alternatively, are there any potential risks or limitations associated with the overreliance on these assessments in the career counseling process?

CLASS ACTIVITIES

1. **Exploring the O*NET IP:** This activity aims to enhance students' understanding of their career interests and how tools like the O*NET IP can guide their career decisions.

    - Access the O*NET IP at www.mynextmove.org/explore/ip.
    - Completing the Profiler: Complete the O*NET IP. Take note of your results for later discussion.
    - Group Discussion: Form small groups. Each student will share their O*NET IP results and discuss their interests and potential career paths.
    - Class Reflection: Gather as a whole class and allow each group to share their key takeaways from the activity.

2. **Career Assessment Tools:** This activity aims to familiarize students with the use and interpretation of popular career assessment tools, and help them understand their potential applications in career development and counseling.

- Divide into small groups. Assign each group one widely used career assessment tool (such as the SII).
- Each group is to research their assigned tool, focusing on its purpose, the theory behind it, how it's administered, and how to interpret the results.
- After researching, each group will present their findings to the class.
- As a class, discuss the potential applications of these tools in career counseling and development. What are some limitations or critiques of these tools?

PERSPECTIVE FROM THE FIELD

The goal of this chapter was to provide an overview of career and occupational assessments and interest inventories. Listen to Brian M. Montalvo for more insights on these assessments and valuable tips for counselors. Brian, the assistant vice president of the Career Center at Florida Atlantic University, is dedicated to the career development profession. He is actively involved with the National Career Development Association (NCDA) and was chosen for NCDA's Leadership Academy. Brian also served as a Trustee for Higher Education Career Coaches and Specialists on the board of directors for NCDA. NCDA named him the National Practitioner of the Year in 2021. Besides his role in career services, Brian teaches career development and career counseling theory at graduate and undergraduate levels. He has authored articles, essays, and a book chapter on various career development topics. Brian is a national certified counselor and a certified career counselor.

Access podcasts via the QR code or http://connect.springerpub.com/content/book/978-0-8261-8913-4/chapter/ch00.

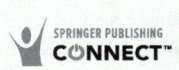 A robust set of instructor resources designed to supplement this text is located at http://connect.springerpub.com/content/book/978-0-8261-8913-4. Qualifying instructors may request access by emailing textbook@springerpub.com.

REFERENCES

Ainspan, N. D. (2011). From deployment to employment. *U.S. Naval Institute Proceedings, 137*, 44–49. https://www.usni.org/magazines/proceedings/2011/february/deployment-employment

Assouline, M., & Meir, E. I. (1987). Meta-analysis of the relationship between congruence and well-being measures. *Journal of Vocational Behavior, 31*(3), 319–332. https://doi.org/10.1016/0001-8791(87)90046-7

Bartone, P. T. (2006). Resilience under military operational stress: Can leaders influence hardiness? *Military Psychology, 18*(1), 131–148. https://doi.org/10.1207/s15327876mp1803s_10

Blustein, D. L., & Ellis, M. V. (2000). The cultural context of career assessment. *Journal of Career Assessment, 8*(4), 379–390. https://doi.org/10.1177/106907270000800407

Burke, C. (2004). *Camp All-American, Hanoi Jane, and the high and tight: Gender, folklore, and changing military culture*. Beacon Press.

Buzzetta, M., & Rowe, S. (2012, November). *Today's veterans: Utilizing cognitive information processing (CIP) approach to build upon their career dreams*. Career Convergence: Web Magazine. http://www.ncda.org

Campbell, D. P. (1974). *Manual for the Strong-Campbell Interest Inventory*. Stanford University Press.

Chan, F., Reid, C., Roldan, G., Kaskel, L., Rahimi, M., & Mpofu, E. (1997). Vocational assessment and evaluation of people with disabilities. *Physical Medicine and Rehabilitation Clinics of North America, 8*(2), 311–325. https://doi.org/10.1016/S1047-9651(18)30328-0

Coll, J. E., Weiss, E. L., & Yarvis, J. S. (2011). No one leaves unchanged: Insights for civilian mental health care professionals into the military experience and culture. *Social Work in Health Care, 50*(7), 487–500. https://doi.org/10.1080/00981389.2010.528727

Council for Accreditation of Counseling and Related Educational Programs. (2023). *2024 CACREP standards*. https://www.cacrep.org/wp-content/uploads/2023/06/Combined-version-6.21.23.pdf

Donnay, D. A. C. (1997). E. K. Strong's legacy and beyond: 70 years of the Strong Interest Inventory. *The Career Development Quarterly, 46*(1), 2–22. https://doi.org/10.1002/j.2161-0045.1997.tb00688.x

Donnay, D. A. C., Morris, M. L., Schaubhut, N. A., & Thompson, R. C. (2005). *Strong Interest Inventory® manual*. The Myers-Briggs Company.

Donnay, D. A. C., Thompson, R. C., Morris, M. L., & Schaubhut, N. A. (2004). *Technical brief for the newly revised Strong Interest Inventory Assessment: Content, reliability, and validity*. https://www.cpp.com/Pdfs/StrongTechnicalBrief.pdf

Elnitsky, C. A., Blevins, C. L., Fisher, M. P., & Magruder, K. (2017). Military service member and veteran reintegration: A critical review and adapted ecological model. *American Journal of Orthopsychiatry, 87*(2), 114–128. https://doi.org/10.1037/ort0000244

Farnsworth, K., Field, J., Field, T., Griffin, S., Jayne, K., & Van de Bittner, S. (2005). *The quick desk reference for forensic rehabilitation consultants*. Elliott & Fitzpatrick.

Feller, R., Hardin, P., Cunningham, T., Whichard, J., & Long, J. (2014). Assessing aptitudes and YOUSCIENCE: Enhancing career development for learners of all ages. *Career Planning and Adult Development Journal, 30*(4), 209–233.

Flynn, L., Krause-Parello, C., Chase, S., Connelly, C., Decker, J., Duffy, S., Danet Lapiz-Bluym, M. D., Walsh, P., & Weglicki, L. (2019). Toward veteran-centered research: A veteran-focused community engagement project. *Journal of Veterans Studies, 4*(2), 265–277. https://doi.org/10.21061/jvs.v4i2.119

Gottfredson, G. D., & Holland, J. L. (1975). Vocational choices of men and women: A comparison of predictors from the self-directed search. *Journal of Counseling Psychology, 22*, 28–34. https://doi.org/10.1037/h0076150

Grojean, M. J., & Thomas, J. L. (2006). From values to performance: It's the journey that changes the traveler. In T. W. Britt, A. B. Adler, & C. A. Castro (Eds.), *Military life: The psychology of serving in peace combat* (pp. 35–59). Praeger.

Haselden, M., Brister, T., Robinson, S., Covell, N., Pauselli, L., & Dixon, L. (2019). Effectiveness of the NAMI homefront program for military and veteran families: In-person and online benefits. *Psychiatric Services, 70*(10), 935–939. https://doi.org/10.1176/appi.ps.201800573

Hayden, S., & Buzzetta, M. (2014). HOPE for the FUTURE: Career counseling for military personnel and veterans with disabilities. *Career Planning and Adult Development Journal, 30*(3), 52–64.

Higate, P. R. (2003). *Military masculinities: Identity and the state*. Praeger.

Hoff, K. A., Song, Q. C., Wee, C. J., Phan, W. M. J., & Rounds, J. (2020). Interest fit and job satisfaction: A systematic review and meta-analysis. *Journal of Vocational Behavior, 123*, 103503. https://doi.org/10.1016/j.jvb.2020.103503

Hoge, C. W., Auchterlonie, J. L., & Milliken, C. S. (2006). Mental health problems, use of mental health services, and attrition from military service after returning from deployment to Iraq or Afghanistan. *JAMA, 295*(9), 1023–1032. https://doi.org/10.1001/jama.295.9.1023

Holland, J. L. (1959). A theory of vocational choice. *Journal of Counseling Psychology, 6*(1), 35–45. https://doi.org/10.1037/h0040767

Holland, J. L. (1997). *Making vocational choices: A theory of vocational personalities and work environments* (3rd ed.). Psychological Assessment Resources.

Hunniecutt, J. R. (2022). My veteran identity (Crisis): Suicides and reintegration. In J. R. Hunniecutt (Ed.), *Rethinking reintegration and veteran identity* (pp. 37–73). Springer International Publishing. https://doi.org/10.1007/978-3-030-93754-6_2

Hunter-Johnson, Y., Niu, Y., Smith, S., Whitaker, B., Wells, R., & Charkasova, A. (2020). The veteran employees: Recruitment, career development, engagement, and job satisfaction of veterans transitioning to the civilian workforce. *New Directions for Adult and Continuing Education, 2020*(166), 139–150. https://doi.org/10.1002/ace.20389

Individuals with Disabilities Education Act, 20 U.S.C. § 1400 (2004).

Kintzle, S., Barr, N., Corletto, G., & Castro, C. A. (2018). PTSD in U.S. veterans: The role of social connectedness, combat experience and discharge. *Healthcare, 6*(3), 102. https://doi.org/10.3390/healthcare6030102

Krane, N. E. R., & Tirre, W. C. (2005). Ability assessment in career counseling. In S. D. Brown & R. W. Lent (Eds.), *Career development and counseling: Putting theory and research to work* (pp. 330–352). John Wiley & Sons, Inc.

Langi, F., Oberoi, A., Balcazar, F., & Awsumb, J. (2017). Vocational rehabilitation of transition-age youth with disabilities: A propensity-score matched study. *Journal of Occupational Rehabilitation, 27*(1), 15–23. https://doi.org/10.1007/s10926-016-9627-4

McCormack, L., & Ell, L. (2017). Complex psychosocial distress post-deployment in veterans: Reintegration identity disruption and challenged moral integrity. *Traumatology, 23*(3), 240–249. https://doi.org/10.1037/trm0000107

McKee-Ryan, F. M., Song, Z., Wanberg, C. R., & Kinicki, A. J. (2005). Psychological and physical well-being during unemployment: A meta-analytic study. *Journal of Applied Psychology, 90*(1), 53–76. https://doi.org/10.1037/0021-9010.90.1.53

Messer, M. A., Greene, J. A., & Holland, J. L. (2013). *The veterans and military occupations finder*. Psychological Assessment Resources.

Nye, C. D., Su, R., Rounds, J., & Drasgow, F. (2012). Vocational interests and performance: A quantitative summary of over 60 years of research. *Perspectives on Psychological Science, 7*(4), 384–403. https://doi.org/10.1177/1745691612449021

Oertle, K. M., & O'Leary, S. (2017). The importance of career development in constructing vocational rehabilitation transition policies and practices. *Journal of Vocational Rehabilitation, 46*(3), 407–423. https://doi.org/10.3233/JVR-170877

Parsons, F. (1909). *Choosing a vocation*. Houghton Mifflin.

Petrovich, J. (2012). Culturally competent social work practice with veterans: An overview of the US military. *Journal of Human Behavior in the Social Environment, 22*(7), 863–874. http://doi.org/10.1080/10911359.2012.707927

Phillips, K. M., Clark, M. E., Gironda, R. J., McGarity, S., Kerns, R. W., Elnitsky, C. A., Andresen, E. M., & Collins, R. C. (2016). Pain and psychiatric comorbidities among two groups of Iraq and Afghanistan era veterans. *Journal of Rehabilitation Research and Development, 53*, 413–432. http://doi.org/10.1682/JRRD.2014.05.0126

Pyne, J. M., Rabalais, A., & Sullivan, S. (2019). Mental health clinician and community clergy collaboration to address moral injury in veterans and the role of the veterans affairs chaplain. *Journal of Health Care Chaplaincy, 25*(1), 1–19. https://doi.org/10.1080/08854726.2018.1474997

Roessler, R. T., Baker, R. J., & Williams, B. (1998). Vocational evaluation. In R. T. Roessler & S. E. Rubin (Eds.), *Case management and rehabilitation counseling: Procedures and techniques* (3rd ed., pp. 83–98). Pro-Ed.

Rounds, J. (1995). Vocational interests: Evaluating structural hypotheses. In D. J. Lubinski & R. V. Dawis (Eds.), *Assessing individual differences in human behavior: New concepts, methods, and findings* (pp. 177–232). Davies-Black Publishing.

Rounds, J., Armstrong, P. I., Liao, H.-Y., Lewis, P., & Rivkin, D. (2008, June). *Second generation occupational interest profiles for the O*NET system: Summary*. The National Center for O*NET Development. https://www.onetcenter.org/reports/SecondOIP_Summary.html

Rounds, J., Hoff, K., & Lewis, P. (2021). *O*NET® Interest Profiler manual*. The National Center for O*NET Development. https://www.onetcenter.org/dl_files/IP_Manual.pdf

Rubin, S. E., & Roessler, R. T. (2008). *Foundations of the vocational rehabilitation process* (6th ed.). Pro-Ed.

Sampson, J. P., Jr., Reardon, R. C., Peterson, G. W., & Lenz, J. G. (2004). *Career counseling & services: A cognitive information processing approach.* Brooks/Cole.

Sargent, A. (2014). A proposed guide for assisting veterans in constructing civilian résumés. *Career Planning & Adult Development Journal, 30*(3), 251–256.

Savickas, M. L., & Porfeli, E. J. (2012). Career Adapt-Abilities Scale: Construction, reliability, and measurement equivalence across 13 countries. *Journal of Vocational Behavior, 80*(3), 661–673. https://doi.org/10.1016/j.jvb.2012.01.011

Strauser, D. R. (2021). *Career development, employment, and disability in rehabilitation: From theory to practice.* Springer Publishing Company.

Strong, E. K., Jr. (1927a). Differentiation of certified public accountants from other occupational groups. *Journal of Educational Psychology, 18*, 227–238. https://doi.org/10.1037/h0070090

Strong, E. K., Jr. (1927b). *Vocational interest blank.* Stanford University Press.

Strong, J., Ray, K., Findley, P. A., Torres, R., Pickett, L., & Byrne, R. J. (2014). Psychosocial concerns of veterans of Operation Enduring Freedom/Operation Iraqi Freedom. *Health and Social Work, 39*, 17–24. https://doi.org/10.1093/hsw/hlu002

Su, R., Rounds, J., & Armstrong, P. I. (2009). Men and things, women and people: A meta-analysis of sex differences in interests. *Psychological Bulletin, 135*(6), 859–884. https://doi.org/10.1037/a0017364

Su, R., Stoll, G., & Rounds, J. (2018). The nature of interests: Toward a unifying theory of trait-situation interest dynamics. In C. D. Nye & J. Rounds (Eds.), *Vocational interests: Rethinking their role in understanding workplace behavior and practice* (pp. 11–38). Taylor & Francis/Routledge.

Su, R., Tay, L., Liao, H.-Y., Zhang, Q., & Rounds, J. (2019). Toward a dimensional model of vocational interests. *Journal of Applied Psychology, 104*(5), 690–714. https://doi.org/10.1037/apl0000373

Tranberg, M., Slane, S., & Ekeberg, S. E. (1993). The relation between interest congruence and satisfaction: A metaanalysis. *Journal of Vocational Behavior, 42*(3), 253–264. https://doi.org/10.1006/jvbe.1993.1018

Troutman, K., & Gagnon, J. (2014). The role of professional coaching and resume writing in successful veteran transitions. *Career Planning & Adult Development Journal, 30*(3), 210–214.

Tsabari, O., Tziner, A., & Meir, E. I. (2005). Updated meta-analysis on the relationship between congruence and satisfaction. *Journal of Career Assessment, 13*(2), 216–232. https://doi.org/10.1177/1069072704273165

U.S. Department of Labor. (2018). *Employment and training administration O*NET® data collection program, 2018.* https://www.onetcenter.org/dl_files/omb2018/Supporting_StatementA.pdf

U.S. Department of Veterans Affairs. (2015). *Profile of post-9/11 veterans: 2013.* National Center for Veterans Analysis and Statistics. http://www.va.gov/vetdata/docs/SpecialReports/Post_911_Veterans_Profile_2013.pdf

Wehman, P., Targett, P., West, M., & Kregel, J. (2005). Productive work and employment for persons with traumatic brain injury: What have we learned after 20 years? *Journal of Head Trauma Rehabilitation, 20*, 115–127. https://doi.org/10.1097/00001199-200503000-00001

Zalaquett, C. (2010). Career and mental health. *Career Planning and Adult Development Journal, 25*, 119–133.

Zalaquett, C. P., & Chatters, S. J. (2016). Veterans' mental health and career development: Key issues for practice. *Career Planning & Adult Development Journal, 32*(1), 86–99.

10

Clinical Assessments and Personality Testing

REBECCA NELSON AND KELLY EMELIANCHIK-KEY

2024 CACREP STANDARD

3.G.10. use of structured interviewing, symptom checklists, and personality and psychological testing

Personality assessments can often be scary and intimidating for clients. There are often parts of ourselves that we subconsciously may not want to explore, although personality assessments give counselors insight into a client's world and can assist a counselor in helping clients reach their goals. As counselors, we need to always remember that it is our job to find ways to reduce client anxiety around testing, be flexible, and explore all the tools. I once worked with a young adult client who didn't want to take a personality assessment, so I handed my client a set of art supplies. I asked him to create a visual representation of his emotions. As the client painted, he revealed layers of his feelings and experiences that words couldn't capture. The unconventional method allowed Jake to express himself authentically and gave me tremendous insight into his personality and inner world, while also demonstrating that profound insights can emerge when clients are given the freedom to convey their inner world in unconventional ways.

CLINICAL ASSESSMENTS IN COUNSELING

Clinical assessment is a systematic and thorough process used in counseling, psychology, psychiatry, social work, and other fields. It aims to evaluate and diagnose an individual's mental health, emotional well-being, and psychologic functioning. The main objective of clinical assessment is to assess mental health disorders and associated conditions. Additionally, clinical assessments play vital roles, such as informing treatment planning decisions (such as if a client needs a higher level of care), monitoring progress during therapy or the intervention period, gauging risk and protective factors, or assisting in research studies to provide valuable data. Once a need is determined based on the client's problem and intake information, goals can be set, and clinical assessments to assist in the treatment planning process must be decided on.

Clinical Assessment Formats

Clinical assessments can come in various formats. Formats for clinical and personality measures include self-report tests, Q-sort tests, ratings and judgments by others, biological measures, behavioral observations, clinical interviews, expressive behavior, document analysis, projective tests, and demographics and lifestyle measures (Friedman & Schustack, 2009). Each assessment type is commonly used in mental health agencies, schools, rehabilitation counseling, and private practice. Many of these methods have been discussed in Chapter 4. Of all forms of assessment, *self-reporting* is the most commonly used type of clinical assessment. Self-reporting begins informally with the client sharing information about what brings them into the counseling process, then continues into the intake information and biopsychosocial spiritual assessment process, and later on in many of the formal assessments that might be selected for use with the client. Self-report tests allow clients to share information about their thoughts, feelings, behaviors, and experiences in response to a standardized and specific set of questions or statements depending on the self-report test being utilized. Commonly used examples of self-report tests that assess for a variety of clinical disorders include, but are not limited to, the Minnesota Multiphasic Personality Inventory (MMPI; Ben-Porath & Tellegen, 2020); the Beck Depression Inventory (BDI; Beck et al., 1961); the Generalized Anxiety Disorder 7 (GAD-7; Spitzer et al., 2006); the Millon Clinical Multiaxial Inventory (MCMI; Millon et al., 2015); and the Posttraumatic Stress Disorder Checklist for *DSM-5* (PCL-5; Blevins et al., 2015), which specifically assesses the symptoms of posttraumatic stress disorder (PTSD) as described by the fifth edition of the *Diagnostic and Statistical Manual of Mental Disorders* (*DSM-5*; American Psychiatric Association, 2013). They are helpful in providing direct insights from the individual, enhancing self-awareness, and highlighting relevant clinical topics for further exploration, assessment, and treatment. It is essential for counselors to carefully consider the strengths and limitations of any assessment tool used in the clinical setting. Furthermore, counselors are encouraged to consider using any assessment tool with other clinically indicated assessment methods. Selected tools should be based on the specific treatment goals of the client.

Clinical Assessments and Use in Various Settings

Clinical assessments are commonly used across mental health counseling settings, from community agencies to private practice, to provide a structured and systematic approach to evaluating and addressing the mental health needs of individuals seeking counseling services. When working in agency settings, it is essential to use various assessment tools and techniques to provide a comprehensive view of a client's mental health. Qualified mental health professionals administer and interpret these assessments to ensure that clients receive the appropriate care and support for their unique needs. Clinical assessments have several common uses in schools to support students' academic, emotional, and psychologic well-being. School counselors use clinical assessments for several reasons, some of which include identifying learning disabilities, assisting in developing Individualized Education Programs (IEPs), identifying exceptionally gifted students for accelerated educational programs, providing behaviors or emotional assessments, helping students with career choices, and monitoring student progress. It's important to note that clinical assessments in schools should be conducted by qualified professionals, such as school psychologists, counselors, and other specialists, to ensure accurate and ethical use of assessment tools and data. Schools must also balance the benefits of assessments with considerations for student well-being, privacy, and the potential for stress associated with testing.

Clinical assessments play a significant role in the field of rehabilitation counseling. They serve several crucial purposes in helping individuals with disabilities overcome challenges, improve their functioning, and lead more fulfilling lives. In rehabilitation counseling, the focus is empowering individuals with disabilities to maximize their potential and improve their quality of life. Clinical assessments provide the foundation for tailored interventions, treatment plans, and support services that address each client's unique needs and goals. Common uses of clinical evaluations are similar to those of clinical mental health counselors, but also include determining assistive technology needs, eligibility for services and disability benefits, vocational assessment, identifying accommodations, and client advocacy and reintegration needs.

Personality Assessments

Personality assessments support clinicians with several essential tasks across the counseling process. *Personality tests* are specific clinical assessments used to evaluate and measure various aspects of an individual's personality, including their traits, characteristics, behaviors, and psychologic attributes. Personality assessments most often used in clinical settings fall into two categories: objective assessments and subjective assessments. Objective assessments are measurements that do not depend on the individual making the assessment, whereas subjective assessments rely on the interpretations of the individual administering the assessment. Personality assessments can be used for a variety of purposes, some of which include clinical utility. Some of these uses include but are not limited to personal growth and self-insight, career development and matching personality traits to potential career paths, hiring and recruitment to select the ideal candidate for jobs, therapy and counseling to aid in the assessment and treatment of mental health conditions, and conflict resolution. Within education, they help educators understand their students' learning styles, preferences, and potential challenges. For counselors working with individuals, couples, or families, personality tests serve several essential tasks across the counseling process. Personality tests offer all clinicians a starting point that informs the treatment planning process. Clinicians can tailor treatment and interventions to target the issues identified through initial and repeated personality measures across the treatment process.

Personality assessment can also reveal additional information about treatment needs that may not be apparent in a client's presentation and informal assessment alone. These additional insights can clarify a hierarchy of treatment priorities. Personality assessments can also enrich therapeutic rapport, as reviewing and discussing assessment results may strengthen trust in the therapeutic alliance and increase commitment to the treatment process. Lastly, personality assessments provide clinicians with empirical data that support ethical practice and can minimize clinician bias or inaccurate interpretation of informal self-reporting by clients. There are many personality assessment tools; some are described in the text that follows and others are listed in Table 10.1 (by no means is the list exhaustive but it highlights common assessment measures).

Some can group *self-concept measures* with personality assessments, yet they are unique. While personality assessments examine a person's responses and identify patterns that emerge from thoughts and behaviors, self-concept and self-esteem assessments examine a person's perception, performance, or feelings about themselves that make up self-worth. There are numerous assessments of self-concept and self-worth, such as the Coopersmith Self-Esteem Inventory (CSEI or SEI; Coopersmith, 1981/1987, 2002). Self-esteem assessments are helpful to assist counselors in identifying areas of intrapersonal challenge for the clients who may need attention and guidance, in addition to appropriate therapeutic techniques and interventions to combat the issue.

MINNESOTA MULTIPHASIC PERSONALITY INVENTORY-3

One example of an objective personality test is the *Minnesota Multiphasic Personality Inventory-3* (MMPI-3; Ben-Porath & Tellegen, 2020). The MMPI is a commonly used assessment tool that consists of a series of statements to which individuals respond with "True" or "False." It is designed to measure various aspects of personality and psychopathology and is used in clinical settings

TABLE 10.1 **COMMON PERSONALITY AND SELF-ESTEEM ASSESSMENTS**

Assessment Tool	Purpose	Scales/Subscales	Number of Items	Normed Population	Strengths	Limitations
16 Personality Factors (16PF; Cattell & Mead, 2008)	The 16PF assesses an individual's personality traits across 16 primary factors. It is used in clinical, occupational, and research settings.	16 primary factors, including warmth, reasoning, emotional stability, dominance, and others	187 items	General adult population	Provides a detailed assessment of personality traits. Used for career development and clinical assessment. Offers a well-defined personality profile.	Requires interpretation by professionals. Limited for assessing specific clinical disorders.
California Psychological Inventory (CPI; Gough, 1956)	The CPI assesses personality traits and psychosocial characteristics for personal and career development. It is commonly used in organizational settings.	Various scales measuring interpersonal, motivation, and mental health factors	434 items	General adult population	Provides insights for personal and career development. Offers a broad range of psychosocial assessments. Useful for vocational and clinical counseling.	Lengthy administration time. Interpretation may require expertise.
Personality Assessment Inventory (PAI; Morey, 1991)	The PAI assesses a wide range of personality and psychopathological constructs. It is used in clinical and forensic contexts.	Multiple scales (e.g., validity scales, clinical scales)	344 items	Diverse clinical populations	Provides complete psychometric assessment. Useful in clinical and forensic evaluations. Covers a range of personality and clinical constructs.	Lengthy to administer. Requires professional interpretation.
Tennessee Self-Concept Scale (TSCS; TSCS-2; Fitts, 1965; Fitts et al., 1996)	The TSCS is a self-report measure designed to capture internal and external aspects of self-concept.	15 dimensions measuring aspects of self-concept (physical, social, emotional, academic, family, moral-ethical, religious, personal, vocational, interpersonal, general)	100 items	Children, adolescent, and adults	Child and adult forms available. Can be used for mental health, research, and academic assessment. Can be used to track changes in self-concept over time and/or in response to clinical interventions. Takes 10–20 minutes to complete.	Self-report may be subject to individual bias. Not a diagnostic tool. Requires professional interpretation.

Note: This list is not exhaustive and citations noted are often for the original citation and may not reflect that of revised instruments.

to aid in diagnosis and treatment planning. The MMPI-3 is objective because it relies on standardized scoring and interpretation procedures, reducing subjective bias in assessment results.

The MMPI-3 contains 335 items, with 263 items remaining from the MMPI-2. The MMPI-3 includes 52 scales, which collapse within validity, higher-order, restructured clinical, somatic/cognitive, internalizing, externalizing, interpersonal, and personality psychopathology scales. There are 72 new and 24 revised items in the MMPI-3 that have created new scales and improved existing ones. The MMPI has been normed with many populations since it was first created, including clinical and nonclinical samples. The MMPI-3 was normed with a new, nationally representative sample, which matches projections for race and ethnicity, education, and age, additionally featuring Spanish language norms available for use with the U.S. Spanish-Language Translation of the MMPI-3. Scoring and interpreting the MMPI is a detailed process that requires training to interpret the results accurately. There are graphs to plot the results with the X-axis containing four content scales and 10 clinical scales. It is important to note there is also the Minnesota Multiphasic Personality Inventory-Adolescent (MMPI-A; Archer et al., 2006), a self-report instrument to assess clinical conditions in adolescents (ages 14–18) consisting of 478 true-false items that are adolescent-specific scales.

MILLON CLINICAL MULTIAXIAL INVENTORY

The Millon Clinical Multiaxial Inventory (MCMI-IV; Millon et al., 2015) is a personality assessment and psychopathology assessment tool that provides diagnoses of specific *DSM-5* disorders (American Psychiatric Association, 2013) for individuals age 18 and older. The assessment is grounded in Theodore Millon's evolutionary theory of personality and has been normed with clinical populations. The MCMI-IV consists of five validity scales, 15 personality scales that examine personality patterns and disorders, and 10 clinical syndrome scales; modifying indices are Disclosure, Desirability, and Debasement. These correction factors are applied to clinical scale scores to diminish the test taker's ability to alter responses. It consists of four strange and improbable items that attempt to detect careless responses. It is scored with a base rate score for interpretation and reporting, where a score of 60 is the median, and those that score over 74 indicate a personality style, disorder, or syndrome.

MYERS-BRIGGS TYPE INDICATOR

The Myers-Briggs Type Indicator® (MBTI®; Myers et al., 2018) was initially published in 1944 and has undergone multiple revisions over the years. The most recent versions, known as Form M and Form Q, utilize scoring and item selection based on item response theory. To gain a comprehensive understanding of an individual's personality, the MBTI measures psychologic preferences of the test taker and how they perceive the world and make choices. Based on Carl Jung's theory of psychologic type, this assessment evaluates four dichotomies: Extraversion-Introversion, Sensing-Intuition, Thinking-Feeling, and Judging-Perceiving. The scale produces eight scores, each corresponding to one of the personality types, which can be analyzed in relation to four opposing typological categories. The MBTI has been published exclusively by the Myers-Briggs Company since 1975 and is highly regarded as the most extensively utilized personality evaluation worldwide. In a clinical setting, this assessment can assist individuals in developing an awareness of their strengths and limitations, as well as understanding the variations that may exist between them and others. It is highly beneficial for individuals and teams as they navigate various obstacles, such as effective communication, conflict resolution, adaptability to change, decision-making processes, leadership skills, and career transitions. The Myers-Briggs Company has an extensive amount of information such as manuals, guides, other written materials, and workshops and seminars to assist with the administration of the instrument by professionals (www.themyersbriggs.com). The 16 personality scores or traits yielded from the MBTI are listed in Table 10.2, along

TABLE 10.2 MBTI 16 CATEGORY MEANINGS AND EXAMPLES

Personality Type	Meaning	Celebrity Example[a]
ISTJ	Quiet, serious, responsible, and practical. Logically makes goals and works toward achievement. Values organization and loyalty.	George Washington
ISFJ	Quiet, sociable, reliable, and conscientious. Reliable in getting things done with accuracy and loyal to those who are important. Enjoys harmony and accord in life.	Mother Teresa
INFJ	Quiet, mystical, idealistic, and sensitive. Inquisitive into the motivations of others and committed to values. Organized and works toward needs of a group.	Martin Luther King Jr.
INTJ	Independent, original, analytical, and determined. Looks for patterns and tries to come up with solutions. High standards and an independent thinker.	Elon Musk
ISTP	Cool and tolerant onlooker, quiet, and analytical. Solution oriented and can get to the root of problems. Very logical thinker.	Clint Eastwood
ISFP	Gentle, caring, sociable, and compassionate. Is present in the here and now and enjoys working on their own schedule. Committed and loyal to those deemed important. Does not like discord.	Bob Dylan
INFP	Optimistic people who are faithful to their values and those of importance. Congruence in life and values is critical. Works to understand others and be flexible unless values are compromised.	J. R. R. Tolkien
INTP	Logical, original, creative thinkers who are inquisitive and quiet. Usually like to solve problems, can be skeptical of things that are unknown, and can adapt.	Albert Einstein
ESTP	Energetic, action-oriented, tolerant, and fun-loving. Is focused on the present moment and has a realistic attitude regarding what is spontaneous, flexible, and fun. Learns by engaging and doing.	Madonna
ESFP	Sociable, realistic, sensible, and adaptable. Likes working collaboratively, adapts to new situations, and enjoys the comfort of others and things.	Marilyn Monroe
ENFP	Enthusiastic, creative, and outgoing. Confident can make connections with others and likes validation from others. Can be flexible and spontaneous.	Robin Williams
ENTP	Inventive, outspoken, enthusiastic, and strategic. Solves problems easily and enjoys a challenge. Analytical and can read other people. Likes new challenges.	Steve Jobs
ESTJ	Reasonable, rational, realistic, and decisive. Makes decisions quickly and can be organized and efficient in getting things done. Is logical and forceful applying plans into action.	Judge Judy
ESFJ	Friendly, conscientious, empathetic, approachable, and responsible. Likes everyone to get along and is loyal. Responsive to others' needs. Likes to be appreciated.	Taylor Swift
ENFJ	Warm, empathetic, responsive, and responsible. Aware of others' emotions and sees the value in those around them. Understands positive and negative feedback and works well in a group. Capable of leadership and inspiring others.	Oprah Winfrey
ENTJ	Blunt, influential, and ready to lead others. Finds solutions to organizational problems and enjoys setting goals. Well informed on subjects and likes to learn. Shares ideas with authority.	Margaret Thatcher

Note: Personality types listed in the table reflect the following preference pairs: Extraversion (E) or Introversion (I), Sensing (S) or Intuition (N), Thinking (T) or Feeling (F), and Judging (J) or Perceiving (P).

[a]These are estimations of personality features to the best of the author's ability and are not based on factual MBTI test scores for these celebrities.

MBTI, Myers-Briggs Type Indicator.

with a celebrity example of each personality type. Remember, these are just a few examples, and no one person will fit neatly into one personality type. These are estimations to the best of the author's ability and are not based on the person's actual test scores.

NEO-PERSONALITY INVENTORY-3

The Revised NEO Personality Inventory-3 (NEO-PI-3; Costa & McCrae, 2008) is a widely used and comprehensive assessment tool that measures the Five Factor Model of personality (also known as Big Five Factor personality traits). These five areas are Neuroticism, Extraversion, Openness, Agreeableness, and Conscientiousness. The NEO-PI-3 measures six subscale areas of refined facets of the five major personality domains. It is used as a measure of personality and within career counseling, within research, and other settings to provide a comprehensive and detailed assessment of an individual's personality structure. The NEO-PI-3 has been standardized and normed in various populations and demonstrates strong psychometric properties. The NEO-PI-3 uses T-scores for scoring and interpretation and compares individual scores to the norm samples. When scoring, a geographical representation of score characteristics is available for the five factors and 30 facets to help visualize and understand the person's profile and how it compares to the norm population group.

Subjective or Unstructured Personality Assessments

Projective tests are assessments that allow clinicians to measure various aspects of personality traits, behaviors, and emotions without participants' knowledge. Projective tests present clients with ambiguous stimuli, which can be words or pictures. They then ask clients to react and answer prompts about the stimuli, allowing the clinician to gain insight into unconscious thoughts and feelings. The responses can be analyzed for meaning, and participants can be asked additional follow-up questions for clarity. They are the opposite of objective tests, which have presupposed meaning. Projective assessments stem from psychoanalytic theory and the concepts of unconscious thoughts that a person is unaware of and has no control over. Psychoanalytic theory is based on the school of thought that if presented with ambiguous stimuli, a person's unconscious thoughts will guide the behaviors and actions that take place in response to the stimuli. Projective tests are created so the person taking the test must interpret something intentionally ambiguous and the responses are guided by the person's thoughts that try to bring structure and meaning based on the person's inner world.

Projective tests are beneficial for counselors and have various strengths. Projective means of assessments can assist in rapport building; they can often be engaging for clients and offer an alternative means for assessment that does not have to be all about talking. Projective assessments can be a valuable tool for clients of all ages who may not be verbally expressive, have limited insight or self-awareness, or may not have strong reading abilities. There are no correct and incorrect answers, which may alleviate some pressure perceived by the person completing the assessment. In some settings, projective assessments are viewed as informal, which may reduce stress and anxiety to get the correct answer or score in some way that is "normal." For this same reason, clients are less likely to respond with response bias or socially desirable answers if the techniques are subjective.

Five groups or classifications of projective tests are described in Table 10.3 and include construction, completion, arrangement, and drawing/projection techniques. Many of these techniques, such as drawing techniques, have become popular over the last 50 years because of their simplicity and easy adaptability to various populations. These techniques vary in the degree of skill required to administer these tests. Counselors can administer many projective tests, but must be mindful of the level of education and training needed

TABLE 10.3 DESCRIPTION OF TYPES OF PROJECTIVE TECHNIQUES

Technique	Definition	Common Examples	Strengths	Limitations
Association Projective Techniques	Individuals are presented stimuli, such as words, images, or other prompts, to elicit the first word, thought, or phrase that comes to mind. Facilitates connecting to the individual's unconscious thoughts and associations that may not be readily apparent through more direct forms of questioning.	Word Association Test (Eriksen & Lazarus, 1952) Rorschach Inkblot Test (Rorschach, 1921)	Provides insight into an individual's subconscious associations. Can uncover hidden or repressed thoughts. Can be used in clinical and research settings.	Responses can be highly subjective and open to interpretation. Limited in its ability to provide a comprehensive picture of the individual's psychologic state.
Construction Projective Techniques (sometimes called picture story techniques)	In this technique, individuals are asked to create something, such as a story, drawing, or collage, in response to a stimulus. The constructed response can provide insights into the individual's inner world and emotions.	Thematic Apperception Test (TAT; Murray, 1943) Draw-a-Person Test (Goodenough, 1926)	Encourages creativity and self-expression. Can reveal underlying emotions and conflicts. Allows for in-depth exploration of the individual's perspective.	Interpretation can be subjective and reliant on the assessor's judgment. Limited standardization and reliability in scoring.
Completion Projective Techniques	Completion projective techniques involve presenting individuals with an incomplete verbal stimulus, such as an unfinished sentence, phrase, scenario, or a partial image, and asking them to complete it. The goal is to tap into their unconscious thoughts and feelings.	Rotter Incomplete Sentences Blank (RISB; Rotter & Rafferty, 1950; Rotter et al., 1992) Rosenzweig Picture-Frustration (Rosenzweig, 1945)	Provides insight into individual's attitudes, beliefs, and thought patterns. Structured format allows for easier interpretation and scoring. Can be used in clinical and research settings.	Limited in its ability to assess deep unconscious content compared to other projective techniques. Responses may vary based on individual interpretation.
Arrangement Projective Techniques	This technique asks individuals to arrange or organize a set of items or objects in a specific way. It can reveal their priorities, preferences, and symbolic meanings they assign to the items.	Sandtray Therapy (Homeyer & Sweeney, 2011), Tomkins-Horn Picture Arrangement Test (Tomkins, 1952)	Offers a creative and nonverbal approach to self-expression. Choice is very important. Can help individuals explore and resolve emotional issues. Can be tailored to the individual's unique symbols and meanings.	Requires specialized training to administer and interpret. Interpretation can be influenced by the assessor's biases.

(continued)

TABLE 10.3 **DESCRIPTION OF TYPES OF PROJECTIVE TECHNIQUES** (*continued*)

Technique	Definition	Common Examples	Strengths	Limitations
Drawing/ Expression Techniques	Drawing techniques involve the use of drawings or visual representations created by individuals to explore their thoughts, emotions, and psychologic well-being.	Kinetic Family Drawings (K-F-D; Burns & Kaufman, 1970) – Kinetic House-Tree-Person (KHTP; Burns, 1987) Draw a Person Test (DAP; Kendig, 1963)	Allow for nonverbal expression of thoughts and emotions. Encourage creativity and self-expression. Can be especially useful for individuals who may have difficulty expressing themselves verbally. Provide insight into a person's perception of self, relationships, and emotional state.	Interpretation can be subjective and reliant on the assessor's judgment. Limited standardization, which can affect reliability and validity. May require specialized training to administer and interpret effectively. The accuracy of interpretations can vary depending on an individual's artistic skill and comfort with drawing.

to administer some projective tests. Projective techniques sometimes lack clearly defined protocols, scoring keys, and interpretation manuals. Not all projective tests lack guidelines, but they offer more flexibility and subjectivity in scoring compared to standardized tests. As you probably remember from Chapter 7, this leads to decreased levels of reliability or consistency in the test and those providing the tests. This means scoring can yield very different results. It is critical for counselors or test administrators to be reliable with interpretations and to follow any offered protocols and guidelines for interpretation, while not allowing personal bias or feelings to play a role in interpretation. Therefore, it is essential to have a structure you follow, or training received by those counselors in settings that offer projective assessments.

RORSCHACH INKBLOT TEST

The Rorschach Inkblot Test (Rorschach, 1921) was created by a Swiss psychiatrist named Hermann Rorschach, who described the test in a book he wrote in 1921. The Rorschach has become the most infamous example of a projective association technique. In this test, clients are presented with a series of 10 ambiguous, prescribed inkblot images and asked about what they see in the inkblot or what comes to mind when they see the inkblot. The responses are then analyzed for patterns, themes, and associations that may provide insights into the individual's personality, thought processes, and feelings. Analysis of responses to inkblots is also hypothesized to reveal deeper and unconscious processes of the individual's psyche. The Rorschach Inkblot Test does not have a universal response guide for scoring, as the responses are open to analysis. However, thorough analysis typically involves coding individual responses across five important categories: (1) location, (2) determinant, (3) form quality, (4) content, and (5) popular, the results of which comprise a final Structural

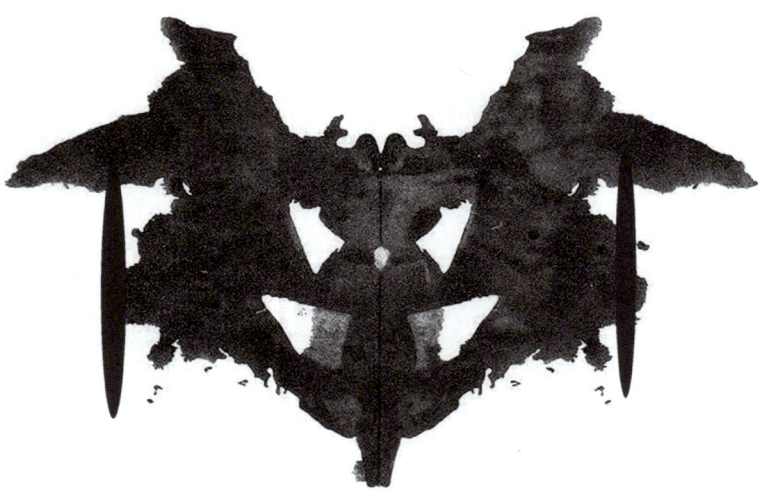

FIGURE 10.1. **Similar Rorschach inkblot sample.**
Source: Hermann Rorschach.

Summary (Exner, 2003). Location refers to which feature(s) of the inkblot the individual responds to (e.g., the whole inkblot or a part of the inkblot; Exner, 2003). Determinant refers to the aspects of an inkblot believed to inform an individual's response, such as color, form, and movement of the inkblot (Exner, 2003). Form quality evaluates if the described response is appropriate for the inkblot contours used (Exner, 2003). Content refers to the name or class of objects in an individual's response, such as nature, human features, and animal features (Exner, 2003). The popular category evaluates whether the response occurs at a high frequency among the general population (Exner, 2003). Rorschach Inkblot Test interpretation is cumulatively based on observed and communicated responses and behaviors during the test-taking time. For these reasons, the Rorschach test remains a controversial projective test (Garb et al., 2005). See Figure 10.1 for a sample image of a Rorschach-like inkblot.

THEMATIC APPERCEPTION TEST

The Thematic Apperception Test (TAT; Murray, 1943) was developed in the 1930s by Henry A. Murray and Christiana D. Morgan at Harvard University. It is an example of a constructive projective technique. The test is comprised of 31 cards (sample in Figure 10.2) with vague pictures. Eight or more cards are selected, and the subject is asked to create a story with a beginning, middle, and end about each card. The interpretation of the responses depends on the judgment and expertise of the evaluator, making it a subjective assessment because different evaluators may draw different conclusions from the same set of responses; however, the goal is to gain insight into the client's world, their needs, and environmental factors. Clear results emerge from objective tests, whereas subjective test outcomes will vary according to the interpretation.

ROTTER INCOMPLETE SENTENCES BLANK COMPLETION

The Rotter Incomplete Sentences Blank (RISB; Rotter & Rafferty, 1950; Rotter et al., 1992) was developed by Julian B. Rotter and Janet E. Rafferty in 1950 and is a verbal completion technique. The RISB is a semistructured technique that asks participants to fill in or finish a sentence fragment for which only a few words are supplied. It comes in three forms for different age groups and comprises 40 incomplete sentences, usually only 1 to 2 words long, such as "I regret . . . " and "Most girls . . . ." The test is designed to detect psychologic maladjustment. It is assumed that the subject reflects their own wishes, desires, fears, and attitudes in the

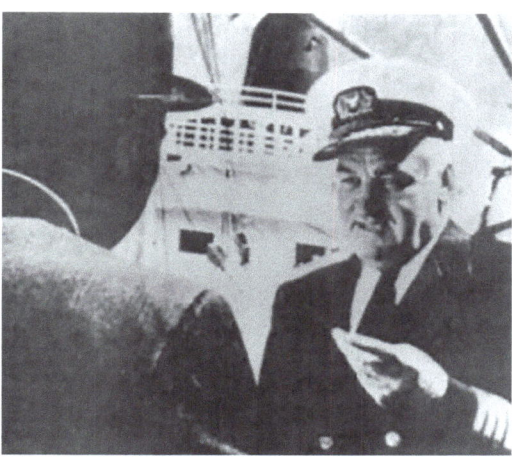

FIGURE 10.2. **Thematic Apperception Test example image.**
Source: Smith, C. P. (1992). *Motivation and personality: Handbook of thematic content analysis.* Cambridge University Press.

sentences they complete. The responses are then scored by comparing them against typical items in empirically derived scoring manuals for men and women and assigning a scale value from 0 to 6 to each response. The total score serves as an index of maladjustment. The RISB is used to assess overall adjustment in adolescents and adults and has been found to have construct validity in detecting psychologic maladjustment. The test is administered by professionals with specific training in the comprehensive system guidelines for RISB administration to ensure accurate and ethical administration and interpretation of the results.

SANDTRAY

Sandtray is an example of a choice arrangement technique. Choice arrangement techniques ask clients to arrange things and examine those arrangements for conscious or unconscious thoughts. Sandtray is traditionally a play therapy technique, and there has been debate about sandtray use for personality testing. Sandtray is just as it sounds: It is a projective arrangement technique using a large tray filled with sand where you allow clients to select from any objects you present and place the objects in the sand to represent a specific scene or prompt you may provide. For example, you can ask the client to show you what an average day in their family looks like. The client then selects any items and arranges them in the sand to set the scene. This hands-on technique is often used to help clients work through conscious or unconscious memories, particularly those who have experienced trauma or grief. Specific and commonly used sandtray techniques include the World Technique (Lowenfeld, 1979) and the Picture Arrangement Test. Evaluating and interpreting sandtrays in therapy is a subjective process that provides for understanding of the client's arrangements and representations. Additionally, you can ask the client specific questions to gain understanding, but you should not put your interpretation on the questions asked. The counselor's role is to help the client express and explore their thoughts and conscious and subconscious motivations directing the sandtray.

KINETIC HOUSE-TREE-PERSON

The Kinetic-House-Tree-Person (KHTP; Burns, 1987; see Figure 10.3) is a common expressive drawing technique adapted from Buck's (1948) House-Tree-Person, where the drawing measures self-perceptions and attitudes. The person is instructed to draw a house, tree, and person on the same page. The person's cognitive, emotional, and social functioning is examined based on the interpretations of the drawing. The KHTP takes the original activity further to

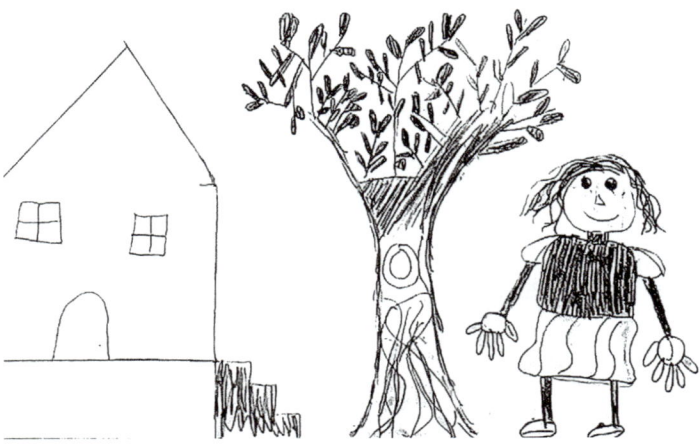

FIGURE 10.3. Sample Kinetic House-Tree-Person.

explore the interaction between the house, the tree, and the person. The KHTP can identify fears, insecurities, self-esteem issues, and social-emotional functioning. The interpretations are subjective and should be conducted by someone who is trained and familiar with the KHTP. Common interpretations are found in the interpretive manual (Burns, 1987), including the house representing family relationships, values, and protection. The tree can represent parts of ego and personality features, while the person is the director and represents self-image. Details like the size of the objects are considered in the interpretations.

OTHER TYPES OF CLINICAL ASSESSMENTS

There are many types of clinical assessments available for counselors to use. Many of them correspond with the various clinical diagnoses in the *DSM-5-TR* (American Psychiatric Association, 2022) and others correspond to traits, states, emotions, behaviors, and measures of symptomology. Counselors use multiple assessment methods and sources to gather a well-rounded and comprehensive understanding of the client's situation. This approach helps in maintaining standardization by ensuring that various aspects of the client's condition are assessed thoroughly. It is critical to use various sources of information before selecting which clinical assessments should be used with your clients, so you are not overwhelming the client with unnecessary testing.

Assessment of Depression and Bipolar Disorder

In the *DSM-5-TR* (American Psychiatric Association, 2022), depression and bipolar are considered mood disorders which are characterized by disturbances or changes in a person's emotional state or mood. Mood disorders can cause increases or decreases in mood, sleep, eating habits, energy levels, thoughts, impulsive behaviors, loss of interest or pleasure in activities, and confusion. Mood disorders, such as depression and bipolar disorder, can tremendously impact a person's well-being and level of day-to-day functioning (American Psychological Association [APA] & APA Task Force on Psychological Assessment and Evaluation Guidelines, 2020). Depression is the most common mental health disorder that is diagnosed in the United States, with the Centers for Disease Control and Prevention (CDC) reporting rates near 19% for adults over 18 years of age (Lee et al., 2023) and depression being the number one risk factor for suicide (CDC, 2013). Many commonly used assessments for depression are regularly used in clinical settings. These assessments enable clinicians to determine the presence of depressive symptoms and evaluate symptom severity. While specific questionnaires vary in their content and structure, there are many common factors frequently assessed across common depression measures, such as mood and affect; sleep patterns; appetite and weight changes; feelings of guilt, helplessness, hopelessness, and worthlessness; presence of suicidality; irritability; general mood; and cognitive function. The duration of these symptoms is also evaluated.

There are now seven distinct bipolar disorder diagnoses in the *DSM-5-TR* (Bipolar I Disorder, Bipolar II Disorder, Cyclothymic Disorder, Substance/Medication-Induced Bipolar and Related Disorder, Bipolar and Related Disorder Due to Another Medical Condition, Other Specified Bipolar and Related Disorder, and Unspecified Bipolar and Related Disorder), each with their own nuanced distinctions (American Psychiatric Association, 2022). The diagnosis of bipolar disorder can be multilayered and challenging for many clinicians, which makes a comprehensive holistic assessment approach critical. Combination approaches can include a systematic evaluation of an individual's personal and family history, an understanding of emotional and psychologic state to examine the severity and nature of mood-related issues, a thorough medical evaluation referral, and clinical interviews and observational assessment. Commonly used depression and bipolar assessments are found in Table 10.4.

BECK DEPRESSION INVENTORY

The most commonly used depression inventory is a standardized and quantitative measure created by Aaron T. Beck, Robert A. Steer, and Gregory K. Brown in 1961. The BDI is a 21-item self-report measure designed to assess the severity of depression in adolescents and adults. It helps clinicians and researchers determine the severity of depression, track changes over time, and evaluate treatment outcomes. It is a multiple-choice questionnaire that individuals complete by selecting the statement that best describes their experience over the past 2 weeks. The BDI has undergone revisions and updates and has strong psychometric properties. The most commonly used version is the Beck Depression Inventory, Second Edition (BDI-II; Beck et al., 1996).

Assessment of Anxiety, Phobias, and Fear

According to the APA (n.d.), anxiety is an emotion distinguished by feelings of tension, worry, and physical symptoms like increased blood pressure. There are several types of anxiety related disorders, such as general anxiety, social anxiety, panic disorders, and phobias. Each of these are marked with their own specific nuances and definitions. For example, a phobia is an ongoing and irrational fear of a specific situation, object, or activity accompanied by remarkable distress, whereas fear is an intense and strong emotion when someone feels threatened or in danger (APA, n.d.). Numerous assessments are frequently employed in various settings to evaluate anxiety and related disorders that assist clients in understanding their anxiety symptoms and that help guide treatment planning and interventions. These tools assist counselors in identifying the presence of anxiety symptoms, frequency, severity, pervasiveness, and intensity. Like depression assessments, the choice of an appropriate anxiety assessment depends on factors such as the target population and specific evaluation objectives. Counselors should always use additional methods of evaluation to narrow down the types of anxiety present before selecting which anxiety assessment would be the most appropriate and valuable to assist the client.

TABLE 10.4 **COMMON DEPRESSION AND BIPOLAR ASSESSMENTS**

Assessment	Description	Number of Items	Normed Population	Strengths	Limitations
Patient Health Questionnaire-9 (PHQ-9; Kroenke & Spitzer, 2002)	Assessment of the presence and severity of depressive symptoms. Rates the frequency of symptoms and has one item that screens for suicidal ideation.	9 items	General adult population	Quick and easy to administer. Well-suited for primary care settings. Strongly associated with clinical diagnoses.	Self-report format may be subject to response bias. Limited in capturing the full range of depression symptoms.
Center for Epidemiologic Studies Depression Scale (CES-D) and Scale for Children (CES-DC; Radloff, 1977; Weissman et al., 1980)	Measures the frequency and severity of depressive symptoms in the general population.	20 items on adult and child versions	General adult population and children	Commonly used in epidemiologic research. Assesses a broad range of depressive symptoms in children and adults.	Self-report format may be subject to response bias. Lengthy for some applications.
Geriatric Depression Scale (GDS; Yesavage, 1982)	Screens for depression in older adults.	15 (GDS-S) or 30 items (GDS-L)	Older adult population	Specifically designed for older adults. Offers short and long forms for flexibility.	May not be as sensitive to mild depressive symptoms. Limited utility for younger populations.
Children's Depression Rating Scale (CDRS; Poznanski et al., 1979)	Evaluates the severity of depressive symptoms in children and adolescents.	Variable (typically around 17 items)	Children and adolescent population	Clinician-administered, providing an objective assessment. Focuses on depressive symptoms in youth.	Lengthy for routine clinical use with children. Requires trained clinicians.
Mood Disorder Questionnaire (MDQ; Hirschfeld et al., 2000)	The MDQ is a self-report screening tool that helps identify individuals who may have bipolar disorder. It assesses the presence of specific symptoms and their impact on functioning.	13 items	General adult population	Quick and easy to administer. Can assist in early detection. High sensitivity in identifying potential cases.	Limited specificity (may lead to false positives). Should be followed up with clinical evaluation for diagnosis.

(continued)

TABLE 10.4 **COMMON DEPRESSION AND BIPOLAR ASSESSMENTS** (*continued*)

Assessment	Description	Number of Items	Normed Population	Strengths	Limitations
Young Mania Rating Scale (YMRS; Young et al., 1978)	The YMRS is a clinician-administered scale used to assess the severity of manic symptoms in individuals with bipolar disorder. It includes items related to mood, energy, and behavior.	11 items	Bipolar disorder patients	Designed specifically to measure manic symptoms. Provides an objective assessment by a trained clinician.	Requires a clinician for administration. Limited to assessing manic symptoms only.
Hamilton Depression Rating Scale (HAM-D; Hamilton, 1960)	The HAM-D is a widely used clinician-administered scale to assess the severity of depressive symptoms, including those experienced by individuals with bipolar disorder during depressive episodes.	17–21 items	General adult population	A comprehensive tool to assess the severity of depressive symptoms. Provides an objective assessment by a trained clinician.	Requires a clinician for administration. Limited to assessing depressive symptoms only.
Bipolar Spectrum Diagnostic Scale (BSDS; Ghaemi et al., 2005)	The BSDS is a self-report screening tool designed to identify individuals at risk for bipolar spectrum disorders. It includes questions about mood, energy, and behavior.	19 items	General adult population	Self-administered and can be completed by individuals. Can help identify potential cases of bipolar spectrum disorders. Provides a dimensional assessment, not categorical.	Limited specificity (may lead to false positives). Requires clinical evaluation for a definitive diagnosis.

Note: This list is not exhaustive, and citations noted are often for the original citation and may not reflect that of revised instruments.

GENERAL ANXIETY DISORDER 7 ITEM

The most common anxiety assessment used in school counseling, mental health counseling, and rehabilitation counseling settings is the GAD-7 item (Spitzer et al., 2006) scale. The GAD-7 measures the pervasiveness of generalized anxiety disorder (GAD) symptoms. It is a self-report scale that consists of seven items examining the symptoms of anxiety, such as feeling nervous or worried. It has been validated in various populations and has strong psychometric properties. It can also be used as a screening tool for other common anxiety disorders, such as panic disorder and social anxiety disorder (Spitzer et al., 2006). Several other commonly used anxiety assessment instruments are noted in Table 10.5.

TABLE 10.5 **COMMON ANXIETY DISORDER ASSESSMENTS**

Assessment	Description	Number of Items	Normed Population	Strengths	Limitations
Beck Anxiety Inventory (BAI; Beck et al., 1988)	A self-report questionnaire designed to assess the severity of anxiety symptoms in adults and adolescents.	21 items	General adult and adolescent populations	Measures a broad range of anxiety symptoms. Well-validated and widely used.	Self-report format may be subject to response bias. Limited in distinguishing between different anxiety disorders.
State-Trait Anxiety Inventory (STAI) and Inventory for Children (STAI-CH; Spielberger et al., 1973, 1983)	Assesses both state anxiety (current or temporary anxiety) and trait anxiety (general predisposition to anxiety) in adults. The child and adolescent version addresses the state and trait anxiety in youth.	40 items (20 for state anxiety, 20 for trait anxiety)	General adult population and children (STAI-CH)	Differentiates between state and trait anxiety. Provides a comprehensive assessment of anxiety.	Longer than some other anxiety scales. Self-report format may be subject to response bias.
Social Phobia Inventory (SPIN; Connor et al., 2006)	Evaluates the severity of social anxiety symptoms in adults.	17 items	General adult population	Focuses on social anxiety, including its cognitive and behavioral aspects. Reliable and valid for assessing social anxiety.	May not capture other anxiety disorders. Self-report format may be subject to response bias.
Screen for Child Anxiety Related Disorders (SCARED; Birmaher et al., 1997)	A self-report assessment designed for children and adolescents to screen for and evaluate anxiety disorders.	41 items	Children and adolescent population	Comprehensive assessment of childhood anxiety disorders. Differentiates between specific anxiety disorders.	Longer and more comprehensive than some other anxiety scales for youth. Self-report format may be subject to response bias.

Assessment of Eating Disorders

Assessments for eating disorders are frequently employed by mental health professionals, researchers, and healthcare providers to evaluate, diagnose, and track individuals with eating disorders or those who may be at risk. Eating disorder assessments are available for all of the *DSM-5-TR* disorders (American Psychiatric Association, 2022), including Anorexia Nervosa (AN), Bulimia Nervosa (BN), Binge Eating Disorder (BED), Other Specified Feeding and Eating Disorder (OSFED), Pica, Rumination Disorder, Avoidant/Restrictive Food Intake Disorder (ARFID), and Unspecified Feeding or Eating Disorder (UFED). Symptoms of an eating disorder do not automatically imply or necessitate a diagnosis to be warranted. Many clients could have disordered eating patterns and behaviors, but the severity is not present. Like other disorders, eating disorders require specific criteria to be met, inclusive of severity and frequency, which can be measured using assessments and additional physical and biological markers. Eating disorder screenings help identify eating disorder concerns early, promoting better treatment outcomes and improved quality of life. By utilizing specific assessment tools, professionals can gain valuable insights into their clients' experiences and tailor treatment plans accordingly. Commonly used eating disorder screenings and assessments are in Table 10.6. It is important to consider personal thoughts and biases that you may have associated with eating disorders before choosing to assess or not assess. Eating disorders are found in many populations and are not caused by or strictly associated with any one single factor or characteristic (National Eating Disorders Association [NEDA], n.d.). Eating disorders arise from long-standing behavioral, biological, emotional, psychologic, interpersonal, and social factors. Due to these biases that exist, eating disorders are often undiagnosed in many populations. A point to also consider during the assessment process of eating disorders is that people's relationship with food can often be part of their cultural

TABLE 10.6 **COMMON EATING DISORDER ASSESSMENTS**

Assessment Tool	Description	Number of Items	Normed Population	Strengths	Limitations
Eating Disorder Inventory (EDI-3; Garner, 2004)	A self-report questionnaire that assesses psychologic traits and behaviors related to eating disorders, including drive for thinness, bulimia, and body dissatisfaction.	91 items	Adolescents and adults	Measures a broad range of eating disorder-related traits. Used in research and clinical settings.	Lengthy and may be time-consuming. Self-report format may be subject to response bias.
Eating Attitudes Test (EAT-26; Garner et al., 1982)	A self-report questionnaire assessing eating attitudes and behaviors, including concerns about dieting, food, and body image.	26 items	General population, adolescents, adults	Quick and easy to administer. Widely used for screening.	Self-report format may be subject to response bias. Limited to screening for eating attitudes.
Eating Disorder Examination (EDE-Q; Fairburn & Beglin, 1994)	A structured interview that assesses eating disorder symptoms, including dietary restraint, eating concerns, weight and shape concerns, and binge eating.	28 items	General population, adolescents, adults	Clinically validated. Assesses various aspects of eating disorders.	Self-report could lead to response bias. Normative data not available for all populations.

(continued)

TABLE 10.6 **COMMON EATING DISORDER ASSESSMENTS** (*continued*)

Assessment Tool	Description	Number of Items	Normed Population	Strengths	Limitations
Child Eating Attitudes Test (ChEAT; Maloney et al., 1988)	A self-report questionnaire designed for children and adolescents to assess attitudes and behaviors related to eating and body image.	26 items	Children and adolescents	Specifically designed for younger populations. Identifies concerns and behaviors related to eating and body image.	Self-report format may be subject to response bias. Limited to assessing attitudes and behaviors in children and adolescents.
Pica, ARFID, and Rumination Disorder Interview (PARDI; Bryant-Waugh et al., 2019)	An interview-based assessment tool designed to evaluate and diagnose Pica, Avoidant/Restrictive Food Intake Disorder (ARFID), and Rumination Disorder in individuals.	Variable (depending on criteria assessed)	Children, adolescents, and adults	Focuses on diagnosing specific eating disorders. Provides a structured format for assessment.	Requires trained clinician for administration. Limited to assessing specific eating disorders.

norms and background. The counselor should always consider cultural rituals and attitudes toward food, even if the formal assessment does not cover it. The most significant environmental factor to the development of eating disorders is the sociocultural idealization of thinness of body size (Culbert et al., 2015).

Assessment of Obsessive-Compulsive and Related Disorders

Obsessive-compulsive disorders are categorized in the *DSM-5-TR* (American Psychiatric Association, 2022) as Uncontrollable and Frequently Occurring Thoughts (Obsessions) and/or Recurring or Repetitive Behaviors (Compulsions) that clients are not able to stop themselves from engaging in (APA, n.d.). Disorders grouped in this category all share the common features of obsessive preoccupation and repetitive behaviors. These disorders include Obsessive-Compulsive Disorder, Body Dysmorphic Disorder, Hoarding Disorder, Trichotillomania (hair-pulling), and Excoriation (skin-picking) Disorders. Obsessions cause extreme distress and include things such as fear of germs, fear of losing control, and constant worry about body features. Compulsions often involve rituals such as excessive handwashing, gathering of items (hoarding), picking skin, and others. Diagnosing these disorders involves discussing thoughts, feelings, symptoms, and behavior patterns to determine the presence of obsessions or compulsive behaviors that interfere with quality of life. Additionally, assessment should include a comprehensive assessment related to the frequency, severity, and pervasiveness of the impact on the person's functioning in addition to a comprehensive approach of diagnostic interviews, clinician-administered inventories, psychologic evaluations, and consideration of diagnostic criteria. A few common assessments in this category are noted in Table 10.7.

TABLE 10.7 **COMMON OBSESSIVE-COMPULSIVE AND RELATED DISORDER ASSESSMENT TOOLS**

Assessment Tool	Description	Number of Items	Normed Population	Strengths	Limitations
Obsessive-Compulsive Inventory-Revised (OCI-R; Foa et al., 1998)	Assessing obsessive-compulsive symptoms and distress	18	Clinically diverse samples	Well-established measure for OCD assessment. Covers a range of OCD symptomatology.	Self-report, subject to response biases. Primarily focused on OCD symptoms.
The Yale-Brown Obsessive Compulsive Scale (Y-BOCS; Goodman et al., 1989)	Assessing the severity and type of OCD symptoms, with emphasis on reflecting changes in severity across treatment	10 items plus a client symptom checklist	General adult population	Most widely used rating scale for OCD. Symptom checklist details target symptoms and can be used to inform treatment planning.	Not a diagnostic tool. Self-report, subject to response biases.
Saving Inventory-Revised (SIR; Frost et al., 2004)	Examines hoarding behavior and related beliefs	23	Community and clinical samples	Comprehensive assessment of hoarding behaviors. Assesses cognitive aspects of hoarding.	Self-report, subject to response biases. Limited focus on other OCD symptoms.
Body Dysmorphic Disorder Symptom Scale (BDD-SS; Phillips et al., 1997)	Assessing the severity of symptoms related to body dysmorphic disorder symptoms	9	Clinical samples	Specific to body dysmorphic disorder. Brief and easy to administer.	Limited coverage of broader psychologic issues. Self-report may be influenced by denial or lack of insight.

OCD, obsessive-compulsive disorder.

Assessment of Neurodevelopmental Disorders

Assessments for neurodevelopmental disorders involve a comprehensive evaluation of an individual's abilities, difficulties, and needs related to their neurodevelopment. These assessments aim to identify and diagnose the following conditions: Intellectual Developmental Disorders (Intellectual Disability and Global Delay), Communication Disorders (Language Disorder, Speech Sound Disorder, Childhood-Onset Fluency Disorder [stuttering], and Social [pragmatic] Communication Disorder), Autism Spectrum Disorder (ASD), Attention Deficit Hyperactivity Disorder (ADHD), Specific Learning Disorder, and Motor Disorders (Developmental Coordination Disorder, Stereotypic Movement Disorder, Tic Disorders). Some of the most common for counselors to assess are ASD and ADHD. Counselors should be aware of the different assessments available for neurodevelopmental disorders, their limitations, and the importance of early intervention and screening (Rutherford et al., 2021). There can be barriers to accessing assessment and diagnosis for clients with neurodevelopmental disorders. Diagnosing ASD can be especially difficult because there is no single medical test or assessment to simply diagnose the disorder. Screenings for ASD are common to start the process of assessment. A combination approach of methods is needed to make a formal diagnosis. The process involves developmental monitoring, formal developmental evaluation, and ongoing and routine assessment (CDC, n.d.), including collaboration with other professionals, such as doctors, psychologists, school counselors, and teachers, to ensure that a comprehensive evaluation is being completed. The client's age and developmental level are considered when choosing an appropriate assessment tool. Table 10.8 contains some common neurodevelopmental disorder screening and assessment tools. Remember that this list is not comprehensive, and instruments often include many limitations.

TABLE 10.8 COMMON ASSESSMENTS FOR NEURODEVELOPMENTAL DISORDERS

Assessment Tool	Description	Number of Items	Normed Population	Strengths	Limitations
ADHD Rating Scale-5 (ADHD-RS-5; DuPaul et al., 2016)	A parent or teacher rating scale used to assess the severity of ADHD symptoms in children and adolescents.	18 items	Children and adolescents	Quick and easy to administer. Helps diagnose and monitor ADHD.	Limited to assessing symptom severity. Requires multiple informants.
Conners' Rating Scales (CRS, Conners 4; Conners, 1999)	There is a short and a long version, as well as a parent, teacher, and self-report form, along with an adult scale. The questionnaire asks about behavior, work or schoolwork, and social life. The responses indicate if ADHD symptoms are present and their pervasiveness.	Varies by version	Children, adolescents, and adults	Offers multiple perspectives (parents, teachers, self). Assesses a wide range of behavioral issues.	Lengthy and may require multiple informants. Self-report can be subjective.
Vanderbilt ADHD Rating Scales (Wolraich et al., 1996, 2003)	Examines ADHD as well as other conditions such as oppositional defiance disorder, anxiety, and depression and is 43 items. Parent rating scale (VADPRS) and teacher rating scale (VADTRS) available.	Varies by version	Children and adolescents	Widely used in research and clinical practice. Assesses core ADHD symptoms.	May not capture the full spectrum of impairment. Requires informant input.

(continued)

TABLE 10.8 COMMON ASSESSMENTS FOR NEURODEVELOPMENTAL DISORDERS (*continued*)

Assessment Tool	Description	Number of Items	Normed Population	Strengths	Limitations
Autism Diagnostic Observation Schedule (ADOS-2; Lord et al., 2012)	ADOS assesses and diagnoses autism in children and adults. It focuses on behavior in three main areas: reciprocal social interaction, communication and language, and restricted and repetitive, stereotyped interests and behaviors.	Varies by module	Children, adolescents, and adults	Provides a structured and standardized evaluation. Assesses social communication and interaction.	Requires specialized training for administration. Time-consuming.
Childhood Autism Rating Scale (CARS-2; Schopler et al., 2010)	A clinician-administered rating scale used to assess the severity of autism symptoms in children. It includes items related to social and communication behaviors.	15 items	Children	Useful for diagnosing and monitoring autism. Provides a structured assessment.	Requires trained clinicians for administration. Limited to children.
Peabody Picture Vocabulary Test (PPVT; Dunn, 2019)	A widely used assessment of receptive vocabulary that evaluates an individual's understanding of spoken words.	170 items	Children and adults	Provides a comprehensive measure of receptive vocabulary. Useful in diagnosing language disorders.	Lengthy and may require significant time to administer. Limited to vocabulary assessment.
Developmental Behavior Checklist (DBC; Einfeld & Tonge, 1995)	The assessment of emotional and behavioral challenges in children and adolescents with intellectual and developmental disabilities.	96 items	Children and adolescents	Provides quick and accurate results. Software available to enter, score, and store DBC checklist data, and to provide raw and percentile scores, on-screen or as a printer report.	Not definitive and should be used in conjunction with other diagnostic methods to make a diagnosis.

ADHD, attention deficit hyperactivity disorder.

Assessment of Psychotic Disorders and Related Disorders

Assessment for psychotic disorders, such as schizophrenia and related disorders (schizoaffective disorder, schizophreniform disorder, and delusional disorder), in counseling typically involves a comprehensive evaluation to determine the presence of symptoms and the impact of those symptoms on an individual's functioning and well-being. Many of these disorders are only provided to adults and include symptoms of delusions, hallucinations, disorganized thinking, disorganized thoughts and behaviors, and other negative symptoms. The assessment of psychotic disorders is a multilayered process. It should include standardized assessment tools, clinical interviews, a complete evaluation of symptoms of functioning, and medical evaluations and physical exams to ensure a medical problem is not causing the symptoms. A recommended assessment for psychotic symptoms is the *Structured Clinical Interview for* DSM-5 (First, 2015), which is a comprehensive diagnostic interview that assesses the presence of psychotic symptoms, along with other mental health disorders, to reach a formal diagnosis. Keep in mind that these disorders can be challenging to diagnose correctly, and outside consultation is always recommended. Gill et al. (2024) note that psychotic disorders can be diagnosed by counselors, but it is often uncommon for many counselors.

Other Common Clinical Assessments

There are numerous other areas of clinical assessments and screenings that relate to the major *DSM-5-TR* diagnoses (American Psychiatric Association, 2022) or assessments of symptoms, behaviors, traits, and states (such as assessments of anger, well-being, violence, delusions, stress, self-esteem, resilience, etc.). Some additional assessments commonly used in counseling are located in Table 10.9. These assessments all provide insight into a person's psychologic state, personality, symptoms, and well-being. It is up to the counselor to ensure that they are using the correct assessments that will allow them to gain the most insight into the client's situation or problem, or assist in reaching their goals.

TABLE 10.9 **OTHER COMMONLY USED CLINICAL ASSESSMENTS IN COUNSELING**

Assessment Tool	General Description of Use
WHO-5 Well-Being Index (World Health Organization, 1998)	The WHO-5 is a self-report questionnaire that assesses an individual's general well-being and emotional health. It measures positive psychologic well-being and is often used in clinical and research settings to evaluate overall mental health and well-being.
Symptom Checklist-90-Revised (SCL-90-R; Derogatis, 1994)	The SCL-90-R is a self-report inventory that assesses various psychologic symptoms and distress. It evaluates psychologic distress, identifies psychopathology, and monitors treatment progress in clinical and research settings.
Brief Symptom Inventory (BSI; Derogatis, 1982)	The BSI is a shorter version of the SCL-90-R and is designed to assess an individual's psychologic symptoms and distress. It is commonly used in clinical practice and research to measure psychologic distress and identify emotional and psychologic issues.
Child Behavior Checklist (CBCL; Achenbach, 1999)	The CBCL is a parent- or caregiver-completed questionnaire that assesses emotional and behavioral problems in children and adolescents. It is used to identify a range of behavioral and emotional issues in children and help guide clinical evaluation and intervention.

(continued)

TABLE 10.9 **OTHER COMMONLY USED CLINICAL ASSESSMENTS IN COUNSELING** (*continued*)

Assessment Tool	General Description of Use
Inventory of Common Problems (ICP; Hoffman & Weiss, 1986)	The ICP is a self-report questionnaire designed to assess common problems and concerns in individuals' lives. It is used to gather information about an individual's problems and concerns for various purposes, including treatment planning and research.
The Depression Anxiety and Stress Scales (DASS; Lovibond & Lovibond, 1995)	The DASS is a self-report assessment developed to measure the negative emotional states of depression, anxiety, and stress. DASS is available in two versions: the DASS-42 and the DASS-21 (shorter version). Both are well-known assessments used in clinical and research settings with strong psychometrics.

CHECKING IN WITH SARAH

Sarah starts seeing a counselor outside of school because her parents feel she needs additional support. Sarah's counselor is getting her to open up a bit more, but she is concerned with Sarah's continued weight loss. Sarah's counselor tries not to discuss her weight much because she can see that Sarah is uncomfortable talking about it, but she becomes concerned because Sarah shares that her hair has been falling out lately and that she often feels dizzy at cheerleading practice. Her counselor recommends that her parents seek a physical evaluation to check Sarah's health. In the meantime, the counselor wants to keep things light for now because she does not feel like she can push Sarah too hard at this point. She wants to use a fun technique to explore Sarah's world and her inner thoughts and also knows that she must assess her eating.

1. What projective test might be an engaging and effective assessment for Sarah to do in counseling that will also provide her counselor with additional information that would be helpful as they continue to work in therapy? What strengths could this assessment provide?

2. What eating disorder assessment would you provide to Sarah? Would you use a combination approach with other interventions or categories of assessments? If so, which ones and how would they be helpful?

3. We never want to overload a client with assessments. But, if you could provide any assessments you want, what other clinical or personality assessments would be useful to use with Sarah and why?

END-OF-CHAPTER RESOURCES

DISCUSSION QUESTIONS

1. What are some strengths and limitations of projective assessment techniques in counseling? What are some ways that counselors can utilize projective techniques, while implementing strategies to reduce the limitations of these instruments?

240 ■ III: ASSESSMENT TYPES

2. Search personality assessments and find a few that a school counselor might use to help a student identify their strengths and career goals. How could school counselors use these assessments to help students make informed decisions about their goals and future plans?

3. Name two strengths and two limitations of using the BDI with clients. Why do you think the BDI is still the most widely used depression scale?

CLASS ACTIVITIES

1. Divide the class into small groups and assign each group a different clinical or personality assessment tool, such as the BDI, the MMPI, or the NEO-PI-R. Have each group research the assessment tool and present on its key features, including its purpose, administration, scoring, and interpretation. Then, have each group share their thoughts on the strengths and limitations of their assigned assessment tool and how they might find it useful in their future counseling practice.

2. Assign students in pairs and have them role-play how they would go about administering a projective test, such as a drawing technique with a client in session. Practice nondirective interpretation and asking the client open-ended questions. Explore the results with the mock client.

3. Select one of the case vignettes from Chapter 1 of this textbook. Ask the students to break into small groups and conceptualize the client and then select and critically evaluate the appropriateness of assessment tools based on the client's unique needs and the specific information they aim to gather.

 ## PERSPECTIVE FROM THE FIELD

The goal of this chapter was to provide an overview, purpose, and utility of the clinical assessments most often used in clinical settings, such as mental health agencies or private practice. In this podcast, we discuss clinical assessments in general, describing how to get client buy-in and assess client comfortability with the instruments. Dr. Ali Cunningham Abbott speaks to neurodivergence and autism spectrum disorder (ASD) assessments specifically, covering related assessments and introducing results with humility. Dr. Abbott is the program director and an associate professor at Lynn University in Boca Raton, Florida. Dr. Abbott was a visiting assistant professor at Florida Atlantic University and an assistant director for the Center for Autism & Related Disabilities (CARD). She currently provides individual counseling for adolescents and adults at the Center for the Treatment of Anxiety & Mood Disorders. She has published and presented on the topic of clinical assessment. Her focus on clinical assessment began with the publication of a book chapter on childhood assessment in *Couple & Family Assessment*. She also wrote a book entitled *Counseling Adults With Autism: A Comprehensive Toolkit* which offers assessment and treatment guidance for clinicians working with autistic clients. Over her career she has presented on the topics of clinical assessment with children, adolescents, and adults across settings including professional organizations, international conferences, and local, grassroots organizations.

Access podcasts via the QR code or http://connect.springerpub.com/content/book/978-0-8261-8913-4/chapter/ch00.

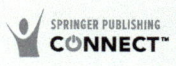

A robust set of instructor resources designed to supplement this text is located at http://connect.springerpub.com/content/book/978-0-8261-8913-4. Qualifying instructors may request access by emailing textbook@springerpub.com.

REFERENCES

Achenbach, T. M. (1999). The child behavior checklist and related instruments. In M. E. Maruish (Ed.), *The use of psychological testing for treatment planning and outcomes assessment* (pp. 429–466). Lawrence Erlbaum Associates Publishers.

American Psychiatric Association. (2013). *Diagnostic and statistical manual of mental disorders* (5th ed.). https://doi.org/10.1176/appi.books.9780890425596

American Psychiatric Association. (2022). *Diagnostic and statistical manual of mental disorders* (5th ed., text rev.). https://doi.org/10.1176/appi.books.9780890425787

American Psychological Association. (n.d.). *APA dictionary of psychology*. Author.

American Psychological Association & APA Task Force on Psychological Assessment and Evaluation Guidelines. (2020). *APA guidelines for psychological assessment and evaluation*. American Psychological Association. https://www.apa.org/about/policy/guidelines-psychological-assessment-evaluation.pdf

Archer, R. P., Zoby, M., & Stredny, R. V. (2006). The Minnesota Multiphasic Personality Inventory-Adolescent. In R. P. Archer (Ed.), *Forensic uses of clinical assessment instruments* (pp. 57–87). Lawrence Erlbaum Associates Publishers.

Beck, A. T., Epstein, N., Brown, G., & Steer, R. (1988). *Beck Anxiety Inventory* [Database record]. APA PsycTests. https://doi.org/10.1037/t02025-000

Beck, A. T., Steer, R. A., & Brown, G. (1996). *Beck Depression Inventory (BDI-II)* [Database record]. APA PsycTests. https://doi.org/10.1037/t00742-000

Beck, A. T., Ward, C. H., Mendelson, M., Mock, J., & Erbaugh, J. (1961). An inventory for measuring depression. *Archives of General Psychiatry, 4*, 561–571. https://doi.org/10.1001/archpsyc.1961.01710120031004

Ben-Porath, Y. S., & Tellegen, A. (2020). *Minnesota Multiphasic Personality Inventory-3 (MMPI-3): Manual for administration, scoring, and interpretation*. University of Minnesota Press.

Birmaher, B., Khetarpal, S., Brent, D., Cully, M., Balach, L., Kaufman, J., & Neer, S. M. (1997). The Screen for Child Anxiety Related Emotional Disorders (SCARED): Scale construction and psychometric characteristics. *Journal of the American Academy of Child & Adolescent Psychiatry, 36*(4), 545–553. https://doi.org/10.1097/00004583-199704000-00018

Blevins, C. A., Weathers, F. W., Davis, M. T., Witte, T. K., & Domino, J. L. (2015). The posttraumatic stress disorder checklist for *DSM-5* (PCL-5): Development and initial psychometric evaluation. *Journal of Traumatic Stress, 28*(6), 489–498. https://doi.org/10.1002/jts.22059

Bryant-Waugh, R., Micali, N., Cooke, L., Lawson, E. A., Eddy, K. T., & Thomas, J. J. (2019). *Pica, ARFID, and Rumination Disorder Interview (PARDI)* [Database record]. APA PsycTests. https://doi.org/10.1037/t76465-000

Buck, J. N. (1948). The H-T-P test. *Journal of Clinical Psychology, 4*, 151–159. https://doi.org/10.1002/1097-4679(194804)4:2<151::AID-JCLP2270040203>3.0.CO;2-O

Burns, R. C. (1987). *Kinetic-House-Tree-Person drawings (KHTP): An interpretative manual*. Brunner/Mazel.

Burns, R. C., & Kaufman, S. H. (1970). *Kinetic family drawings (K-F-D): An introduction to understanding children through kinetic drawings*. Brunner/Mazel.

Cattell, H. E. P., & Mead, A. D. (2008). The Sixteen Personality Factor Questionnaire (16PF). In G. J. Boyle, G. Matthews, & D. H. Saklofske (Eds.), *The SAGE handbook of personality theory and assessment: Vol. 2. Personality measurement and testing* (pp. 135–159). Sage Publications, Inc. https://doi.org/10.4135/9781849200479.n7

Centers for Disease Control and Prevention. (n.d.). *Screening for autism spectrum disorder*. Updated May 16, 2024. https://www.cdc.gov/autism/diagnosis

Centers for Disease Control and Prevention. (2013). *Web-Based Injury Statistics Query and Reporting System (WISQARS)* [Online]. National Center for Injury Prevention and Control. https://www.cdc.gov/injury/wisqars/fatal_help/faq.html

Conners, C. K. (1999). Clinical use of rating scales in diagnosis and treatment of attention-deficit/hyperactivity disorder. *Pediatric Clinics of North America, 46*(5), 857–870. https://doi.org/10.1016/s0031-3955(05)70159-0

Connor, K. M., Davidson, J. R. T., Churchill, L. E., Sherwood, A., Foa, E., & Weisler, R. H. (2006). *Social Phobia Inventory (SPIN)* [Database record]. APA PsycTests. https://doi.org/10.1037/t03804-000

Coopersmith, S. (1987). *Self-esteem inventories*. Consulting Psychologists Press. (Original work published 1981)

Coopersmith, S. (2002). *Revised Coopersmith self-esteem inventory manual*. Mind Garden.

Costa, P. T., Jr., & McCrae, R. R. (2008). The Revised NEO Personality Inventory (NEO-PI-R). In G. J. Boyle, G. Matthews, & D. H. Saklofske (Eds.), *The SAGE handbook of personality theory and assessment: Vol. 2. Personality measurement and testing* (pp. 179–198). Sage Publications, Inc. https://doi.org/10.4135/9781849200479.n9

Council for Accreditation of Counseling and Related Educational Programs. (2023). *2024 CACREP standards*. https://www.cacrep.org/wp-content/uploads/2023/06/Combined-version-6.21.23.pdf

Culbert, K. M., Racine, S. E., & Klump, K. L. (2015). Research review: What we have learned about the causes of eating disorders—a synthesis of sociocultural, psychological, and biological research. *Journal of Child Psychology and Psychiatry, and Allied Disciplines, 56*(11), 1141–1164. https://doi.org/10.1111/jcpp.12441

Derogatis, L. R. (1982). *Brief Symptom Inventory (BSI)* [Database record]. APA PsycTests. https://doi.org/10.1037/t00789-000

Derogatis, L. R. (1994). *SCL-90-R: Administration, scoring and procedures manual* (3rd ed.). NCS Pearson.

Dunn, D. M. (2019). *Peabody picture vocabulary test* (5th ed.). Pearson.

DuPaul, G. J., Power, T. J., Anastopoulos, A. D., & Reid, R. (2016). *ADHD Rating Scale-5 for children and adolescents: Checklists, norms, and clinical interpretation*. Guilford Press.

Einfeld, S. L., & Tonge, B. J. (1995). The Developmental Behavior Checklist: The development and validation of an instrument to assess behavioral and emotional disturbance in children and adolescents with mental retardation. *Journal of Autism and Developmental Disorders, 25*(2), 81–104. https://doi.org/10.1007/BF02178498

Eriksen, C. W., & Lazarus, R. S. (1952). *Word association test* [Database record]. APA PsycTests. https://doi.org/10.1037/t01414-000

Exner, J. E. (2003). *The Rorschach: A comprehensive system* (4th ed.). Wiley.

Fairburn, C. G., & Beglin, S. J. (1994). *Eating Disorder Examination Questionnaire (EDE-Q)* [Database record]. APA PsycTests. https://doi.org/10.1037/t03974-000

First, M. B. (2015). Structured clinical interview for *DSM* (SCID). In R. L. Cautin & S. O. Lilienfeld (Eds.), *The encyclopedia of clinical psychology*. Wiley. https://doi.org/10.1002/9781118625392.wbecp351

Fitts, W. H. (1965). *Tennessee Self-Concept Scale*. Western Psychological Services.

Fitts, W. H., Warren, W. L., & Western Psychological Services (Firm). (1996). *Tennessee Self-Concept Scale: TSCS-2 manual* (2nd ed.). Western Psychological Services.

Foa, E. B., Kozak, M. J., Salkovskis, P. M., Coles, M. E., & Amir, N. (1998). The validation of a new obsessive–compulsive disorder scale: The Obsessive–Compulsive Inventory. *Psychological Assessment, 10*(3), 206–214. https://doi.org/10.1037/1040-3590.10.3.206

Friedman, H. S., & Schustack, M. W. (2009). *Personality: Classic theories and modern research* (M. Limoges, Ed.). Pearson Education.

Frost, R. O., Steketee, G., & Grisham, J. (2004). Measurement of compulsive hoarding: Saving inventory-revised. *Behavior Research and Therapy, 42*(10), 1163–1182. https://doi.org/10.1016/j.brat.2003.07.006

Garb, H. N., Wood, J. M., Lilienfeld, S. O., & Nezworski, M. T. (2005). Roots of the Rorschach controversy. *Clinical Psychology Review, 25*(1), 97–118. https://doi.org/10.1016/j.cpr.2004.09.002

Garner, D. M. (2004). *Eating disorder inventory-3. Professional manual*. Psychological Assessment Resources, Inc.

Garner, D. M., Olmsted, M. P., Bohr, Y., & Garfinkel, P. E. (1982). The eating attitudes test: Psychometric features and clinical correlates. *Psychological Medicine, 12*(4), 871–878. https://doi.org/10.1017/s0033291700049163

Ghaemi, S. N., Miller, C. J., Berv, D. A., Klugman, J., Rosenquist, K. J., & Pies, R. W. (2005). Sensitivity and specificity of a new bipolar spectrum diagnostic scale. *Journal of Affective Disorders, 84*(2-3), 273–277. https://doi.org/10.1016/S0165-0327(03)00196-4

Gill, C. S., Dailey, S. F., Karl, S., & Barrio Minton, C. (2024). DSM-5 *learning companion for counselors*. American Counseling Association.

Goodenough, F. L. (1926). *Measurement of intelligence by drawings*. World Book Company.

Goodman, W. K., Price, L. H., Rasmussen, S. A., Mazure, C., Fleischmann, R. L., Hill, C. L., Heninger, G. R., & Charney, D. S. (1989). The Yale-Brown Obsessive Compulsive Scale: I. Development, use, and reliability. *Archives of General Psychiatry, 46*(11), 1006–1011. https://doi.org/10.1001/archpsyc.1989.01810110048007

Gough, H. G. (1956). *California psychological inventory*. Consulting Psychologists Press.

Hamilton, M. (1960). A rating scale for depression. *Journal of Neurology, Neurosurgery, and Psychiatry, 23*(1), 56–62. https://doi.org/10.1136/jnnp.23.1.56

Hirschfeld, R. M., Williams, J. B., Spitzer, R. L., Calabrese, J. R., Flynn, L., Keck, P. E., Jr., Lewis, L., McElroy, S. L., Post, R. M., Rapport, D. J., Russell, J. M., Sachs, G. S., & Zajecka, J. (2000). Development and validation of a screening instrument for bipolar spectrum disorder: The Mood Disorder Questionnaire. *The American Journal of Psychiatry, 157*(11), 1873–1875. https://doi.org/10.1176/appi.ajp.157.11.1873

Hoffman, J. A., & Weiss, B. (1986). A new system for conceptualizing college students' problems: Types of crises and the inventory of common problems. *Journal of American College Health, 34*(6), 259–266. https://doi.org/10.1080/07448481.1986.9938947

Homeyer, L. E., & Sweeney, D. S. (2011). *Sandtray therapy: A practical manual* (2nd ed.). Routledge/Taylor & Francis Group.

Kendig, I. V. (1963). The Draw-a-Person test. In D. Rosenthal (Ed.), *The Genain quadruplets: A case study and theoretical analysis of heredity and environment in schizophrenia* (pp. 257–268). Basic Books. https://doi.org/10.1037/11420-016

Kroenke, K., & Spitzer, R. L. (2002). The PHQ-9: A new depression diagnostic and severity measure. *Psychiatric Annals, 32*(9), 509–515. http://doi.org/10.3928/0048-5713-20020901-06

Lee, B., Wang, Y., Carlson, S. A., Greenlund, K. J., Lu, H., Liu, Y., Croft, J. B., Eke, P. I., Town, M., & Thomas, C. W. (2023). National, state-level, and county-level prevalence estimates of adults aged ≥18 years self-reporting a lifetime diagnosis of depression—United States, 2020. *MMWR Morbidity Mortality Weekly Report, 72*(24), 644–650. http://doi.org/10.15585/mmwr.mm7224a1

Lord, C., Luyster R. J., Gotham K., & Guthrie, W. (2012). *Autism diagnostic observation schedule, second edition (ADOS-2) manual (Part II): Toddler module*. Western Psychological Services.

Lovibond, P. F., & Lovibond, S. H. (1995). *Depression Anxiety and Stress Scales (DASS-42)* [Database record]. APA PsycTests. https://doi.org/10.1037/t39835-000

Lowenfeld, M. (1979). *Understanding children's sandplay; Lowenfeld's World Technique*. Allen and Unwin.

Maloney, M. J., McGuire, J. B., & Daniels, S. R. (1988). Reliability testing of a children' version of the Eating Attitude Test. *Journal of the American Academy of Child & Adolescent Psychiatry, 27*(5), 541–543. https://doi.org/10.1097/00004583-198809000-00004

Millon, T., Grossman, S., & Millon, C. (2015). *The Millon Clinical Multiaxial Inventory-IV (MCMI-IV)*. Pearson. https://millonpersonality.com/millon-inventories/multiaxial-inventory-iv-mcmi-iv

Morey, L. C. (1991). *Personality Assessment Inventory* [Database record]. APA PsycTests. https://doi.org/10.1037/t03903-000

Murray, H. A. (1943). *Thematic Apperception Test manual*. Harvard University Press

Myers, I. B., McCaulley, M. H., Quenk, N. L., & Hammer, A. L. (2018). *MBTI® manual for the Global Step I and Step II assessments* (4th ed.). The Myers-Briggs Company.

National Eating Disorders Association. (n.d.). *Statistics*. Accessed July 30, 2024. https://www.nationaleatingdisorders.org/statistics/#bipoc-statistics

Phillips, K. A., Hollander, E., Rasmussen, S. A., Aronowitz, B. R., DeCaria, C., & Goodman, W. K. (1997). A severity rating scale for body dysmorphic disorder: Development, reliability, and validity of a modified version of the Yale-Brown Obsessive Compulsive Scale. *Psychopharmacology Bulletin, 33*(1), 17–22. PMID: 9133747.

Poznanski, E. O., Cook, S. C., & Carroll, B. J. (1979). A depression rating scale for children. *Pediatrics, 64*(4), 442–450. PMID: 492809.

Radloff, L. S. (1977). The CES-D scale: A self-report depression scale for research in the general population. *Applied Psychological Measurements, 1*, 385–401. https://doi.org/10.1177/014662167700100306

Rorschach, H. (1921). *Psychodiagnostik* (H. Huber, Trans.). Bern Bircher.

Rosenzweig, S. (1945). The picture-association method and its application in a study of reactions to frustration. *Journal of Personality, 14*, 3–23. https://doi.org/10.1111/j.1467-6494.1945.tb01036.x

Rotter, J. B., Lah, M. I., & Rafferty, J. E. (1992). *Rotter Incomplete Sentences Blank manual* (2nd ed.). Psychological Corporation.

Rotter, J. B., & Rafferty, J. E. (1950). *The Rotter Incomplete Sentences Blank: College form*. Psychological Corporation.

Rutherford, M., Maciver, D., Johnston, L., Prior, S., & Forsyth, K. (2021). Development of a pathway for multidisciplinary neurodevelopmental assessment and diagnosis in children and young people. *Children, 8*(11), 1033. https://doi.org/10.3390/children8111033

Schopler, E., Van Bourgondien, M. E., Wellman, G. J., & Love S. R. (2010). *Childhood autism rating scale* (2nd ed.). Western Psychological Services.

Smith, C. P. (1992). *Motivation and personality: Handbook of thematic content analysis*. Cambridge University Press.

Spielberger, C. D., Edwards, C. D., Montouri, J., & Lushene, R. (1973). *State-Trait Anxiety Inventory for Children (STAI-CH)* [Database record]. APA PsycTests. https://doi.org/10.1037/t06497-000

Spielberger, C. D., Gorsuch, R. L., Lushene, R., Vagg, P. R., & Jacobs, G. A. (1983). *Manual for the State-Trait Anxiety Inventory*. Consulting Psychologists Press.

Spitzer, R. L., Kroenke, K., Williams, J. B., & Löwe, B. (2006). A brief measure for assessing generalized anxiety disorder: The GAD-7. *Archives of Internal Medicine, 166*(10), 1092–1097. https://doi.org/10.1001/archinte.166.10.1092

Tomkins, S. S. (1952). The Tomkins-Horn picture arrangement test. *Transactions of the New York Academy of Sciences, 15*, 46–50. https://doi.org/10.1111/j.2164-0947.1952.tb01151.x

Weissman, M. M., Orvaschel, H., & Padian, N. (1980). *Center for Epidemiological Studies Depression Scale for Children (CES-DC)* [Database record]. APA PsycTests. https://doi.org/10.1037/t12228-000

Wolraich, M. L., Hannah, J. N., Pinnock, T. Y., Baumgaertel, A., & Brown, J. (1996). Comparison of diagnostic criteria for attention-deficit hyperactivity disorder in a county-wide sample. *Journal of the American Academy of Child and Adolescent Psychiatry, 35*(3), 319–324. https://doi.org/10.1097/00004583-199603000-00013

Wolraich, M. L., Lambert, W., Doffing, M. A., Bickman, L., Simmons, T., & Worley, K. (2003). Psychometric properties of the Vanderbilt ADHD diagnostic parent rating scale in a referred population. *Journal of Pediatric Psychology, 28*, 559–568. https://doi.org/10.1093/jpepsy/jsg046

World Health Organization. (1998). *Wellbeing measures in primary health care/The DepCare Project: Report on a WHO meeting*. Stockholm, Sweden, February 12–13, 1998. World Health Organization. Regional Office for Europe. https://iris.who.int/handle/10665/349766.

Yesavage, J. A., Brink, T. L., Rose, T. L., Lum, O., Huang, V., Adey, M., & Leirer, V. O. (1982). Development and validation of a geriatric depression screening scale: A preliminary report. *Journal of Psychiatric Research, 17*(1), 37–49. https://doi.org/10.1016/0022-3956(82)90033-4

Young, R. C., Biggs, J. T., Ziegler, V. E., & Meyer, D. A. (1978). A rating scale for mania: Reliability, validity and sensitivity. *The British Journal of Psychiatry: The Journal of Mental Science, 133*, 429–435. https://doi.org/10.1192/bjp.133.5.429

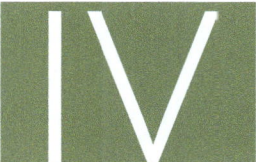

Applying and Integrating Assessments in Various Settings

11

Trauma, Harm, and Substance Abuse Assessments

CARMAN S. GILL, AYSE TORRES, AND KELLY EMELIANCHIK-KEY

2024 CACREP STANDARDS

3.G.12. procedures to identify substance use, addictions, and co-occurring conditions

3.G.13. procedures for assessing and responding to risk of aggression or danger to others, self-inflicted harm, and suicide

3.G.14. procedures for assessing clients' experience of trauma

3.G.15. procedures for identifying and reporting signs of abuse and neglect

Addiction Counseling

5.A.3. assessment for symptoms of psychoactive substance toxicity, intoxication, and withdrawal

5.A.6. evaluating and identifying individualized strategies and treatment modalities relative to substance use disorder severity, stages of change, or recovery

I still remember this situation so vividly. I was an intern working in a residential psychiatric facility. I was in session with a client, and she was getting terribly upset and anxious. At this point, I didn't have many tools in my toolbox, so I tried a grounding technique. She very calmly stated, "I know what would help," and she took the pen that she was using and pressed it into her skin so hard that she bled. I yelled for help, and she dropped the pen stating that she was fine and felt better. She received help, but from that moment on, my interest and need to learn more about self-harming behaviors peaked.

INTRODUCTION

In this chapter, we focus on assessments that are used across counseling settings and are crucial for determining level of care, diagnosis, and treatment needs and goals. Trauma and trauma history play a critical role in many mental health issues. Accurate identification of trauma history and impact on the client's presenting problems will enhance diagnosis and treatment goals. Likewise, thorough, accurate risk and suicide assessment complies with the spirit of nonmaleficence, which is ethically mandated by the American Counseling Association's (ACA's) Code of Ethics (ACA, 2014), and may result in life-saving interventions

UNDERSTANDING AND ASSESSING TRAUMA

Whereas most people will experience a traumatic event in their lifetime, individuals react differently to similar events, and most will not develop long-term mental health problems. Researchers report 89.7% of people will experience trauma in their lifetime (Kilpatrick et al, 2013). *Trauma* is defined as "involving an emotional, mental, and physical response to a powerfully negative experience or series of situations in which people perceive that they or a loved one experienced serious psychologic, physical or emotional harm" (Duffey & Haberstroh, 2020, p. 2). More recently, the neurobiological nature of trauma has come to the forefront, particularly in terms of one or more traumatic events. *Traumatic events* can include war, sexual assault, car accidents, abuse, and exposure to natural or human-caused disasters (American Psychiatric Association, 2022). A study by Benjet et al. (2016) found that the most frequently reported types of traumas include accidents/injuries, unexpected death of a loved one, witnessing death or serious injury, life-threatening illness, and collective violence, accounting for 51% of traumatic events. Derived from the words *bad stars*, *disaster* refers to large scale, mass events, in which there is massive destruction often including the loss of human life.

Stress, the mental tension related to difficult situations (World Health Organization [WHO], n.d.), is inherent to everyday life. Stress may be chronic or acute, developmentally related, or situational in nature. Stressor events can lead to changes in functioning that manifest in a variety of ways, including the engagement of coping mechanisms. A *crisis* occurs when the individual coping is overwhelmed; they perceive their efforts to deal with stress have failed, and they experience internal confusion and anxiety, resulting in diminished functioning. With support and intervention, crisis can facilitate adaptation, resilience, and increase in coping skills, but there is a danger that, without appropriate intervention and support, the individual will experience diminished functioning, negative mental symptoms, and life-impairing illness. *Posttraumatic stress* (PTS) is the most extreme type of stress. Posttraumatic Stress Disorder (PTSD) is the *DSM-5-TR* (American Psychiatric Association, 2022) diagnosis assigned to life-impairing responses to PTS. Stress, PTS, and disorders related to trauma and stress are often conceptualized on a continuum (see Figure 11.1).

Following exposure to a traumatic event, the symptoms related to PTSD may include intrusive memories and dreams, or even flashbacks and dissociation. Individuals may actively avoid any reminders of the event and/or become hypervigilant, easily aroused, or

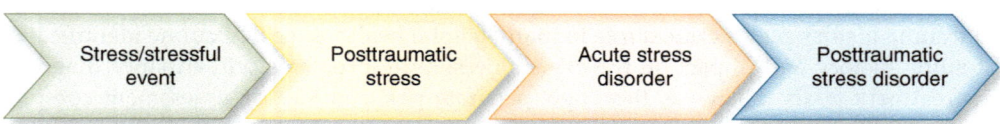

FIGURE 11.1. **Stress and trauma continuum.**

startled; experience angry outbursts or sleep disturbance; endure concentration and memory problems; and engage in reckless behavior. Further, cognition and mood may be negatively affected, resulting in symptoms such as fractured memory, decreased self-esteem, self-blame, decreased interest in activities, and difficulty or inability to experience positive emotions (American Psychiatric Association, 2022). Because of the deleterious nature of trauma, autism spectrum disorder (ASD), and PTSD, counselors must effectively assess the client's trauma history, current symptoms, and impact on the person's functioning. Additionally, counselors need to understand and assess other types of traumas, including secondary trauma and vicarious trauma. For all levels and types of traumas, appropriate, thorough, and accurate assessment is key to providing effective interventions. While we will cover specific assessments, including traumatic events-focused and PTSD symptomology-focused assessments, along with strengths-based, growth-oriented assessments, such as the Posttraumatic Growth Inventory (PTGI), we also include resources for other helpful instruments.

Initial Risk and Trauma Assessment

Clients present to treatment experiencing various levels of symptomology and distress. Assessment begins when counselors initially engage with the client, meeting for the first time. As indicated in Chapter 4, observation is often the first method of assessment. Counselors are mindful of physical indications of trauma response, even in the first meeting. For example, clients who are struggling with symptoms of acute or intense trauma may appear withdrawn, detached from reality and/or the experience, or appear easily startled and scared. Remember, trauma symptomology occurs in terms of avoidance and/or reactivity. Counselors can take note of these physical reactions and engage in assessment based on these cues. Clients may present with symptoms that are extreme enough that the counselor needs to assess the distress level the person is experiencing in the moment.

When interacting with clients for the first time and if changes in functioning are present, counselors can assess the level of distress, and changes in the level of distress, to form a foundation regarding how to proceed. One method for doing is the *Subjective Units of Distress (SUD)* scale. Based on behavioral theory and attributed to Wolpe in 1969, the goal of this assessment is to determine the level of anxiety response a client has related to specific stimuli. For example, the counselor may employ these scaling questions to determine the client's current level of anxiety related to responding to or discussing questions or topics about trauma history. SUDs are usually measured on a scale of 1 to 10, with 10 representing the most severe anxiety response. The client is asked to consider this scale and determine a number that best represents their current experience of the construct. Whereas this informal assessment does give the counselor some data to work with, measurement error is introduced as a result of multiple factors, one of which is self-report from the client. If the SUD number is extremely elevated and/or the counselor becomes aware of physical reactions indicating difficulty continuing with the assessment, immediate intervention, such as grounding techniques, may be necessary.

At intake, a full biopsychosocial-spiritual (BPSS) interview typically occurs, as described in Chapter 4. During the first session, counselors assess the level of risk associated with the client's symptomology. In addition to demographics, the presenting problem and current functioning, basic logistics, and orientation, counselors will monitor for the potential for crisis and any signs of risk for harm to the client, to others, and/or to the community (Duffey & Haberstroh, 2020). There are formal and informal methods for obtaining this information. Informally, during the intake session, the counselor may ask the client specific questions related to trauma, suicidality, NSSI, and homicidal ideation. Counselors in training and beginning counselors may feel uncomfortable asking these types of questions. Not only is this an ethical mandate, but we have a legal obligation to protect our clients and the community if safety is a concern. Approaching the client with honesty and genuine concern lessens the barriers to this type of assessment. Counselors can ask the client about their trauma history using open-ended questions such as, "Have you experienced events in your past that are traumatic in nature?" and "What experiences of trauma, if any, have you endured in your life?"

CHECKING IN WITH JOHN

Reflect on the case of John, a 37-year-old veteran, who served his country with distinction since he was 21 years old. He was wounded in combat and lost two friends in the incident as well. John continues to experience nightmares related to this event and difficulty sleeping as a result. He has a spinal cord injury, extreme back pain, and difficulties with balance and walking. John was diagnosed with PTSD and depressive disorder. Now, over a year into his retirement, despite his desire to work, John's physical disability, a direct consequence of his service-related injury, presents further obstacles in his job search. He worries that his disability may limit his career options and hinder his chances of finding meaningful employment in the civilian sector. On a personal note, John is married and has an 8-year-old daughter who brings him joy and motivation.

1. What questions might a counselor ask John to determine the nature and extent of his experience of trauma?

2. How could the SUD scale be incorporated and how could this be integrated into a BPSS?

3. How could a counselor proceed in terms of questions related to trauma, suicidality, NSSI, and homicidal ideation?

4. What are John's strengths and protective factors? How could a counselor further investigate these?

FORMAL ASSESSMENT OF TRAUMA EVENTS

The U.S. Department of Veteran Affairs and the International Society for Traumatic Stress Studies (ISTSS) provide a wealth of trauma assessment resources on their websites. These resources are highlighted in our reference list at the end of this chapter. Here we will cover the Life Events for *DSM-5* (LEC-5; American Psychiatric Association, 2013; Weathers et al., 2013b) checklist for identifying potentially traumatic events, and the Adverse Childhood Experiences (ACE; Felitti et al., 1998) questionnaire prior to the discussion of primary and secondary traumatic stress scales and growth-oriented instruments.

The LEC-5 checklist (Weathers et al., 2013b) is a 17-item assessment designed to determine whether or not an individual has experienced one or more traumatic life events. For each of the 16 categories, or types of events, the client is asked to endorse one of six choices, specifically whether they experienced an event in the category, witnessed it, learned about it, if the event is part of their job, if it does not apply, or if they are unsure about the event. For example, item #3 asks the client to respond to "Transportation accident (for example, car accident, boat accident, train wreck, plane crash)" using one of the six response choices that were previously identified. The instrument includes a final question related to stressful event(s) not covered by the previous questions, with the same choices available to the client. The instrument offers instructions in the form of a prompt to use with the client and states that the client should consider their entire life span when responding. The measure does not result in a score for the client and there are no psychometrics available for this version. Rather, the intention is to identify any *DSM-5* Criterion A traumatic event (American Psychiatric Association, 2013), begin an ongoing assessment that may include additional instruments such as the Clinician-Administered PTSD Scale for *DSM-5* (CAPS-5; American Psychiatric Association, 2013; Weathers et al., 2013a), and form a plan for diagnosis and treatment. The instrument can be downloaded from the VA website at www.ptsd.va.gov/professional/assessment/te-measures/life_events_checklist.asp, which offers three versions: the standard self-report, extended self-report, and an interview format with abuse ratings.

The ACE questionnaire (Felitti et al., 1998) is used to assess childhood trauma retrospectively or in the moment. This questionnaire is based on a longitudinal study of the experience of childhood abuse and risk factors and incidence of disease, healthcare utilization, decreased quality of life, and mortality in adults. The instrument itself is 10 items with yes/no answers, and includes domains such as abuse, household dysfunction, and physical and psychologic neglect (Felitti et al., 1998). Scoring can be completed in less than 5 minutes by tallying the positive responses. Lower scores (1–3/10) indicate lower risk of the negative outcomes associated with ACE. Individuals who score between 4–6/10 are at moderate risk, and those who score 7 or higher are at high risk for adverse adult outcomes. Examples of these outcomes include increased risk of mental illnesses, incarceration, chronic disease, and early death (Centers for Disease Control and Prevention [CDC] 2024b). Perhaps due to strong psychometric properties and ease of use, ACE is administered frequently when engaging in trauma screening, case conceptualization, and intervention. A downloadable copy of this instrument is located at https://novopsych.com.au/wp-content/uploads/2023/03/Adverse-Childhood-Experiences-Questionnaire-ACE-ACE-q-trauma-assessment.pdf. Dube et al. (2004) provided evidence of test-retest reliability of scores through kappa coefficients. They noted that kappa coefficients indicted "good agreement" and "moderate to substantial agreement" (Dube et al., 2004, p. 100). Counselors can find the questionnaire at www.acesaware.org/wp-content/uploads/2022/07/ACE-Questionnaire-for-Adults-Identified-English-rev.7.26.22.pdf.

PRIMARY AND SECONDARY TRAUMA SYMPTOM–RELATED ASSESSMENTS

In addition to formal assessment of trauma events, measures for symptoms related to PTSD, compassion fatigue, and quality of life are available for the counselor to use. In this section, we describe the CAPS-5 (Weathers et al., 2013a), the Professional Quality of Life Scale Version 5 (ProQOL-5; Stamm, 2010), and the PTGI (Tedeschi & Calhoun, 1996). These represent just a small number of the formal assessments available.

The CAPS-5 (Weathers et al., 2015) is a 30-item, evidence-based, structured interview assessment of symptoms consistent with the *DSM-5* updated PTSD criteria (American Psychiatric Association, 2013). Because a diagnosis of PTSD requires exposure to a traumatic event, this assessment begins with identification of PTSD Criterion A and provides prompts for obtaining key information regarding the traumatic event. Consistent with Criterion B, the counselor is given prompts for obtaining information regarding not only the frequency of intrusive experiences that the client is enduring but also toward determining the level of distress these intrusive experiences are causing. For example, Item 1 (B1) directs the clinician to ask, "In the past month, have you had any unwanted memories of (EVENT) while you were awake, so not counting dreams?" (Weathers et al., 2015, p. 5). The client is asked to report how remembering starts to happen, how bothersome these memories are, if the client is able to ignore them, and the frequency of the memory. Based on this information, the counselor can determine a rating on the scale of 0 to 4, using the severity and frequency criterion provided within the instrument. There are five similar items related to Criterion B, followed by two items related to Criterion C (persistent avoidance), which are presented in the same format. Authors include seven questions related to Criterion D, which follow the same pattern and comprise negative changes in mood and cognition related to the traumatic event. Six questions with the same format encompass Criterion E, significant changes in reactivity and arousal related to the traumatic event. Two questions are related to the duration of the disturbances, and the rating scale does not apply here. Rather, the counselor will ask specific questions regarding more than 1 month or delay in symptom onset. The three questions related to Criterion G have unique rating scales and cover clinical significance of the disturbance in terms of occupational, social, or other life impairment. Items 26 to 28 are considered global ratings, and the counselor is asked to estimate the validity of responses, severity of symptoms, and any improvement in functioning noted. The final two question categories for the client address depersonalization and derealization. These are scored on a 0 to 4 scale, consistent with the first 20 items (Weathers et al., 2015). A summary sheet and simplified information for scoring are both provided within the instrument.

Frequently referred to as the "gold standard" in PTSD assessments (ISTSS, 2023), this instrument has been widely used and demonstrates strong evidence of reliability and validity (Weathers et al., 2018). The measure is free for qualified clinicians who have a graduate degree and are trained in the use of psychodiagnostic assessments. The U.S. Department of Veterans Affairs provides methods for requesting these assessments, as well as training materials, on their website at www.ptsd.va.gov/professional/assessment/adult-int/caps.asp#obtain. Counselors should note that there are multiple versions of this assessment and select the instrument most appropriate for their needs. For example, the CAPS-5 Past Week instrument is recommended for symptom tracking and routine outcome monitoring purposes, not for diagnosing PTSD (Weathers et al., 2015).

To this point in the chapter, we have discussed primary trauma and related assessment. The ProQOL-5 (Stamm, 2009) focuses on secondary trauma exposure. Secondary traumatic stress refers to the mental health impact experienced by those who work with trauma survivors. Examples include first responders, nurses, firefighters, and mental healthcare providers, including counselors. In 1982, Figley identified symptoms of "the cost of caring" or compassion fatigue in helping professionals. Compassion fatigue, often associated with vicarious trauma, is defined by ACA as the "emotional residue of exposure that counselors have from working with people as they are hearing their trauma stories and become witnesses to the pain, fear, and terror that trauma survivors have endured" (ACA, n.d., p. 1). This construct differs from burnout, in that burnout refers to exhaustion and frustration related to the workplace, rather than the type of work. Further, this construct reflects only one end of the trauma spectrum. Posttraumatic growth outcomes, such as compassion satisfaction, or the satisfaction the helpers experience as a positive result of the individual and societal impact of caring for others, can also be a result of this process.

The ProQOL-5 is designed to measure quality of life in three distinct scales: burnout, secondary traumatic stress, and compassion satisfaction. This 30-item, self-report instrument is one of the most commonly used measures of perceived positive and negative outcomes associated with working in the helping professions. The wording is broad, using *help, helping,* and *helpers,* and normative data are provided for comparison. Users are asked to respond to the items on a 5-point Likertscale, with 5 reflecting "very often" and 1 being "never." Thus, the range of raw scores is 30 to 150. The introductory prompt requests that the user respond honestly, based on frequency of experience over the last month. For example, item #30 states "I am happy that I chose to do this work," and the authors of this book would reply "5–Very Often." Compassion satisfaction is scored using items 3, 6, 12, 16, 18, 20, 22, 24, 27, and 30; burnout is scored using items 1, 4, 8, 10, 15, 17, 19, 21, 26, and 29; and secondary traumatic stress scores are derived from items 2, 5, 7, 9, 11, 13, 14, 23, 25, and 28. In terms of scoring the instrument, some items are reverse scored and must be adjusted accordingly. Following this, the scales are summed and converted from raw score to T-scores. In addition to specific directions for scoring, the *Concise Manual for the Professional Quality of Life Scale* (Stamm, 2010), a free download, includes definitions, directions for use, psychometrics, cut scores, guidance for interpretation, instructions for routine outcome monitoring, and handouts. Alphas are reported by scale as follows: Compassion satisfaction = .88; burnout = .75; and secondary traumatic stress = .81. The ProQOL-5 is normed for a variety of populations and is translated into 28 languages. The instrument, in multiple versions, along with the manual and supplemental material is located at the https://proqol.org website. It is free to use, provided the format is not changed, the author is credited, and it is not sold (The Center for Victims of Torture, 2021). Additionally, the ISTSS provides a Vicarious Trauma Toolkit, available on their website at https://istss.org/clinical-resources/treating-trauma/vicarious-trauma-toolkit.

Posttraumatic growth is the opportunity offered by crisis. When individuals experience a traumatic event, they may develop negative symptoms as previously described. Whether these symptoms occur, or do not occur, that individual may also grow from the event, becoming more resilient, gaining more effective coping skills, and increasing self-awareness and overall mental health. Positive psychologic response after a traumatic experience is called posttraumatic growth (Tedeschi & Calhoun, 1996). The PTGI (Tedeschi & Calhoun, 1996) was designed to measure this construct. The PTGI is a 21-item, self-report assessment of five factors related to posttraumatic growth as follows: appreciation of life, relationship with others, new possibilities in life, personal strength, and spiritual change. Each statement is rated on a scale of 0 ("I did not experience a change as the result of my crisis") to 6 ("I experienced this change to a very great degree as a result of my crisis"; Tedeschi & Calhoun, 1996, p. 459). The statements correspond directly to the five factors and the instrument is scored by adding the ratings on each factor, as well as totaling the numbers for an entire scale score. Tedeschi and Calhoun (1996) found an overall internal consistency of the instrument at .90. Scale specific reliability ranged from .85 to .67. Test-retest reliability for a 2-month time period was .71 for the entire scale. Further, these researchers also reported evidence of a modest relationship with optimism and extraversion. The scale is recommended for understanding growth after stressor events and to inform clients and others in terms of assessment, scope, and planning for ongoing personal growth (Tedeschi & Calhoun, 1996).

UNDERSTANDING AND ASSESSING HARM

In this section, we continue our discussion of risk by covering suicide, NSSI, and risk of harm to others. We cover commonly used tools for assessing and responding to suicide, NSSI, and/or risk of aggression to others. Additional resources for counselors to use in practice are provided as well.

Suicide

Suicide refers to the act of intentionally ending one's own life and is a leading cause of death in the United States (CDC, 2023). In 2021, 48,183 Americans died at their own hands, a substantial increase from the previous year (CDC, 2023). Further, *suicidal behavior* is defined as "potentially self-injurious behavior with at least some intent to die" (American Psychiatric Association, 2022, p. x). Intent to die is associated with suicidal thoughts, which include considering or ruminating about intentionally ending one's life. The CDC reports that, in 2021, 12.3 million people in the United States seriously considered suicide, 3.5 million endorsed creating a plan, and 1.7 million people attempted suicide (CDC, 2023). *Suicide attempt* refers to the act of intentionally trying to end one's life. These terms differ from NSSI, which is described by Emelianchik-Key and La Guardia (2019) as "self-inflicted tissue damage that is intentional, direct, socially unacceptable, and without suicidal intent" (p. xiv).

INITIAL AND ONGOING ASSESSMENT

The first step in effective suicide prevention and intervention is a thorough and accurate assessment. Earlier in this chapter, we covered some initial assessment for intake, first session, and ongoing work with the client. We noted that counselors must ask clients questions regarding suicide, suicidal ideation, and intent. Counselors can make clients aware of the prevalence of suicide and association with certain symptoms and diagnoses, as well as the deleterious nature of suicide for the loved ones, as part of this process. For example, counselors might say, "You are expressing a lot of severe emotional distress and depression. Have you had thoughts of hurting or killing yourself?" Remember that, as stated in Chapter 4, these questions follow a discussion of informed consent, so that the client is aware of potential outcomes of their answers. As a counselor, you have a duty to act to protect the life of the client if necessary.

Paladino (2020) notes that there are two factors for suicide assessment: suicidal risk factors and a lethality assessment. We introduced some specific questions regarding suicidal ideation. However, if the client answers in the affirmative, follow-up for both factors is necessary. In terms of suicide risk factors, counselors need to fully assess thoughts of harm/suicide, history of these thoughts and any suicidal behavior, and current intent. Lethality includes a plan and availability of means to act on that plan. Examples of follow-up questions, by category, are provided in Table 11.1.

Counselors should note that, throughout this assessment, there are opportunities for active listening, responding, and the instillation of hope. Paladino states, "Counselors are aware of the role of disconnection and the use of the counseling relationship to foster growth and connection. The relationship enhances a sense of safety, mutual empathy, and understanding" (2020, p. 146). The client can benefit from hearing the seriousness of the words associated with the act of suicide (i.e., *kill* and *die*), as well as the empathy communicated by the counselor. Genuine empathy and caring are the foundations of an ongoing working alliance that can serve as a protective factor.

When conducting a suicide assessment, counselors need to consider risk factors as well. Risk factors can fall into multiple levels, such as individual, relationship, community, and society (CDC, 2024a). Although there is currently no single strong predictor of suicide on the individual level, people with previous attempts are 25% to 30% more likely to try again (American Psychiatric Association, 2022). The presence or history of mental illness, such as depression, bipolar disorder, trauma-related disorders, eating disorders, and/or anxiety, is considered a risk factor, as are serious medical illness and chronic pain. Occupational issues and/or loss of a job, legal problems, and substance-related issues are also associated with higher risk. Additional individual risk factors include impulsive tendencies, perpetration of violence, feelings of hope, victimization, and childhood trauma/multiple ACEs (CDC, 2024a). Age is also a risk factor, as suicide is the second leading cause of death for Americans ages 25 to 34 and third for those 15 to 24 years old. Further, while women engage in suicidal behavior more frequently than do men, males tend to use more lethal means, such as firearms, resulting in a higher completion rate (American Psychiatric Association, 2022).

TABLE 11.1 **EXAMPLE QUESTIONS**

Suicidal Ideation (if the client responds in the affirmative to questions regarding suicide)	You are thinking of ending your life. How frequently do these thoughts occur and how long have you been having them?
	What precipitates or prompts these thoughts?
	When did these thoughts begin?
History	Have you ever had thoughts of killing yourself before now?
	If so, what happened when you had these thoughts? Did you act on them?
	What prevented you from acting on them? -or- What happened when you tried to act on suicidal thoughts?
	How many times has this happened for you?
Current Intent	When was the last time you thought about suicide?
	On a scale of 1 to 10, with 10 being very likely, how likely are you to try to kill yourself after you leave today?
	How likely are you to act on these thoughts?
Plan	Have you thought about what you would do to end your life?
	Have you made a plan for completing suicide?
	What steps are you considering taking?
Means	How would you act on that plan or carry out those steps?
	Do you own or have access to a gun or other weapon?
	Do you have access to pills that might harm you?

At a relationship level, individuals who experience struggles such as isolation, loss of a loved one or close relationship, relationships that are high in conflict, a loved one who completes suicide, and bullying are at higher risk. Further, community issues, such as systemic discrimination, difficulty with acculturation, and historical trauma, increase risk. Suicide rates are higher for non-Hispanic American Indian/Alaska Native and middle-aged adults (35–64 years), as well as veterans and young people who identify as LGBTQ+. At particular risk of suicidal behavior are individuals who identify as sexual minorities, with more than 1 in 5 high school students identifying as sexual minorities reporting at least one suicide attempt (CDC, 2023). Communities that lack resources for healthcare, have high rates of community violence, and experience suicide clusters increase risk. Societal factors such as stigma surrounding help-seeking, easy access to weapons, and social and other media portrayals of suicide should be considered as well (CDC, 2024a).

Consistent with the previously described risk factors, the SAD PERSONS scale (Patterson et al., 1983) is a 10-item clinical rating scale, designed to determine one's suicide risk. SAD PERSONS is an acronym for **S**ex, **A**ge, **D**epression, **P**rior history, **E**thanol (alcohol abuse), **R**ational thinking loss, **S**upport system loss, **O**rganized plan, **N**o significant other, and **S**ickness. For each of these items, a description is given for context. For instance, item one is sex and the associated description states, "Men typically use more lethal suicide methods (e.g., guns, cars) than do women (Hoberman & Garfinkel, 1988; Shaffer, 1988). Therefore, men are identified within this scale as being at increased risk" (Juhnke, 1996, p. 252). This is in keeping with the risk factors described earlier, as are other items on this assessment.

Counselors who are clinically concerned about their client's decompensating mental health symptoms, or any other indication that the person may be at risk, may use the SAD PERSONS scale to assist in making level of care determinations. One point is assigned for each of these answers and summed to obtain a total scale score. This assessment provides a scoring system for risk wherein a score of 0 to 2 represents no discernible issues and a recommendation for referral and monitoring is given. For a score of 3 to 4, a recommendation is given to send the client home with more frequent check-ins. For scores of 5 to 6, consideration is given to hospitalization if there are concerns that the client will not return for ongoing care. For scores falling into the 7 to 10 range, hospitalization is warranted (Patterson et al., 1983).

Hockberger and Rothstein (1988) reported that a modified version of the SAD PERSONS scale, the MSPS, in which four items were weighted (assigned 2 points for each item), determined the necessity of hospitalization for scores at or greater than 6, with a sensitivity of 94% and a specificity of 71% for clients endorsing suicidal ideation in general. Modifications included 2 points for depression, rational thinking loss, organized or serious attempt, and stated future intent. For age, they specified those under 19 and over 45 are more at risk. In addition, they added an A for availability of lethal means, weighted 2 points, resulting in the SAD PERSONAS Scale. In follow-up emergency department studies, the SAD PERSONS scale and the MSPS demonstrated overall poor ability to predict suicide. However, researchers identified five items that were predictive of future suicide attempts when presenting within 6 months with a 94% sensitivity rate, Bolton et al. stated: a previous attempt or history of psychiatric care, substance abuse, suicidal intent, ages 19 to 45 years, and an absence of rational thinking (Bolton et al., 2012). Significant association between high-risk scores and a two- to threefold increase in risk of suicide over the 5-year follow-up period were uncovered as well (Katz et al., 2017). In terms of utility, clients who are experiencing distress may be more likely to respond to this interview form, rather than formal assessments. The counselor can then gain crucial information for determining level of care. As with other assessments, counselors must use clinical judgment and consider all factors involved in making these decisions, understanding that some items, such as pain, may be of more concern than others (Juhnke, 1994).

FORMAL INVENTORIES

For a thorough suicide assessment, clinicians can use formal inventories, along with interviews and rating scales. There are multiple instruments available for clinical use. We cover two of these in the text that follows, in addition to the Suicide Assessment Five-Step Evaluation and Triage (SAFE-T), designed to assist counselors when taking the next steps. Keep in mind that formal suicide assessments to address risk are often something we may have to do in the moment, so understanding the signs and risk factors for suicidality is often critical in suicide assessment.

The Suicide Probability Scale (SPS; Cull & Gill, 1992) is a 36-item, self-report measure for assessing suicide risk in adolescents and adults, 14 and older. The instrument takes about 5 to 10 minutes to administer, and the manual and tests are available for a fee. Based on dimensions of coping behavior and subjective well-being, this instrument includes four clinical scales, as follows: hostility, negative self-evaluation, suicide ideation, and hopelessness. The instrument administered to test takers does not include the word *suicide* in the title, and counselors are encouraged not to indicate the purpose of the assessment (Erford et al., 2018). Counselors ask the client to respond to statements on a 4-point Likert scale, with 1 corresponding to "none or a little of the time" and 4 to "most or all of the time." Scores are produced in two ways. Counselors can sum subscale scores for an overall instrument score, or electronic scoring is available through Western Psychological Services (WPS; www.wpspublish.com/sps-suicide-probability-scale). Raw scores range between 36 and 144 with higher scores indicating higher suicide probability. Counselors can calculate the normalized T-score, or WPS provides a report that includes this score, a total weighted score, and a suicide probability score.

The SPS is restricted in use to Level C qualifications, requiring appropriate training and knowledge, as well as a clinical license and master or doctoral degree. The instrument has strong psychometric properties including evidence of reliability and validity, as well as population norms. A meta-analysis conducted by Erford et al. reported strong internal consistencies across 10 studies with total instrument alpha at .91, and test-retest reliability of .71 (2018). Multiple studies have addressed validity for this instrument using consistent convergent correlations with inventories such as the Suicide Resiliency Inventory (SRI), the Beck Depression Inventory (BDI), and the Center for Epidemiological Studies–Depression scale (CES-D). For hospitalized youth, the weighted SPS score demonstrates strong predictive value for postdischarge suicide attempts (Huth-Bocks et al., 2007).

The Columbia-Suicide Severity Rating Scale (C-SSRS; The Columbia Lighthouse Project, 2016), also known as the Columbia Protocol, is a self-report assessment that is intended to be a quick, plain-language questionnaire for predicting suicidal behavior in adults and youth. The assessment is available in multiple languages and versions for free on The Columbia Lighthouse Project website (https://cssrs.columbia.edu). We cover the C-SSRS full-lifetime/recent, which includes four parts. The first part, questions 1 and 2, attempts to determine if suicidal ideation exists. If the client answers in the affirmative to question 2, "Have you actually had thoughts about killing yourself?", the clinician proceeds to more direct questions regarding severity. The second part, questions 3 to 5, includes items that examine the severity level (Erford et al., 2018). For example, question 3 states, "Have you been thinking about how you might do this?" and directs the clinician to ask for a description if the answer is yes. If the client answers negative to the first two assessment questions, the counselor can proceed to the third section, in which the questions are directly related to suicidal ideation. This section includes scaling questions regarding severity, frequency, duration, controllability, deterrents, and rationale. For example, in terms of frequency, the counselor would ask, "How many times have you had thoughts?", with the scale ranging from 1 (less than once a week) to 5 (more than 8 hours/persistent or continuous).

The final section addresses actual attempts including NSSI behavior, interrupted attempts, aborted attempts, and preparatory behavior. This section asks for lifetime data and that from the past 3 months, gives examples, and seeks to collect historical information on suicide attempts. The assessment is scored by summing positive responses. Any positive response is considered an indication of suicidal ideation. Posner et al. (2011) reported internal consistencies from three studies for the intensity subscale. The initial study included two intervals: since last visit ($\alpha = 0.937$) and past week ($\alpha = 0.946$). Further, the internal consistency for this subscale in the additional studies was 0.73, which is moderate. Evidence of good convergent and divergent validity was established using other suicidal ideation and behavior assessments (Posner et al., 2011). Giddens et al. (2014) note that, while the U.S. Food and Drug Administration (FDA) refers to this instrument as the gold standard for suicide assessments, some of the major limitations that apply to suicide assessments also apply to this instrument, including difficulty with full inclusion of all suicide characteristics, limited range of ideation and behavior, and ambiguous wording. More recently, the instrument has been paired with the SAFE-T protocol to assist clinicians with the next steps.

The SAFE-T (Substance Abuse and Mental Health Services Administration [SAMHSA], 2009) provides five concrete steps for determining and responding to the level of risk for suicide for adults and adolescents, based on recommendations from the American Psychiatric Association's Practice Guideline (American Psychiatric Association Work Group on Suicidal Behaviors, 2003). The five steps are: identifying risk factors, identifying protective factors, conducting a suicide assessment, determining risk and intervention needs, and documenting the process. SAMHSA provides a form integration in which SAFE-T risk factors (step 1) are the indications of suicidal ideation severity from the C-SSRS (first and second parts), followed by the suicidal behavior question. In addition, counselors collect information regarding mood and diagnosis, symptoms, family history, precipitants, and changes in treatment level. Clinicians are directed to ask specifically about access to lethal means.

Step 2 determines any internal or external protective factors the person may have. On this form, step 3 is consistent with the C-SSRS third section, five questions regarding suicidal ideation intensity, as previously described, for 48 hours, for a month, and for a lifetime. This section includes rating scales for a total scale score (range 0–25) and a notes section for specific behaviors. Step 4 provides the counselor with detailed guidance as to the level of risk and possible interventions. Documenting the level of risk and associated rationale, as well as intervention and a follow-up plan, occurs on the form in step 5. The assessment form includes a straightforward format for recording this information. The SAFE-T guidance form is located on the SAMHSA website (https://store.samhsa.gov/product/SAFE-T-Pocket-Card-Suicide-Assessment-Five-Step-Evaluation-and-Triage-for-Clinicians/sma09-4432) and further guidance is available at https://cssrs.wpengine.com/the-columbia-scale-c-ssrs/cssrs-for-communities-and-healthcare/#filter=.general-use.english.

Additional resources for suicide assessment are provided in Table 11.2. It is incumbent upon the counselor to understand the importance of suicide and risk assessment, have tools for multidimensional assessment, and know how to follow with appropriate interventions for all levels of care resulting from assessment, prior to engaging with clients. Ongoing supervision and self-reflection are crucial to providing clients in distress with the most effective care.

TABLE 11.2 **SUICIDE ASSESSMENT RESOURCES**

Website Name	Description	Link
Digital Shareables on Suicide Prevention (NIMH)	People can download and share informational graphics, social media messages, and videos to help raise awareness about suicide prevention.	www.nimh.nih.gov/get-involved/digital-shareables/shareable-resources-on-suicide-prevention
Suicide Prevention Resource Center online library	This resource provides information and personal stories on mental health and suicide prevention and links to resources.	https://sprc.org/online-library
Suicide Prevention (NIMH)	On this site people can learn about suicide prevention, including helpline numbers, warning signs, risk factors, treatments and therapies, and resources for more information.	www.nimh.nih.gov/health/topics/suicide-prevention
Screening for and Addressing Suicide Risk in Clinical Settings Toolkit (Rural Health Information Hub)	This resource describes screening tools, interventions, and follow-up for suicide risk and how these services can be implemented in rural areas.	www.ruralhealthinfo.org/toolkits/suicide
Help Prevent Suicide (SAMHSA)	This website has resources, videos aimed at helping high-risk populations, and a help line for suicide prevention.	www.samhsa.gov/suicide
American Foundation for Suicide Prevention (AFSP)	AFSP engages in mental health initiatives to raise awareness for and support mental health.	https://afsp.org/

AFSP, American Foundation for Suicide Prevention; NIMH, National Institute of Mental Health; SAMHSA, Substance Abuse and Mental Health Services Administration.

Nonsuicidal Self-Injury

Nonsuicidal self-injury (NSSI) refers to self-inflicted, intentional wounds directly to the tissues of the body via various methods (cutting, burning, scratching, hitting, and punching) without suicidal intent (Emelianchik-Key & LaGuardia, 2019; Nock, 2010). The term NSSI is often used synonymously with self-injurious behavior and deliberate self-harm. NSSI can be challenging to conceptualize and assess because cases are all vastly different based on factors like age, ethnicity, and gender, in addition to clinical and nonclinical populations that engage in NSSI behaviors. With the recent changes in the *DSM-5-TR*, diagnostic codes were added for suicidal behavior and NSSI. These changes are located in Section 2, the "Other Conditions That May Be a Focus of Clinical Attention" chapter (American Psychiatric Association, 2022). The rationale for adding these codes is to bring consideration to self-injury, which is commonly seen in clinical practice settings, and to provide a uniform way for clinicians to document these issues as they arrive in session. This change in the *DSM-5-TR* will help interprofessional collaboration and allow for improved estimation of risk factors for suicide. To be clear, NSSI is different than suicide attempts, which means the behavior must thoroughly and accurately be assessed.

INITIAL AND ONGOING ASSESSMENT OF NONSUICIDALSELF-INJURY

The Interpersonal-Psychological Theory of Suicide (IPTS; Joiner, 2005) provides a theoretical framework for why some people engage in suicidal behavior while others who are also at high risk do not. The theory uses the concepts of thwarted belongingness (the feeling of "I am alone") and perceived burdensomeness (the feeling "I am a burden"), which merge with the acquired capability for suicide. The acquired capability for suicide is the ability to withstand physical pain and suffering. NSSI would be viewed as a risk factor for suicide, allowing someone the acquired capability to tolerate pain. With repeated NSSI, the physical tolerance for pain will increase and the fear of death and emotional pain will decrease, increasing risk for suicide (even if that is not the intent). This framework is critical in assessing suicide risk with those who self-injure, but it is important to note this is not a predictive model for suicide. As counselors, we cannot assume that all people who self-injure will automatically be at risk for suicide. This is why assessment of NSSI is essential and we must examine risk and protective factors when working with those who engage in NSSI (Emelianchik-Key, 2019).

Simply asking about NSSI behaviors is not enough to fully capture the depth of NSSI in clients. There are formal assessments (which we will discuss shortly) that provide time-specific information, as well as severity and frequency information, which is needed to clearly assist in assessing critical aspects of NSSI. However, these cannot replace the importance of building rapport with your client and examining risk and protective factors. Emelianchik-Key (2019) notes that counselors should respond nonjudgmentally, immediately, and directly; avoid shock or emotional displays; avoid minimizing the situation; and reinforce that you are there to assist the client. Additionally, counselors should strive to understand the complexity of the self,consider ethical codes, assist in healthy coping strategies, and continue in ongoing evaluation while ensuring that medical referrals are not needed.

INFORMAL ASSESSMENTS

During an initial assessment of self-injurious behavior, it is crucial to ask open-ended questions and to include questions that examine risk and protective factors. This will assist in beginning the informal assessment process. The first thing to consider is to determine the intent behind the self-injurious behavior. Clearly ask if there was intent to die. Check for prior suicide attempts. As noted earlier, a history of suicide attempts or suicidal ideations is associated with higher risk when assessing. Once it is clear that the self-injury is not an attempt to die, gather more information related to risk. If the counselor is experienced with working with NSSI, informal questions that may be asked to begin the conversation around NSSI behaviors are as follows (Emelianchik-Key, 2019):

- Can you recall what prompted or triggered the urge to self-injure?
- Is there a common spot on your body that you inflict injury? Why this location?
- Did you engage in any specific patterns or rituals before injuring?
- Is there a particular location that makes you feel safe to self-injure or do you do it as needed in any location?
- How does injuring provide relief at that moment, and what emotions followed the injury?
- What alerts you that it is time to stop he self-harming behavior?
- Is there a specific feeling when you know you are done?
- Typically, how much time passes before you start feeling better after harming yourself?
- Have you ever sustained injuries from the self injurious behavior that warranted medical attention?
- How frequently do you engage in self-harm?
- Are there environments or places where you can resist the urge to harm yourself (i.e., school, work)?
- Can you describe instances when you wanted to harm yourself but didn't? What gave you the strength to refrain?
- Who in your life is aware of your self-harming behavior? How do they support you? If no one knows, can you think of someone you might feel comfortable telling?

If the counselor is not experienced with NSSI interviews, there are some other informal methods of use to assist in the assessment process if the questions do not come naturally. The HIRE model and the SOARS model are flexible approaches using acronyms to help the clinician remember to assess each domain. The HIRE acronym is as follows: H = History, I = Interest in change, R = Reasons behind behavior, and E = Exposure to risk (Buser & Buser, 2013). The SOARS model (Westers et al., 2016) was designed for physicians who see NSSI when examining patients and gives specific questions that can be asked with each letter. The S = Suicidal ideation; O = Onset, frequency, and methods; A = Aftercare; R = Reasons for the self-injury; and S = Stage of change, referring to Prochaska's model of readiness for change, which is described as part of substance use assessments later in this chapter.

FORMAL ASSESSMENTS

Understanding the function, intention, and purpose of self-injury in a client's life is necessary before choosing a formal assessment. When the intent is suspected to be suicide, assessments like the *Direct and Indirect Self-Harm Inventory* (Green et al., 2017) will be helpful to differentiate or determine if suicide is a consideration. Many existing suicide scales fail to entirely rule out NSSI with a suicide attempt, but many NSSI scales do consider suicidal ideation. When selecting an assessment tool, it is critical that clinicians understand the assessment tool itself, as well as how to administerand score it and interpret the results. Understanding risk factors (i.e., other mental health disorders) and protective factors (i.e., supportive environment) are critical for those who engage in NSSI. Assessing impulsivity prior to selecting an assessment is important because ritualistic or episodic NSSI would be addressed and assessed differently. There are numerous formal assessments to assist with the assessment of NSSI. Some of those assessments are listed in Table 11.3.

The *Deliberate Self-Harm Inventory* (DSHI; Gratz, 2001; Gratz et al., 2012) has 17 self-report items that are behaviorally based and assess aspects of deliberate self-harm such as frequency, severity, and duration of self-harming behavior. The instrument has high internal consistency; adequate construct, convergent, and discriminant validity; and adequate test-retest reliability. The DSHI is one of the first instruments that clearly defines self-harm, which allows researchers to measure precise behaviors to ensure participants do not only report those of interest to researchers.

The NSSI–Assessment Tool (NSSI-AT; Whitlock et al., 2014) assesses the frequency and function of NSSI including NSSI habituation, functions, age of onset, wound locations, motivations, severity, practice patterns, and perceived life interference. The NSSI-AT contains 12 modules across 39 items. When administered, the entire sample is given the first module, but remaining modules are visible to only those who screen positive for NSSI. The NSSI-AT is web-based, which allows for some flexible and customized questions and response options based on earlier responses. This means that comprehensive, distinct questions are asked to clients with relevant experiences, rather than by all who take the assessment.

TABLE 11.3 **NONSUICIDAL SELF-INJURY INVENTORIES**

Assessment Tool	Target Population	Strengths	Limitations
The Inventory of Statements About Self-Injury (ISAS)	Adolescents and adults	Describes various features of NSSI behaviors and intent	Restricted information on frequency and severity; limited generalizability to diverse populations
The Functional Assessment of Self-Mutilation (FASM)	Adolescents and adults	Stresses the purpose of self-mutilation	Limited generalizability to diverse populations
Self-Harm Inventory (SHI)	Adolescents and adults	Short and easy to administer	Limited information on functions
Self-Injurious Thoughts and Behaviors Interview (SITBI)	Adolescents and adults	Structured interview format with thorough assessment	Time-consuming and may require training
Self-Harm Behavior Questionnaire (SHBQ)	Adolescents and adults	Contains diverse self-harm behaviors and methods	Limited information on functions and intentions
The Self-Injury Questionnaire (SIQ)	Adolescents	Brief and easily administered	Limited coverage of self-harm functions

NSSI, nonsuicidal self-injury.

INTEGRATED APPROACHES

Integrated approaches to the assessment of self-injury consider various aspects of self-injury behavior, including the physical act of self-injury, as well as the underlying psychologic distress, motivations behind the behavior, and psychosocial factors. These methods provide a thorough picture of self-injury, which can help guide treatment planning and intervention strategies. Integrated approaches use a combination of observational methods, semistructured clinical interviews, and formal assessments. These methods can include monitoring the individual's behavior over time, looking for signs of self-injury, and observing their interactions with others. An integrated approach to self-injury assessment should also consider the individual's social and environmental context. This can include factors such as the individual's relationships with others, their living situation, and any stressors or challenges they may be facing in their life. Craigen et al. (2010) have a two-tier integrated approach to assess self-injury that includes formal assessment for self-injury and other diagnoses, coupled with informal assessment techniques that gain access to psychosocial information.

Risk of Harm to Others/Homicidal Risk

Assessing and managing the risk of harm is a crucial aspect of mental health counseling. This assessment plays a vital role in ensuring safe and effective care and making informed decisions about transitioning between services. It is important to acknowledge that complete elimination of risk is not feasible in the realm of mental health. Risk is an inherent part of our environment and human behavior. Mental health professionals focus on evaluating, managing, and mitigating risks rather than eradicating them altogether (Royal College of Psychiatrists, 2016). Gaining an understanding of a client's history of violence or risk toward others is pivotal in identifying patterns and escalating risks. In a broader sense, risk management involves the careful planning and implementation of strategies to prevent violence and other forms of harmful behavior.

The field of violence risk assessment has experienced significant growth in recent decades. Researchers have developed over 400 diverse tools designed to evaluate the risk of violence and offending (Viljoen et al., 2018). The widespread adoption of these risk assessment tools is driven by the belief that they can assist professionals in effectively managing and ultimately reducing risk. Various professionals, including mental health professionals, probation officers, nurses, psychiatrists, and police, widely utilize these tools. Moreover, risk assessment tools find common application in forensic psychiatric facilities (Singh et al., 2014), general psychiatric hospitals, treatment programs, correctional centers, and various court evaluations. These tools play a crucial role in not only treatment approaches, such as therapy, but also in strategies like supervision, case management, and placement decisions. Risk assessment tools serve as a standardized means of evaluating individuals for potential violence, thereby ensuring that healthcare providers share a common frame of reference. In doing so, the likelihood of misinterpreting communications about a person's propensity for violence is reduced (CDC, n.d.).

Nevertheless, the use of these tools has sparked controversy within the mental health field. While some argue that they are indispensable for effective risk management, others contend that they are biased and unreliable. Critics assert that such tools may perpetuate stereotypes and disproportionately affect specific populations (e.g., those from economically disadvantaged backgrounds). Moreover, there are concerns that an overreliance on these tools may detract from the crucial role of clinical judgment and personalized treatment plans in risk management. Despite facing criticism, risk assessment tools have become widely used in various fields. In fact, their implementation is often legally required for certain populations, such as individuals on probation or parole. For example, in the United

States, risk assessment tools are employed by at least 20 states to determine sentencing for offenders (Starr, 2014), and 28 states utilize them to determine an offender's eligibility for parole (Harcourt, 2007). In the realm of youth probation, all 50 states have adopted the use of risk assessment tools, with 34 states mandating their application on a statewide basis (Wachter, 2015). Given that over 4.5 million American adults and adolescents are placed on probation or parole annually, and more than 1.5 million Americans are incarcerated, these tools are employed extensively (Viljoen et al., 2018).

INITIAL AND ONGOING ASSESSMENT

Risk formulation encompasses both initial and ongoing assessment, playing a pivotal role in guiding decision-making processes when evaluating and addressing potential harm. This critical process aims to answer key questions: What is the severity and immediacy of the risk? Is it specific or general? How volatile is it? What indicators suggest an escalating risk? Furthermore, risk formulation seeks to identify the most suitable treatment and management plan to effectively mitigate the risk. Risk formulation involves assessing the following factors (Royal College of Psychiatrists, 2016):

- *Risk factors*: Risk assessment involves understanding an individual's unique vulnerabilities and strengths within their specific context. These factors are complex and cover various aspects, including the individual and their family, community, and cultural influences. Risk factors can be broadly categorized into two types: static and dynamic. Static risk factors include a history of prior violence, age of first violent incident, conduct issues, and ACE. Dynamic risk factors are changeable and often the main focus of treatment. They include elements such as peer relationships, social support, mental health status, impulse control, attitudes toward interventions and violence, anger, and substance use. Understanding these factors is crucial in comprehending the changing risks of violence throughout an individual's life and serves as the primary targets for intervention.

- *History*: When evaluating risk, it is essential to have an accurate understanding of the history of violent incidents. This valuable information can be obtained by examining records such as past mental health records, school districts, or social services departments, as well as a comprehensive history of criminal offenses. Gathering insights from conversations with other professionals, caregivers, and family members can also provide crucial information. When assessing a history of harm to others, four key components are essential: recentness, severity, frequency, and pattern.

  - The recentness of an event or incident influences the current risk level, with more recent incidents implying a higher risk.

  - Severity is also a key determinant, with incidents resulting in major physical injuries such as fractures, large lacerations, or loss of consciousness being considered as high risk.

  - The frequency of events or incidents also plays a critical role, with persistent and repeated offenses indicating a high risk.

  - The pattern of incidents, such as the context in which they occur, can provide crucial insights into the assessment.

- *Ideation/mental state*: It is crucial to consider current ideation and mental state when assessing the risk of harm. This includes evaluating any recent changes in behavior or thought patterns that may indicate a potential for violence. These include the presence of symptoms like firmly held beliefs of persecution (persecutory delusions) or the perception of external control over one's mind or body (delusions of passivity). Additionally, emotions associated with violence, such as irritability, anger, hostility, and suspiciousness, should be noted. It is also crucial to consider any specific threats made by the client. Finally, command hallucinations, where the client hears voices instructing them to attack a specific person, should be taken into account. It is also essential to determine if there are any underlying mental health conditions that could contribute to violent behavior.

- *Intent*: When an individual makes a statement indicating their intention to cause harm to another person, it is a clear sign of risk that should never be disregarded. The expression of intent, whether it is implied or explicit, holds immense power and serves as the most reliable predictor of future behavior.

- *Planning*: If someone admits to having thoughts of harming others, it's important to determine if they have thought about how they might do so. This can be based on their own statements or other evidence. A higher risk is indicated if they have a specific plan to harm someone. The risk increases further if they also have access to the means to carry out the plan.

METHODS TO ASSESS RISK OF HARM

When assessing harm to others, two main approaches are commonly used: the "actuarial method" and the "clinical approach." *Actuarial risk assessment instruments* (*ARAIs*) are widely used in various fields to estimate the likelihood of individuals engaging in future violent behavior. These instruments are based on extensive research and utilize statistical methods to provide an estimation of the risk of future violence. By considering empirically validated risk factors, ARAIs generate a probability percentage indicating the likelihood of an individual's involvement in violent behavior within a specific timeframe. The benefit of using an actuarial assessment is that human judgment biases are removed from the clinical decision-making process, giving them higher perceived usefulness in legal settings.

It is important to recognize that actuarial tools alone cannot replace professional judgment; instead, they serve as a valuable supplement to inform decision-making. The resulting information derived from ARAIs plays a crucial role in making well-informed decisions regarding treatment, supervision, and management strategies aimed at reducing the potential for violence. By incorporating these evidence-based tools, professionals can enhance their understanding of individual risk profiles and implement targeted interventions to ensure public safety. Commonly used actuarial risk assessment tools are located in Table 11.4.

Structured professional judgment (*SPJ*) is an approach to risk assessment and decision-making that combines evidence-based structured tools with the professional judgment of practitioners. Unlike the unstructured approach that relies on individual impressions and experience, SPJ is a data-driven, systematic approach that promotes transparency and consistency without sacrificing flexibility. This approach includes clear definitions for each rated item and coding rule. It allows for the exercise of professional judgment in determining violence risk and provides guidance to evaluators without strict cutoffs or reliance on algorithms. The SPJ tools are designed for use by professionals in various fields, including general or forensic mental health, corrections, police, social services, and employment settings. These tools represent best practices and assist professionals in gathering and integrating information to make decisions in cases involving violence risk.

The SPJ approach has several advantages compared to other methods. First, SPJs are highly personalized, requiring evaluators to consider the frequency, severity, trajectory, and

TABLE 11.4 **VIOLENCE RISK ASSESSMENTS**

Assessment Tool	Purpose	Number of Items	Strengths	Limitations
Static-99 (Hanson & Thornton, 1999)	Most commonly used assessment for risk of sexual and violent recidivism in adult male sex offenders.	10 items	• Well established and strong psychometrics for adult male sex offenders. • Provides a structured approach to risk assessment.	• Limited applicability to other populations. • Graded risk or severity categories have low utility. • Training needed for administration.
Violence Risk Appraisal Guide-Revised (VRAG-R; Rice et al., 2013)	Assesses the risk of violent recidivism in individuals.	Not specified	• Revised version has improved predictive accuracy. • Provides detailed information about risk factors.	• Specific number of items not specified. • Limited information available on the instrument.
Level of Service Inventory-Revised (LSI-R; Andrews & Bonta, 2000)	Assesses the risk and needs of offenders to guide case management and treatment planning.	54 items in 10 subcomponents	• Comprehensive assessment of risk and needs. • Well-validated for use with offenders.	• Lengthy and takes significant time. • Requires training to administer.
Historical Clinical Risk Management-20 (HCR-20; Douglas & Reeves, 2011)	Assesses the risk of violence in individuals.	20 items	• Integrates historical, clinical, and risk management factors. • Structured approach to risk assessment.	• Requires training to administer. • Items do not predict violence, only risk.

relevance of each risk factor when assessing violence risk. This level of specificity allows for a more detailed and personalized evaluation. Second, SPJs help create risk management plans that go beyond numerical predictions and instead rely on a comprehensive understanding of an individual's history, current condition, and future intentions. Lastly, research has confirmed the effectiveness of SPJs. Comparative studies between actuarial and SPJ measures have shown that assessments using SPJ tools are equally proficient in predicting violence, thereby maintaining consistent ratings among evaluators. This consistency demonstrates the reliability and applicability of the SPJ approach in various professional settings.

Among the SPJ tools commonly employed are the Historical Clinical Risk Management-20 (HCR-20), the Short-Term Assessment of Risk and Treatability (START), and the Structured Assessment of Violence Risk in Youth (SAVRY).

REPORTING ABUSE AND NEGLECT

As a counselor, it's crucial to be aware of the ethical and legal obligations when encountering situations of potential abuse and neglect. Confidentiality is a cornerstone of therapeutic relationships, but it is subject to certain limitations. Despite the confidentiality inherent in the counselor–client relationship, there are situations where disclosure is mandated by law. In all 50 states, if a client poses a danger to themselves or others, or if there is suspicion of child/older adult/person with a disability abuse, counselors are required to report it to the authorities. Each state may have slight variations regarding when mental health professionals must file a report, but many states have duty-to-warn and duty-to-protect laws. It is critical that you know your own state laws as you enter counseling practice. To report incidents, counselors are advised to contact their local child or older adult protective services agency and the police department for guidance on the appropriate filing procedures. It is crucial for counselors to be well-versed in the state laws concerning mandated reporting to ensure compliance.

Child Abuse

Recognizing and addressing child abuse and neglect is a crucial first step in helping affected children. It's important to learn how to identify the signs, as the presence of a single sign may not necessarily indicate abuse, but repeated or combined signs warrant further investigation. If you suspect a child is being harmed, reporting your concerns can protect the child and provide assistance to the family. Anyone can report suspicions of child abuse and neglect, and certain professionals are legally obligated to do so under specific circumstances.

There are several signs that may indicate the presence of child abuse or neglect.

- *Child indicators*: These include sudden changes in behavior or school performance, unaddressed physical or medical issues, learning difficulties without apparent causes, a constant state of vigilance, lack of adult supervision, excessive compliance or withdrawal, and a reluctance to return home after school or activities.

- *Parental indicators*: Parents who show little concern for their child, deny or blame the child for problems, request harsh physical discipline from caregivers, view the child negatively, demand unattainable levels of performance, and rely on the child for emotional support exhibit concerning behaviors.

- *Parent–child relationship*: Signs of a strained parent–child relationship include minimal physical or visual interaction, a consistently negative perception of each other, and verbal expressions of not liking one another.

Abuse of Older Adults or Adults With Disabilities

A vulnerable adult refers to an individual above the age of 18 who faces challenges in meeting their own needs. These challenges can arise from factors such as aging or disabilities. Vulnerable adults are particularly susceptible to abuse, neglect, and financial exploitation due to their limited ability to protect themselves. Signs of abuse or neglect may include:

- indications or insinuations of experiencing abuse made by the individual;

- failure to have basic needs met, such as food, water, or adequate clothing;

- being left unattended for extended periods when a caregiver should be present;

- lack of necessary medical aids, such as glasses, dentures, walkers, medication, or hearing aids;

- failure to receive amenities or essential living essentials when a caregiver has control of their finances;

- sudden changes in behavior or character that are out of character;

- abrupt withdrawal, either voluntarily or due to a caregiver controlling their interactions with others;

- unexplained bruises, scrapes, burns, or other marks; and

- becoming a victim of forgery, fraud, theft, or other financial crimes.

UNDERSTANDING AND ASSESSING SUBSTANCE USE DISORDERS

Substance use screening is a common occurrence in most counseling settings, both at initial contact and in an ongoing manner. The American Society of Addiction Medicine (ASAM) defines *addiction* as "a treatable, chronic medical disease involving complex interactions among brain circuits, genetics, the environment, and an individual's life experiences" (ASAM, 2019, para. 1). With the publication of the *DSM-5*, the way we conceptualize addiction shifted toward a continuum in which abuse and addiction are viewed as part of a fluid, continuous spectrum. Listing 10 classes of drugs, the *DSM-5-TR* includes three substance-related classifications: Use, Intoxication, and Withdrawal (American Psychiatric Association, 2022). Symptoms are shared among substance-related disorders, as well as gambling disorder. These include: use in increasing amounts; unsuccessful attempts to control use; excessive time spent on activities related to use or effects; cravings; neglecting occupational, school, and/or other obligations due to use; interpersonal and social problems related to use; giving up major life activities due to use; engaging in dangerous behavior because of substance use; continued use with knowledge of psychologic or physical consequences; tolerance; and withdrawal (American Psychiatric Association, 2022).

With all substance use disorders, co-occurring disorders are more likely than not. SAMHSA (2021) reported that, in 2020, 6.7% of adults in the United States (about 17 million people) experienced both a mental illness and a substance use disorder. Because clients may use substances to mask, cope with, or manage mental illness symptomology, screening for substance use should include screening for co-occurring mental illness. Of concern are the rising rates of opioid use disorder and related mortality, particularly among young people (Peavy & Banta-Green, 2021). Counselors need tools for comprehensive and effective initial and ongoing assessments. In this section, we describe commonly used substance assessments, including the CAGE (**C**utting down, **A**nnoyance by criticism, **G**uilty feelings, **E**ye-opener), the AWARE (**A**dvanced **WA**rning of **RE**lapse) questionnaire, the Substance Abuse Subtle Screening Inventory-4 (SASSI-4), and the University of Rhode Island Change Assessment (URICA) scale. Additional resources are provided in Table 11.5.

Originally introduced by Ewing and Rouse, the *CAGE* is a four-question assessment with simple "yes" or "no" answers, intended for screening of potential alcohol abuse and addiction (O'Brien, 2008). The acronym includes four questions, based on "cutting down," "annoyance by criticism," "guilty feelings," and "eye-opener." Counselors can ask four questions, beginning with "Have you ever":

TABLE 11.5 ADDITIONAL ASSESSMENTS FOR SUBSTANCE USE DISORDER

Assessment Tool	Target Population	Purpose	Strengths/ Limitations	Additional Information
Alcohol, Smoking and Substance Involvement Screening Test (ASSIST)	At-risk adults	Developed by WHO to identify substance use and related disorders at multiple levels	Based on Motivational Interviewing tenets Brief Administered paper/pencil or electronically ASSIST-Y for young people Not validated for individuals under 18 years of age	WHO ASSIST Working Group (2002) www.who.int/publications/i/item/978924159938-2
Alcohol Use Disorders Identification Test-C (AUDIT-C)	Adults, problem or hazardous drinkers	Identification of hazardous drinking and active substance use disorder	Brief, three questions Easily scored Differing cutoff scores for men and women Strong sensitivity estimates Not validated for individuals under 18 years of age Focused nature may not provide a thorough perspective	Bush et al. (1998) https://pcssnow.org/wp-content/uploads/2017/04/AUDIT-C_Measure-and-Scoring.pdf
Screener and Opioid Assessment for Patients with Pain (SOAPP)© Version	Individuals prescribed or potentially prescribed opioids for pain management	Screening for potential opioid abuse and misuse	Attempts to predict aberrant drug use behavior Brief Easily score Sensitivity lower than other screening tools Focus on individuals who are prescribed opioids for pain	Finkelman et al. (2015) www.mcstap.com/docs/SOAPP-5.pdf

1. tried to cut down on drinking but could not?

2. been annoyed by criticism of your drinking?

3. felt badly or experienced guilt about drinking?

4. begun drinking in the morning to get rid of a hangover or steady your nerves?

Answers in the affirmative for two or three of these questions indicates a "high index of suspicion," and yes to all four is "virtually diagnostic" for alcohol use disorder (AUD; O'Brien, 2008, p. 2054). The CAGE has the advantage of being brief and easily added to the assessment process. Dhalla and Kopec (2007) reported that CAGE scores are associated with evidence of high test-retest reliability and adequate correlation with similar instruments. However, counselors should note that the CAGE was developed prior to *DSM-5* conceptualizations of AUD.

The CAGE was cojoined for use with other substances by adding Adapted to Include Drugs (CAGE-AID; Brown et al., 1998). The counselor is to encourage the client using the prompt, "When thinking about drug use, include illegal drug use and the use of prescription drugs other than as prescribed," followed by the addition of "Or other drug use" to the end of the four previously noted questions (Brown et al., 1998, p. 102). Another adaptation is the Family CAGE-AID, intended to screen non-substance using members for substance dependence within the family (Basu et al., 2016). This assessment cojoins the Family CAGE (Frank et al., 1992) and the CAGE-AID. The Family CAGE adds "or anyone in your family" to the four "have your ever" questions. For example, "Have you ever felt that you or anyone in your family should cut down on your/their drinking?" (Frank et al., 1992). The Family CAGE-AID includes Adapted to Include Drugs to this version. The Family CAGE has evidence of strong internal consistency reliability (coefficient alpha = .84–.89) and offers evidence of construct validity through correlations with similar assessments. Scores on the Family CAGE-AID demonstrated strong correlations with *International Classification of Diseases*, Tenth Edition (*ICD-10*; WHO, 1990) symptom scores (Basu et al., 2016). The CAGE and the CAGE-AID are available online through the American Addiction Centers at https://americanaddictioncenters.org/alcoholism-treatment/cage-questionnaire-assessment.

Developed by Gorski and Miller (1982) for the purpose of predicting potential for relapse, the *Advanced WArning of RElaspe (AWARE) questionnaire 3.0* is a 28-item self-report scale with responses falling on a rating scale of 1 to 7 (Miller & Harris, 2000). Examples of the questionnaire statements include: "I feel nervous or unsure of my ability to stay sober" and "I have many problems in my life." When selecting a number in response to statements, clients would consider "how much this has been true for you," with 1 reflecting "never" and 7 reflecting "always." Scores range from 28 to 196, with high scores representing more warning signs of relapse endorsed by the client. Probability of heavy drinking based on these scores is given for those abstinent for the two prior months and those who are still drinking. Miller and Harris found evidence of good prediction of relapse occurrence ($r = .42$, $p < .001$). The AWARE questionnaire, along with scoring and interpretation, is publicly available through the https://adai.uw.edu/instruments/pdf/Advanced_Warning_of_Relapse_39.pdf.

The *Substance Abuse Subtle Screening Inventory-4* (*SASSI-4*; Lazowski & Geary, 2016) is a 105 question, self-report assessment, intended to identify probability of a substance use disorder, including among those clients who may be defensive or denying symptoms (Balkin & Juhnke, 2018). This assessment includes 74 true or false questions, many of which indirectly, or subtly, address substance abuse and addiction. Thirty-one face-valid questions ask directly about alcohol and other drugs. Additionally, the SASSI-4 breaks down responses on 11 scales, as follows: Face-Valid Alcohol, Face-Valid Other Drug, Symptoms, Obvious Attributes, Subtle Attributes, Defensiveness, Supplemental Addiction Measure, Family versus Control Subjects, Correctional, Random Answering Pattern, and Prescription Drug Abuse. Each of these scales provides the counselor with useful information in terms of the relationship with alcohol and other substances (Balkin & Juhnke, 2018).

Identified as one of the most commonly used alcohol assessments by addiction counselors (Juhnke et al., 2003), this instrument is available in paper/pencil and electronic formats, for a fee. The SASSI-4 is easily hand-scored and electronic versions provide a report that includes a narrative report and a graph of the client's scale scores, along with decision rules outcomes resulting from the client scores (SASSI Institute, 2018). Evidence of reliability and validity are provided on the SASSI Institute website, and both are based on Lazowski and Geary's (2016) study of this instrument. The report concludes that the SASSI-4 has high reliability, demonstrated through internal consistency and test-retest methods. Further, this instrument has high positive predictive power in terms of *DSM* diagnosis of Substance Use Disorder at 97%. Additional information is located on the SASSI website (https://sassi.com/sassi-online-faqs).

The *University of Rhode Island Change Assessment (URICA) scale* (Prochaska & DiClemente et al., 1983), sometimes referred to as the Decisional Balance Scale, aims to identify the stage of change an individual is experiencing related to a specific behavior, such as drinking cessation. Based on Prochaska and DiClemente's grant-funded transtheoretical model (TTM) that identifies the sequence or "stages" that individuals move through when attempting to change their behavior, this assessment is available for alcohol, tobacco, substance, and other targets of behavioral change. The TTM posits that change is a process; within this process, people travel through specific stages when considering if they want to change their behaviors. The stages are: precontemplation, contemplation, preparation, action, maintenance, and termination (Prochaska & DiClemente, 1983). The URICA measures four of these stages, excluding preparation and termination. Precontemplation indicates low readiness for change, whereas action and maintenance indicate higher readiness. The 28-item alcohol version of the URICA is a self-report measure with five possible responses, with ratings from 1 (strongly disagree) to 5 (strongly agree). The resulting range of scores is 28 to 140. Clients are asked to circle the number that describes the extent to which they disagree or agree with the statements. An example statement is, "As far as I'm concerned, I don't have any problems that need changing." For this instrument, the counselor is directed to tell the client that "problems" are those related to drinking. The question numbers are associated with one of the four measured stages of change. When scoring, the numeric responses are listed under the associated stage, with four responses being intentionally omitted, leaving seven responses for each stage. Means are calculated for each stage, giving comparison information. For the final step, the mean for precontemplation is subtracted from the sum of the other three stages for an overall readiness score. Cut-off scores for each stage are provided as well at www.guilford.com/add/miller11_old/urica.pdf?t=1. As stated throughout this book, counselors take a multidimensional approach to assessment and consider data from multiple sources prior to gaining a full understanding of the client's needs, strengths, and worldview.

As discussed in the chapter, the integration of assessment scores into the therapeutic process presents an opportunity to enhance treatment outcomes significantly. Through a comprehensive understanding of the scores and their implications, counselors can tailor their approach to meet the unique needs of their clients, fostering greater efficacy of interventions. By using assessment data for treatment planning and decision-making, counselors encourage a more evidence-based and targeted approach to therapy. The role of communication in the assessment process is also noteworthy. Effective communication can significantly enhance the therapeutic journey's overall outcome from conveying assessment findings to stakeholders to encouraging reflective practices. Communicating assessment findings involves empathy, understanding, and respect for the client's feelings and reactions. Moreover, the report should be comprehensive, clearly highlighting both the strengths and weaknesses while considering the influences of social, ethnic, racial, and cultural variables on the results. The use of assessment results for the formulation of treatment plans, case conceptualization, and routine outcome monitoring underscores the pivotal role of assessments in the counseling process. By making assessment results understandable and accessible to clients, we empower them to actively participate in their therapeutic journey. Furthermore, through case conceptualization, we can develop a structured understanding of the client's situation, helping to guide treatment and anticipate potential challenges. With the aid of progress monitoring tools and routine outcome monitoring, we can continually assess the effectiveness of therapy, making necessary adjustments to ensure optimal outcomes.

END-OF-CHAPTER RESOURCES

DISCUSSION QUESTIONS

Counselors use informal assessment methods for determining trauma history in the first session. They may ask questions such as, "Have you experienced events that caused you acute stress?", "Have these events resulted in dreams or nightmares?", "Have you experienced reliving the event(s) during waking hours?", and "Do you avoid people or locations that remind you of the event?" Many other questions apply to both trauma history and PTS.

1. How would you approach the client with questions related to trauma?

2. What additional questions could you ask?

3. What impact does creating a relationship/forming a bond with the client have on how you approach assessing trauma history?

4. What are the fears that you may have when engaging in this type of discussion?

5. What are the warning signs for suicidal behavior and NSSI? How do these differ?

Counselors use informal assessment methods for determining level of risk in the first session. They may ask, "Have you had thoughts of harming or killing yourself?" or state "You have reported symptoms of depression that are severe. Are you thinking of ending your life?"

6. How would you approach questions related to suicidality?

7. What impact does creating a relationship/forming a bond with the client have when asking these questions?

8. What are the fears that you may have when engaging in this type of discussion?

CLASS ACTIVITIES

1. Split up into groups of three for a role-play. One member will role-play a counselor and another member will role-play a suicidal client. As the role-play unfolds, a third member will document the suicide assessment. Following this role-play, all three members will apply the SAFE-T protocol and determine level of care recommendations.

2. In groups of two or more, take turns describing how you would assess a client for violence or risk of self-harm.

3. Using the PTGI, assess yourself in terms of growth. Do you agree with the scale outcome? In what ways would you like to grow?

4. As a class, we will review the substance abuse screening tools located in Table 11.5. Compare and contrast these instruments with other assessments of substance use disorders.

5. Take a look at the suicide risk factors and screening inventories. Come up with your own acronym that helps you remember what to do when screening for suicidality in clients. Practice using your acronym in a role-play with a partner.

PERSPECTIVE FROM THE FIELD

Chapter 11 covers assessment of trauma, harm, suicidal injuries, and NSSI, as well as substance abuse measures. Dr. Casey A. Barrio Minton reflects on practical methods and strategies for engaging in suicide assessment with different types of clients and a variety of settings. She describes a practice model for assessment and for intervention, and she talks about how to differentiate between suicidal ideation and NSSI. Dr. Barrio Minton covers how to determine degrees of harm and lethality, as well as asking targeted questions which not only provide insight into the client's level of risk but also elicit methods for instilling hope whenever possible. Dr. Barrio Minton is a professor of counselor education and head of the Department of Educational Psychology and Counseling at the University of Tennessee, Knoxville. Her scholarly work focuses on crisis intervention, clinical mental health issues, and professionalization through teaching and leadership. Dr. Barrio Minton is author or editor of several books and was founding editor of the *Journal of Counselor Leadership and Advocacy*, and she is serving as the incoming editor of *Counselor Education and Supervision*. Dr. Barrio Minton is a past-president of Chi Sigma Iota International, the Association for Assessment and Research in Counseling, the Southern Association for Counselor Education and Supervision, and the Association for Counselor Education and Supervision. She is a Fellow of the ACA.

Access podcasts via the QR code or http://connect.springerpub.com/content/book/978-0-8261-8913-4/chapter/ch00.

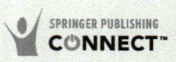 A robust set of instructor resources designed to supplement this text is located at http://connect.springerpub.com/content/book/978-0-8261-8913-4. Qualifying instructors may request access by emailing textbook@springerpub.com.

REFERENCES

American Counseling Association. (n.d.). *Fact Sheet: Vicarious trauma*. California Department of Corrections and Rehabilitation. https://www.cdcr.ca.gov/bph/wp-content/uploads/sites/161/2021/10/Trauma-Fact-Sheets-October-2021.pdf

American Counseling Association. (2014). *2014 ACA code of ethics*. https://www.counseling.org/docs/default-source/default-document-library/ethics/2014-aca-code-of-ethics.pdf

American Psychiatric Association. (2013). *Diagnostic and statistical manual of mental disorders* (5th ed.). https://doi.org/10.1176/appi.books.9780890425596

American Psychiatric Association. (2022). *Diagnostic and statistical manual of mental disorders* (5th ed., text rev.). https://doi.org/10.1176/appi.books.9780890425787

American Psychiatric Association Work Group on Suicidal Behaviors. (2003). *Practice guideline for the assessment and treatment of patients with suicidal behaviors*. American Psychiatric Association. https://psychiatryonline.org/pb/assets/raw/sitewide/practice_guidelines/guidelines/suicide.pdf

American Society of Addiction Medicine. (2019). *Definition of addiction*. https://www.asam.org/quality-care/definition-of-addiction

Andrews, D. A., & Bonta, J. (2000). *The level of service inventory-revised*. Multi-Health Systems.

Balkin, R. S. & Junkie, G. A. (2018). *Assessment in counseling: Practice and application*. Oxford University Press.

Basu, D., Ghosh, A., Hazari, N., & Parakh, P. (2016). Use of Family CAGE-AID questionnaire to screen the family members for diagnosis of substance dependence. *Indian Journal of Medical Research, 143*(6), 722–730. https://doi.org/10.4103/0971-5916.191931

Benjet, C., Bromet, E., Karam, E. G., Kessler, R. C., McLaughlin, K. A., Ruscio, A. M., & Koenen, K. C. (2016). The epidemiology of traumatic event exposure worldwide: Results from the World Mental Health Survey Consortium. *Psychological Medicine, 46*(2), 327–343. https://doi.org/10.1017/S0033291715001981

Bolton, J., Spiwak, R., & Sareen, J. (2012). Predicting suicide attempts with the SAD PERSONS scale: A longitudinal analysis. *The Journal of Clinical Psychiatry, 73*, 735–741. https://doi.org/10.4088/JCP.11m07362

Brown, R. L., Leonard, T., Saunders, L. A., & Papasouliotis, O. (1998). The prevalence and detection of substance use disorders among inpatients ages 18 to 49: An opportunity for prevention. *Prevention Medicine, 27*(1), 101–110. https://doi.org/10.1006/pmed.1997.0250

Buser, T., & Buser, J. (2013). The HIRE model: A tool for the informal assessment of nonsuicidal self-injury. *Journal of Mental Health Counseling, 35*(3), 262–281. https://doi.org/10.17744/mehc.35.3.h27684682833phk1

Bush, K., Kivlahan, D. R., McDonell, M. B., & Bradley, K. A. (1998). The AUDIT Alcohol Consumption Questions (AUDIT-C): An effective brief screening test for problem drinking. *Archives Internal Medicine, 3*, 1789–1795. https://doi.org/10.1001/archinte.158.16.1789

Centers for Disease Control and Prevention. (n.d.). *Violence risk assessment tools*. The National Institute for Occupational Safety and Health. https://wwwn.cdc.gov/WPVHC/Nurses/Course/Slide/Unit6_8

Centers for Disease Control and Prevention. (2023). *Preventing suicide requires a comprehensive approach*. https://www.cdc.gov/suicide/pdf/2023_CDC_SuicidePrevention_Infographic.pdf

Centers for Disease Control and Prevention. (2024a, April 25). *Risk and protective factors for suicide*. https://www.cdc.gov/suicide/risk-factors/index.html

Centers for Disease Control and Prevention. (2024b, May 16). *About adverse childhood experiences*. https://www.cdc.gov/aces/about/index.html

The Center for Victims of Torture. (2021). *Professional Quality of Life*. https://proqol.org

The Columbia Lighthouse Project. (2016). *About the protocol: A unique suicide risk screening tool*. https://cssrs.columbia.edu/the-columbia-scale-c-ssrs/about-the-scale

Council for Accreditation of Counseling and Related Educational Programs. (2023). *2024 CACREP standards*. https://www.cacrep.org/wp-content/uploads/2023/06/Combined-version-6.21.23.pdf

Craigen, L. M., Healey, A. C., Walley, C. T., Byrd, R., & Schuster, J. (2010). Assessment and self-injury: Implications for counselors. *Measurement and Evaluation in Counseling and Development, 43*(1). 3–15. https://doi.org/10.1177/0748175610362237

Cull, J. G., & Gill, W. S. (1992). *Manual for the Suicide Probability Scale*. Western Psychological Services.

Dhalla, S., & Kopec, J. A. (2007). The CAGE questionnaire for alcohol misuse: A review of reliability and validity studies. *Clinical Investigative Medicine, 30*(1), 33–41. https://doi.org/10.25011/cim.v30i1.447

Douglas, K. S., & Reeves, K. A. (2011). Historical Clinical Risk Management-20 (HCR-20) violence risk assessment scheme: Rationale, application, and empirical overview. In K. S. Douglas & R. K. Otto (Eds.), *Handbook of violence risk assessment* (pp. 157–196). Taylor & Francis Group.

Dube, S. R., Williamson, D. F., Thompson, T., Felitti, V. F., & Anda, R., F. (2004). Assessing the reliability of retrospective reports of adverse childhood experiences among adult HMO members attending a primary care clinic. *Child Abuse & Neglect, 28*(7) 729–737. https://doi.org/10.1016/j.chiabu.2003.08.009

Duffey, T., & Haberstroh, S. (2020). *Introduction to crisis and trauma counseling*. American Counseling Association.

Emelianchik-Key, K. E. (2019). Assessment and diagnosis. In K. Emelianchik-Key & A. La Guardia (Eds.), *Nonsuicidal self-injury throughout the lifespan: A clinicians guide for treatment outcomes* (pp. 76–101). Routledge.

Emelianchik-Key, K. E., & La Guardia, A. (2019). *Nonsuicidal self-injury throughout the lifespan: A clinicians guide for treatment outcomes*. Routledge.

Erford, B. T., Jackson, J., Bardhoshi, G., Duncan, K., & Atalay, Z. (2018). Selecting suicide ideation assessment instruments: A meta-analytic review. *Measurement and Evaluation in Counseling and Development, 51*(1), 42–59. https://doi.org/10.1080/07481756.2017.1358062

Felitti, V. J., Anda, R. F., Nordenberg, D., Williamson, D. F., Spitz, A. M., Edwards, V., Koss, M. P., & Marks, J. S. (1998). Relationship of childhood abuse and household dysfunction to many of the leading causes of death in adults. The Adverse Childhood Experiences (ACE) study. *American Journal of Preventive Medicine, 14*(4), 245–258. https://doi.org/10.1016/s0749-3797(98)00017-8

Finkelman, M. D., Kulich, R. J., Zacharoff, K. L., Smits, N., Magnuson, B. E., Dong J., & Butler, S. F. (2015). Shortening the Screener and Opioid Assessment for Patients with Pain-Revised (SOAPP-R): A proof-of-principle study for customized computer-based testing. *Pain Medicine, 16*(12), 2344–2356. https://doi.org/10.1111/pme.12864

Frank, S. H., Graham, A. V., Zyzanski, S. J., & White, S. (1992). Use of the Family CAGE in screening for alcohol problems in primary care. *Archives of Family Medicine, 1*, 209–216. https://doi.org/10.1001/archfami.1.2.209

Giddens, J. M., Sheehan, K. H., & Sheehan, D. V. (2014). The Columbia-Suicide Severity Rating Scale (C-SSRS): Has the "gold standard" become a liability? *Innovations in Clinical Neuroscience, 11*(9–10), 66–80. PMID: 25520890.

Gorski, T. F., & Miller, M. (1982). *Counseling for relapse prevention*. Herald House—Independence Press.

Gratz, K. L. (2001). Measurement of deliberate self-harm: Preliminary data on the Deliberate Self-Harm Inventory. *Journal of Psychopathology and Behavioral Assessment, 23*(4), 253–263. https://doi.org/10.1023/A:1012779403943

Gratz, K. L., Latzman, R. D., Young, J., Heiden, L. J., Damon, J., Hight, T., & Tull, M. T. (2012). Deliberate self-harm among underserved adolescents: The moderating roles of gender, race, and school-level and association with borderline personality features. *Personality Disorders: Theory, Research, and Treatment, 3*(1), 39–54. https://doi.org/10.1037/a0022104

Green, J. D., Hatgis, C., Kearns, J. C., Nock, M. H., & Marx, B. P. (2017). The Direct and Indirect Self-Harm Inventory (DISH): A new measure for assessing high-risk and self-harm behaviors among military veterans. *Psychology of Men & Masculinity, 18*(3), 208–214. https://doi.org/10.1037/men0000116

Hanson, R. K., & Thornton, D. (1999). *Static-99: Improving actuarial risk assessments for sex offenders* (User Report 99-02). Department of the Solicitor General of Canada.

Harcourt, B. E. (2007). *Against prediction: Profiling, policing, and punishing in an actuarial age*. University of Chicago Press.

Hoberman, H. M., & Garfinkel, B. D. (1988). Completed suicide in children and adolescents. *Journal of the American Academy of Child and Adolescent Psychiatry, 27*(6), 689–695. https://doi.org/10.1097/00004583-198811000-00004

Hockberger, R. S., & Rothstein, R. J. (1988). Assessment of suicide potential by non psychiatrists using the SAD PERSONS score. *The Journal of Emergency Medicine, 6*(2), 99–107. https://doi.org/10.1016/0736-4679(88)90147-3

Huth-Bocks, A. C., Kerr, D. C. R., Ivey, A. Z., Kramer, A. C., & King, C. A. (2007). Assessment of psychiatrically hospitalized suicidal adolescents. *Journal of the American Academy of Child & Adolescent Psychiatry, 46*(3), 387–395. https://doi.org/10.1097/chi.0b013e31802b9535

International Society for Traumatic Stress Studies. (2023). *Clinician administered PTSD scale*. https://istss.org/clinical-resources/adult-trauma-assessments/clinician-administered-ptsd-scale

Joiner, Jr., T. E. (2007). *Why people die by suicide*. Harvard University Press.

Juhnke, G. A. (1994). SAD PERSONS scale review. *Measurement & Evaluation in Counseling and Development, 27*(1), 325–327.

Juhnke, G. A. (1996). The adapted-SAD PERSONS: A suicide assessment scale designed for use with children. *Elementary School Guidance & Counseling, 30*(4), 252–258. https://www.jstor.org/stable/42871225

Juhnke, G. A., Vacc, N. A., Curtis, R. C., Coll, K. M., & Paredes, D. M. (2003). Assessment instruments used by addictions counselors. *Journal of Addictions and Offender Counseling, 23*(2), 66–72. https://doi.org/10.1002/j.2161-1874.2003.tb00171.x

Katz, C., Randall, J. R., Sareen, J., Chateau, D., Walld, R., Leslie, W. D., Wang, J. L., & Bolton, J. M. (2017). Predicting suicide with the SAD PERSONS scale. *Depression Anxiety, 34*(9), 809–816. https://doi.org/10.1002/da.22632

Kilpatrick, D. G., Resnick, H. S., Milanak, M. E., Miller, M. W., Keyes, K. M., & Friedman, M. J. (2013). National estimates of exposure to traumatic events and PTSD prevalence using *DSM-IV* and *DSM-5* criteria. *Journal of Traumatic Stress, 26*(5), 537–547. https://doi.org/10.1002/jts.21848

Lazowski, L. E., & Geary, B. B. (2016). Validation of the Adult Substance Abuse Subtle Screening Inventory-4 (SASSI-4). *European Journal of Psychological Assessment, 35*(1), 86–97. http://doi.org/10.1027/1015-5759/a000359

Miller, W. R., & Harris, R. J. (2000). A simple scale of Gorski's warning signs for relapse. *Journal of Studies on Alcohol, 61*, 759–765. https://doi.org/10.15288/jsa.2000.61.759

Nock, M. K. (2010). Self-injury. *Annual Review of Clinical Psychology, 6*, 339–363. https://doi.org/10.1146/annurev.clinpsy.121208.131258

O'Brien, C. P. (2008). The CAGE questionnaire for detection of alcoholism. *JAMA, 300*(17), 2054–2056. https://doi.org/10.1001/jama.2008.570

Paladino, D. A. (2020). Suicide prevention and intervention. In T. Duffey & S. Haberstroh (Eds.), *Introduction to crisis and trauma counseling* (pp. 137–164). American Counseling Association.

Patterson, W. M., Dohn, H. H., Bird, J., & Patterson, G. A. (1983). Evaluation of suicidal patients: The SAD PERSONS score. *Psychosomatics, 24*, 343–349. https://doi.org/10.1016/s0033-3182(83)73213-5

Peavy, K. M., & Banta-Green, C. (2021). *Understanding and supporting adolescents with an opioid use disorder*. Addictions, Drug & Alcohol Institute. http://adai.uw.edu/pubs/pdf/2021AdolescentsOUD.pdf

Posner, K., Brown, G. K., Stanley, B., Brent, D. A., Yershova, K. V., Oquendo, M. A., Currier, G. W., Melvin, G. A., Greenhill, L., Shen, S., & Mann, J. J. (2011). The Columbia-Suicide Severity Rating Scale: Initial validity and internal consistency findings from three multisite studies with adolescents and adults. *American Journal of Psychiatry, 168*, 1266–1277. https://doi.org/10.1176/appi.ajp.2011.10111704

Prochaska, J., & DiClemente, C. (1983). Stages and processes of self-change of smoking: Toward an integrative model of change. *Journal of Consulting and Clinical Psychology, 51*(3), 390–395. https://doi.org/10.1037//0022-006x.51.3.390

Rice, M. E., Harris, G. T., & Lang, C. (2013). Validation of and revision to the VRAG and SORAG: The Violence Risk Appraisal Guide—Revised (VRAG-R). *Psychological Assessment, 25*(3), 951–965. https://doi.org/10.1037/a0032878

Royal College of Psychiatrists. (2016). *Rethinking risk to others in mental health services* (Council Report 201). Author.

SASSI Institute. (2018). *Substance use measures*. https://sassi.com/clinical-faqs

Shaffer, D. (1988). The epidemiology of teen suicide: An examination of risk factors. *The Journal of Clinical Psychiatry, 49*(9, Suppl), 36–41. PMID: 3047106.

Singh, J. P., Desmarais, S. L., Hurducas, C., Arbach-Lucioni, K., Condemarin, C., Dean, K., ... & Otto, R. K. (2014). International perspectives on the practical application of violence risk assessment: A global survey of 44 countries. *International Journal of Forensic Mental Health, 13*(3), 193–206. https://doi.org/10.1080/14999013.2014.922141

Stamm, B. H. (2009). *Professional Quality of Life: Compassion Satisfaction and Fatigue version 5 (ProQOL)*. https://img1.wsimg.com/blobby/go/dfc1e1a0-a1db-4456-9391-18746725179b/downloads/ProQOL_5_English.pdf?ver=1712345351117

Stamm, B. H. (2010). *The concise ProQOL manual* (2nd ed.). ProQOL.org.

Starr, S. (2014). Evidence-based sentencing and the scientific rationalization of discrimination. *Stanford Law Review, 66*(4), 803–872. https://papers.ssrn.com/sol3/papers.cfm?abstract_id=2318940

Substance Abuse and Mental Health Services Administration. (2009). *SAFE-T pocket card.* https://store.samhsa.gov/sites/default/files/sma09-4432.pdf

Substance Abuse and Mental Health Services Administration. (2021). *Key substance use and mental health indicators in the United States: Results from the 2020 National Survey on Drug Use and Health* (HHS Publication No. PEP21-07-01-003, NSDUH Series H-56). https://www.samhsa.gov/data

Tedeschi, R. G., & Calhoun, L. G. (1996). The posttraumatic growth inventory: Measuring the positive legacy of trauma. *Journal of Traumatic Stress, 9*, 455–471. https://doi.org/10.1007/BF02103658

Viljoen, J. L., Cochrane, D. M., & Jonnson, M. R. (2018). Do risk assessment tools help manage and reduce risk of violence and reoffending? A systematic review. *Law and Human Behavior, 42*(3), 181–214. https://doi.org/10.1037/lhb0000280

Wachter, A. (2015). *Statewide risk assessment in juvenile probation.* https://www.ojp.gov/ncjrs/virtual-library/abstracts/statewide-risk-assessment-juvenile-probation

Weathers, F. W., Blake, D. D., Schnurr, P. P., Kaloupek, D. G., Marx, B. P., & Keane, T. M. (2013a). *The Clinician-Administered PTSD Scale for DSM-5 (CAPS-5).* www.ptsd.va.gov

Weathers, F. W., Blake, D. D., Schnurr, P. P., Kaloupek, D. G., Marx, B. P., & Keane, T. M. (2013b). *The Life Events Checklist for DSM-5 (LEC-5)–Standard.* https://www.ptsd.va.gov/professional/assessment/te-measures/life_events_checklist.asp

Weathers, F. W., Blake, D. D., Schnurr, P. P., Kaloupek, D. G., Marx, B. P., & Keane, T. M. (2015). *The Clinician-Administered PTSD Scale for DSM-5 (CAPS-5)–Past week.* https://www.ptsd.va.gov

Weathers, F. W., Bovin, M. J., Lee, D. J., Sloan, D. M., Schnurr, P. P., Kaloupek, D. G., Keane, T. M., & Marx, B. P. (2018). The Clinician-Administered PTSD Scale for *DSM-5* (CAPS-5): Development and initial psychometric evaluation in military veterans. *Psychological Assessment, 30*(3), 383–395. https://doi.org/10.1037/pas0000486

Westers, N. J., Muehlenkamp, J. J., & Lau, M. (2016). SOARS model: Risk assessment of nonsuicidal self-injury. *Contemporary Pediatrics, 33*(7), 25–31. https://www.contemporarypediatrics.com/view/soars-model-risk-assessment-nonsuicidal-self-injury

Whitlock, J., Exner-Cortens, D., & Purington, A. (2014). Assessment of nonsuicidal self-injury: Development and initial validation of the Non-Suicidal Self-Injury (NSSI-AT). *Psychological Assessment, 26*(3), 935. https://doi.org/10.1037/a0036615

WHO ASSIST Working Group. (2002). The Alcohol, Smoking and Substance Involvement Screening Test (ASSIST): Development, reliability, and feasibility. *Addiction, 97*, 1183–1194. http://doi.org/10.1046/j.1360-0443.2002.00185.x

Wolpe, J. (1969). Basic principles and practices of behavior therapy of neuroses. *The American Journal of Psychiatry, 125*(9), 1242–1247. https://doi.org/10.1176/ajp.125.9.1242

World Health Organization. (n.d.). *Stress.* https://www.who.int/news-room/questions-and-answers/item/stress#:~:text=What%20is%20stress%3F,experiences%20stress%20to%20some%20degree

World Health Organization. (1990). *International statistical classification of diseases and related health problems* (10th rev.). https://icd.who.int/browse10/2019/en

12

The Assessment Process in Counseling

AYSE TORRES, CARMAN S. GILL, AND KELLY EMELIANCHIK-KEY

2024 CACREP STANDARD

3.G.17. procedures for using assessment results for referral and consultation

I remember when I completed a nearly perfect biopsychosocial-spiritual. The client and I had really good rapport and she was ready for change. I asked the questions, with solid follow-up, and gathered a ton of information. When she left, I looked at all the information I had gathered and became overwhelmed. What was I going to do with all of this data? How would I make sense of it and make a good plan for her treatment?

INTENTIONALITY IN ASSESSMENT

Determining the direction of counseling and which assessments are necessary can be a bit nebulous for new counselors. Strauser and Greco offer a five-step model, based on problem-solving principles, for rehabilitation counselors toward maximizing therapeutic efficacy (2020). These steps begin with problem orientation, as counselors assess client awareness and readiness for change. Step two includes problem identification, in which both individuals work collaboratively to clearly define the presenting issues. Step three encourages a generation of ideas toward resolving the problem. Here, the client's strengths heavily influence the generation of ideas. Decision-making is the fourth step, in which the counselor and client weigh the likelihood of success for each of the generated ideas, anticipate obstacles, and determine the attractiveness of the idea for the client. The final step, verification, includes a collaboration in which the counselor and client evaluate the process and determine if the problem is diminished or resolved (Strauser & Greco, 2020). Reassessment based on measurable outcomes and preselected instruments is important here.

Based on this problem-solving model and Adler's stages of psychotherapy (establishing a relationship, psychologic investigation, interpretation, reorientation [Sweeney, 2019]), we posit a cyclical model of the assessment process, which encourages counselors to engage in ongoing evaluation and reevaluation in counseling. We encourage a cycle that includes both initial and ongoing assessment, administration of specific measures, communication of findings, co-constructed interpretation, implementation, and routine outcome evaluation (ROM). ROM, which we discuss later in this chapter, is a standard part of counseling practice. Further, competent counselors are not only intentional in terms of the assessment process, but they are also aware of the systemic nature of assessment and intentionally maximize communication and integration of results. Figure 12.1 is a graphic representation of this process.

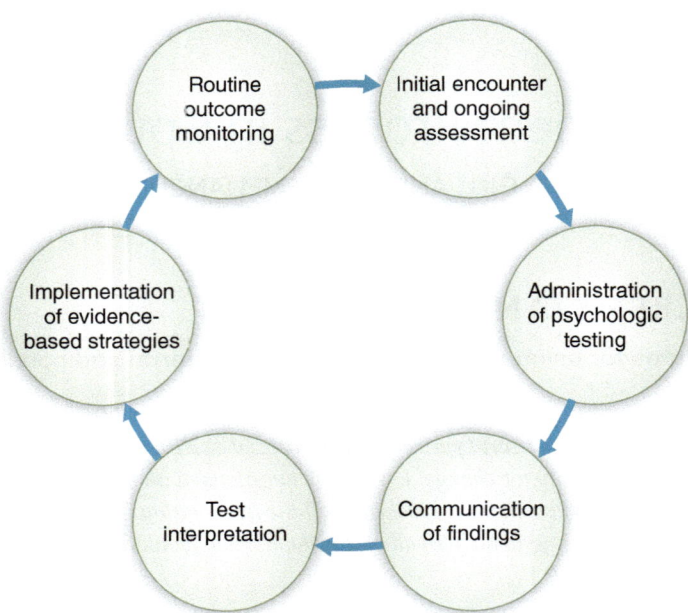

FIGURE 12.1. **Cycle of assessment in counseling.**

AN INTEGRATED APPROACH TO COMMUNICATION

Assessment plays a vital role in the therapeutic process, going beyond mere data collection. Results foster transparency, guide decision-making, and drive continuous improvement throughout the therapeutic journey. The results act as essential tools for understanding a client's strengths, weaknesses, abilities, and areas of concern, ultimately shaping the course of therapeutic intervention. Additionally, assessment results provide a structured, comprehensive, and tangible record of a client's progress over time. It is the counselor's responsibility to effectively communicate the results to individuals entitled to receive the information. Effective communication is crucial in delivering assessment results, as it fosters shared understanding and collaborative decision-making. These reports also serve as reliable references for future sessions and other mental health professionals involved in the client's care. From initial contact to termination of the counseling relationship, counselors engage in the assessment process in some way, and in an ethical manner that is consistent with the counseling process itself. Consider the steps or stages of Adlerian counseling which we discussed earlier. We know as counselors that assessment in general is infused in all client contact. However, counselors' approach to assessment interactions with clients throughout the various stages can contribute to positive treatment outcomes. The common factors theory of counseling may inform this process in terms of establishing and maintaining the relationship. Common factors theorists posit that change occurs due to elements shared by most if not all therapies and that these elements form a transtheoretical model which is the key to helping and healing (Wampold, 2015). These elements include, but are not limited to, the therapeutic alliance, empathy, goal consensus and collaboration, genuineness, positive regard, and mastery (Nahum et al., 2019), as well as emotional experience (Peluso & Freund, 2018), Further, working from a common factors mindset while engaging in assessment for each stage of counseling may result in higher rates of client retention (Luedke et al., 2017), more effective therapeutic interaction, and overall symptom reduction (Nahum et al., 2019). The therapeutic alliance is arguably the most well-researched component of this model and includes tasks, goals, and bonds. Bonds refer to the "real relationship," a genuine relationship, free of transference (Wampold, 2015). It is within this relationship, embedded in empathy and genuine concern for client well-being, that counselors approach clients to collaborate on effective, systemic assessment.

Communicating Assessment Findings

When presenting findings, it can be highly beneficial, and sometimes even essential, to involve additional individuals beyond the client while ensuring confidentiality and adhering to proper consent procedures. This may include not only parents or legal guardians (especially for minors), but also caregivers, teachers, mental health professionals, and other relevant stakeholders who play a significant role in the client's life. By engaging these individuals in the process, a more comprehensive and holistic perspective can be achieved, which ultimately enhances the overall understanding and impact of the findings. Moreover, in cases where clients are required to undergo court-mandated assessments, counselors may need to effectively communicate the assessment results to the court or court officials, ensuring that the information is accurately conveyed and understood within the legal context. Maintaining confidentiality in the communication of assessment results is crucial. It respects and protects an individual's privacy, fostering trust in the professional relationship. Sharing sensitive information can have serious consequences, such as legal implications, damage to reputation, or psychologic harm. Therefore, it is critical to uphold the highest standards of confidentiality when communicating assessment results, ensuring that information is only shared with authorized individuals and contexts. This not only safeguards the individuals involved but also preserves the integrity of the assessment process.

The process of effectively communicating assessment findings involves several key steps that aim to ensure a comprehensive understanding of the results. The initial step to engage in presenting assessment results is to ensure that you create a safe and collaborative environment where clients feel safe engaging in conversation about topics that can sometimes be sensitive in nature. When sharing the assessment outcomes with the client, it is crucial for the counselor to engage in an open and empathetic discussion to gauge the client's feelings and reactions toward the assessment and its administration. By understanding the client's attitudes and perceptions, valuable context can be obtained, which enhances the interpretation of the results. Next, counselors should provide clarity and structure for the interpretation process. This can be achieved by restating the purpose of the assessment and outlining how the scores will be presented. It is important for the counselor to convey this explanation in a language that is accessible and free of complex professional jargon, ensuring that the client fully comprehends the information being conveyed.

When reviewing assessment results, it is vital for counselors and clients to collaborate in examining the actual assessment so clients can feel empowered and take ownership in the process. The counselor should offer a concise yet comprehensive explanation of the implications of the results, emphasizing their significance while also addressing their limitations. This approach is important to avoid any misunderstandings and to ensure that the client fully grasps the meaning and relevance of the assessment outcomes. Sensitivity and empathy are essential throughout this process to create a safe and supportive environment for the client. When the client feels supported, they will be able to engage in self-reflective dialogue and gain new personal insights. Additionally, using a strengths-based framework to facilitate the conversation will allow the client to focus on resources and positive qualities, as opposed to focusing on things they may consider to be negative in the assessment scores. To integrate the assessment results in the therapeutic process, the counselor combines the information collected with other pertinent client information. This holistic approach allows the client to relate the findings to their existing knowledge about the field being assessed, such as their abilities, attitudes, mental health symptoms, career interests, and values. By considering these additional factors, a more comprehensive understanding of the assessment results can be achieved, enabling the client to make informed decisions and plans for the future. Furthermore, assessment results can also contribute to referrals and consultation with other helping professionals, as well as future planning. By utilizing the assessment findings in these ways, the counselor can support the client in further exploration and development, ensuring that the assessment process has a lasting impact on their personal growth and well-being.

Communicating Assessment Results: Writing the Assessment Report

Writing the assessment report is crucial for effective communication. It demands thorough preparation to ensure clarity, readability, and organization. Following the regulations of the Health Insurance Portability and Accountability Act (HIPAA), it is important to write the report in a manner easily understood by the client and any other individuals with whom counselors share the information. It should effectively highlight both strengths and weaknesses. The report should include a statement addressing the validity of the testing situation, taking into account social, ethnic, racial, and cultural variables that may influence the results. Exercise caution when interpreting test results and acknowledge any limitations when necessary. An assessment report comprises the following vital components that collectively provide a comprehensive understanding of the client and their situation. These components are instrumental in formulating an effective and suitable treatment plan, ensuring optimal outcomes.

- Demographic Information: The introduction of the report should provide a descriptive overview of the client, including their name, age, gender, grade or occupation, and relevant background information such as family dynamics or current living situation.

- Purpose and Source of Referral: This section establishes the purpose of the assessment and how it came about. If the client was referred by someone else, it is important to include the referrer's name and role in the referral process.

- Background Information: This section covers the client's personal, social, medical, educational, and vocational history, which may have an impact on their current situation. It is crucial to recognize and document any noteworthy events or experiences that could potentially affect the assessment results in this category (e.g., substance use/abuse).

- Assessment Procedures: This section provides detailed information on the specific tools and procedures employed to gather information about the client. It encompasses a range of methods such as standardized assessments, interviews, behavioral observations, and self-report questionnaires. Scores should be objectively written and conveyed in a way that is understood by any reader, which might include converting the scores (as noted in Chapter 6) or using percentile scores so they are easily understood.

- Behavioral Observations: This section presents comprehensive information about noteworthy behaviors exhibited by the client, including body language, verbal cues, facial expressions, and overall demeanor. It is important to include only relevant observations in this section.

- Assessment Results: This section provides a thorough analysis of the client's test results, including scores and interpretations. The information should be presented in an objective and professional manner, ensuring clarity and precision.

- Clinical Impressions/Diagnosis: Based on the assessment findings and additional gathered data, this section presents the clinician's impression or diagnosis of the client, including potential mental health disorders, developmental delays, or any other concerns that may arise.

- Recommendations: This section provides professional recommendations based on the assessment results and clinical impressions. These recommendations may encompass therapy options, referrals to specialists, or accommodations in an educational setting.

- Conclusions: This section provides a concise overview of the assessment, highlighting key findings with emphasis.

- Additional Resources: This section provides a comprehensive compilation of resources that can benefit the client or their support system. These resources encompass a wide range, including books, websites, and local support groups, specifically tailored to address their unique concerns.

Communicating Assessment Results: Treatment Planning

Counselors effectively utilize assessment results to collaboratively develop comprehensive and tailored treatment plans that address the unique needs of each individual client. This collaborative process involves active participation, open communication, and shared decision-making between the counselor and the client, fostering a trusting and empowering therapeutic relationship. By clearly presenting assessment outcomes and therapeutic objectives, counselors lay the groundwork for mutual understanding and shared treatment goals. When providing assessment results to clients, it is crucial to offer a developmentally appropriate explanation that makes them feel included. This may involve simplifying complex terminology into more accessible language, using metaphors or stories to convey the essence of the treatment plan. Additionally, involving caregivers in a balanced and ethical manner can enhance engagement and investment in counseling. By adopting a transparent and participative approach, counselors empower clients to become active architects of their own healing journey.

In order for clients to effectively advocate for themselves in this collaborative process, it is crucial that they grasp the valuable insights obtained from the assessment phase. Counselors face the delicate task of sharing essential assessment results and clinical impressions with clients. The approach to transparency must be executed ethically and compassionately, taking into account the client's readiness to receive, comprehend, and integrate this information. When providing feedback, counselors should prioritize the client's needs and focus on their strengths. The feedback should not only highlight areas for improvement but also recognize the client's inherent capacities and resources. It is crucial to approach diagnostic labels with sensitivity, emphasizing that they are not defining traits but rather tools for understanding and treatment planning. The process of discussing the results should be interactive, inviting the client's input and collaboration to create a treatment plan that aligns with their goals and values. Transitioning from assessment to action requires a delicate balance of honesty and tact. Counselors need to combine their analytical rigor with deep empathic skills to establish a foundation for successful therapeutic engagement.

The assessment findings provide valuable insights into the client's psychologic landscape, highlighting areas that require targeted intervention. When setting treatment goals, emotional well-being, cognitive functioning, interpersonal relationships, and behavioral patterns should be considered. The SMART methodology is a widely adopted approach for setting goals. SMART stands for Specific, Measurable, Achievable, Relevant, and Time-bound. This framework promotes clarity and attainability in goal setting, ensuring that objectives are well-defined and within reach. The SMART framework brings precision and accountability to the therapeutic process, offering a structured approach to evaluating progress. Another popular methodology is PROIE (Problem, Resources, Objectives, Interventions, and Evaluation), which establishes a comprehensive treatment agenda.

Advancements in technology offer new possibilities to enhance treatment planning. Platforms like TheraNest and SimplePractice come equipped with goal banks and template options, streamlining the planning process. Resource websites, such as Psychology Tools and Therapist Aid, serve as invaluable additions to a clinician's toolkit. These digital tools empower clinicians to create evidence-based, client-centered goals, thus elevating the quality of care and optimizing treatment outcomes. Importantly, just like case conceptualizations, treatment plans and their embedded goals are not static entities. As clients' needs evolve, counselors must dynamically adapt their therapeutic strategies to ensure treatment alignment is maintained. As we devise the best way to create treatment plans, counselors always ensure platforms that are HIPAA compliant and maintain client confidentiality are utilized.

Communicating Assessment Results: Case Conceptualization

Creating a thorough case conceptualization assists in systematically organizing and analyzing assessment findings in a comprehensive and structured manner. The case conceptualization goes beyond being a static document; it is a dynamic narrative that captures the rich nuances of the client's lived experience. Because case conceptualization is "a method and clinical strategy for obtaining and organizing information about a client, understanding and explaining the client's situation and maladaptive patterns, guiding and focusing treatment, anticipating challenges and roadblocks, and preparing for successful termination" (Sperry & Sperry, 2020, p. 4), this document serves as a roadmap for treatment, providing a clear understanding of the client's presenting issues, underlying factors, and potential treatment approaches.

There are numerous methodologies available for structuring the case conceptualization, each with its own unique components and emphasis. These models offer different perspectives and frameworks for understanding the client's concerns and formulating effective treatment plans. Table 12.1 presents various models for case conceptualizations and outlines their respective components. By engaging in a comprehensive case conceptualization process, practitioners can enhance their understanding of the client's needs and tailor interventions that are more aligned with their unique circumstances.

Although case conceptualization models are diverse, stemming from different theoretical orientations, they generally follow a similar structure, based on the scientific method. They typically include five components and may be reminiscent of the Adlerian stages we initially presented. These components usually have a flow resembling the following: problem

TABLE 12.1 **INCORPORATING THEORETICAL MODELS IN CASE CONCEPTUALIZATION**

Model	Target Reporting Areas	Contributors
Biopsychosocial-Spiritual	Biological, psychologic, social, spiritual	Sulmasy (2002)
Five Ps	Presenting issue, predisposing factors, precipitating factors, perpetuating factors, protective factors	Macneil et al. (2012)
Ecological Systems Theory	Microsystem, mesosystem, exosystemic, macrosystem	Bronfenbrenner (1979), Darling (2007)
Integrative Case Conceptualization	Blends elements from multiple theoretical frameworks to offer a comprehensive understanding of the client.	Sperry (2005)
Dialectical Behavior Therapy Case Conceptualization	Client snapshot, diagnosis and comorbidity, target behaviors, biosocial theory, behavioral chain analysis, dialectical dilemmas, solution analysis, strengths and skills, treatment planning	Fitzpatrick & Rizvi (2022), Haynes & O'Brien (2000)
International Classification of Functioning, Disability, and Health (ICF)	I) Functioning and Disability: Body Functions and Body Structures and Activities and Participation II) Contextual Factors: Environmental Factors and Personal Factors.	World Health Organization (2001)

identification through assessment and data collection, identification of the psychologic process through data analysis and organization, synthesis of client data, evidence-based treatment planning and intervention, and reassessment for improvement, obstacles, detection, or termination (Gill et al., 2024). Noteworthy is the integration of assessment in all of these models. In this chapter, we will explore two methods for case conceptualization: Integrative Case Conceptualization (ICC; Sperry, 2005) and the *International Classification of Functioning, Disability, and Health (ICF;* World Health Organization [WHO], 2001). Further, we include the Multitiered Systems of Support (MTSS) framework for K–12 educators. These approaches offer useful frameworks for comprehending and dealing with complex cases, providing insights into the various aspects of individuals' functioning and well-being.

INTEGRATIVE CASE CONCEPTUALIZATION

The ICC model (Sperry & Sperry, 2020) is one of the few models of case conceptualization that incorporates a multicultural component (Ridley et al., 2017) and specifically addresses the spiritual and religious domains (Stoupas et al., 2018). Counselors are asked to identify "level of acculturation, ethnic and gender identification (if relevant)" (Sperry, 2010, p. 113). A counselor also "links presentation to culture versus psychologic factors; [and] anticipates impact of cultural factors on treatment process" (Sperry, 2010, p. 113). Chapter 3 in this book identifies issues with diversity in testing and assessment, and Chapter 4 describes methods for testing that meet the needs of diverse clients, as well as assessing for religion and spirituality. Without this knowledge, counselors will struggle to create a comprehensive case conceptual framework.

The ICC model addresses case conceptualization in terms of functions, components, and elements. Within this model, the theorists identify five functions of case conceptualization. In the first function, the counselor focuses primarily on obtaining essential information and organizing data through diagnostic, clinical and cultural formulation interviews (CFIs). Data are used to formulate hypotheses regarding the client's presenting problem, origination of the problem, and any maladaptive patterns, as well as perpetuants and contributors to this problem (Sperry & Sperry, 2020). The second function, explaining, draws on the data gathered to develop a deeper understanding of the client's stories. Inclusive of individual personalities, needs, sociocultural identities, and worldview, the explaining function begins to form a diagnostic, clinical, and cultural formulation, providing the basis for a third function of guiding and focusing treatment. Within the fourth function, counselors use data to anticipate obstacles and challenges to the treatment process. And finally, the fifth function of the ICC model includes preparation for appropriate termination.

In addition to the five functions of case conceptualization, this model includes four components. Sperry and Sperry underscore the importance of assessment throughout these components, stating, "Assessment is a prerequisite to developing a case conceptualization and a comprehensive assessment is essential in developing a competent and clinically useful case conceptualization" (2020, p. 29). The first component, Diagnostic Formulation, attempts to answer the question "what happened" and relies heavily on data gathered in terms of presentation, precipitants, and pattern. This information is gathered in the diagnostic and clinical assessments, which correspond with Adler's relationship building and psychologic assessment stages described previously in the chapter. Whereas diagnostic and clinical assessments are described in depth in Chapters 4 and 5, counselors may find additional assessments, including genograms and Adlerian early recollections (ERs), helpful for the Diagnostic Formulation. Intended to uncover basic lifestyle patterns, or "rules," ERs provide a wealth of information toward understanding the client's worldview. Further, genograms provide valuable information about the client's system and patterns within this family or other system. These assessments are explored in detail following the ICC components. The information gathered from these assessments contributes to a Diagnostic Formulation that includes three specific elements: presentation, precipitant, and pattern. Pattern here refers to the client's movement regarding others (i.e., toward, away, against, and ambivalent) toward a goal that is related to the movement. For example, the client moves away from others to feel safe. This pattern is typically rigid, pervasive, in response to a precipitant, and contributes in a negative way to the presenting problem. Further, if appropriate, *Diagnostic and Statistical Manual of Mental Disorders* (5th ed., text revision; *DSM-5-TR*; American Psychiatric Association, 2022) diagnosis is considered within this Diagnostic Formulation (Sperry & Sperry, 2020).

Clinical Formulation, the second component, attempts to answer the question, why did this happen? Information gathered through clinical assessments, including assessing predispositions and perpetuants, is key. Predisposition refers to etiological factors and are uncovered through a thorough assessment of biological, sociocultural, and psychologic factors that impact the presenting problem. Perpetuants are factors that serve to maintain maladaptive patterns and include triggers that exacerbate the problem. Along with the precipitant, predispositions and perpetuants contribute to and maintain a system in which the pattern is activated and reinforced. Whereas predispositions and perpetuants form the basis of the clinical formulation, these elements do not exist alone. These and the resultant clinical formulation are embedded in culture (Sperry & Sperry, 2020).

The Cultural Formulation answers, "What role did culture play?" and is the third component in this model. The *DSM-5-TR* defines *culture* as "systems of knowledge, concepts, values, norms, and practices that are learned and transmitted across generations" (American

Psychiatric Association, 2022, p. 860). Elements of Cultural Formulation are cultural identity, acculturation and acculturative stress, cultural explanation, and culture v. personality (Sperry & Sperry, 2020). Here again, a thorough and accurate assessment is crucial. The CFI provided in the *DSM-5-TR* is one method for gathering cultural information. Others include the genogram, described in the text that follows, and formal instruments, such as the Gender Minority Stress and Resilience Measure (Testa et al., 2015) and the Abbreviated Multidimensional Acculturation Scale (Zea et al., 2003). The role spirituality and religion play in the client's culture is important as well, and genograms can be adapted to include related themes (Gill et al., 2019). In addition, counselors can choose from a variety of qualitative and quantitative methods for spiritual assessment, including spiritual ecomaps, timelines, the Spiritual Assessment Scale (SAS; Howden, 1992), and the Brief Religious Coping Scale (BROPE; Pargament et al., 2011), to name a few. As stated in Chapter 3, when assessing culture, counselors must work from a place of multicultural competence and cultural humility.

The final component in the ICC model is the Treatment Formulation. In this component, we attempt to answer, "How can it change?" There are seven elements in this component as follows: treatment goals, focus, strategy, intervention, anticipated obstacles, treatment-cultural, and prognosis. This formulation relies heavily upon accurate Diagnostic, Clinical, and Cultural Formulations. Using the information from these previous components, the counselors create an accurate blueprint toward providing Treatment Formulation in which the counselor works with the client to establish goals. The goals are co-constructed, including evidence-based treatment, methods for outcome assessment, and routine outcomes monitoring. Counselors attempt to anticipate treatment obstacles, particularly those based in the client's pattern. Finally, prognosis is included in this component of the ICC model (Sperry & Sperry, 2020).

Supplemental Assessments: Incorporating a Systems View With Genograms

Integrating a genogram into a biopsychosocial-spiritual clinical intake interview offers a multilayered and dynamic snapshot of a client's familial landscape. Genograms extend beyond the limitations of family trees to delve into intricate relationship dynamics, medical histories, and behavioral patterns. They serve as invaluable assets for identifying hereditary and environmental factors that may impact mental health, thereby enriching the case conceptualization. Additionally, genograms can highlight potential risk factors, such as a family history of substance abuse, mental illness, and suicide, enabling early intervention and more precise treatment planning. In the realm of creativity, counselors can take an interactive approach to genogram construction, perhaps involving clients in the cocreation of their genogram through digital platforms or even art-based methods, thereby tapping into the aesthetic sensibilities of clients. These collaborative and creative endeavors can make the process more engaging, while also fostering a rapport and trust that will set a strong foundation for the therapeutic alliance. Nonetheless, counselors must exercise discretion, as exploring familial histories can sometimes unearth sensitive or traumatic issues. An empathetic approach is essential to navigate these complex dynamics.

Intended to graphically portray the family or other system, the counselor will draw or ask the client to draw their family in terms of basic couple relationships. Symbols are used for each member with a circle to indicate male and a square for female (see McGoldrick et al., 2020). In these relationships, the female is always noted on the right side. Transgender individuals are represented for female to male by a square with a circle inside and male to female with the square inside the circle. Lesbian female is indicated using an upside-down triangle and a gay male using a square box with an upside-down triangle. Triangles are used for pregnancies, stillbirth, miscarriage, and abortions. When an individual is deceased, their representative symbol has an X placed over it. The genogram typically includes family systems for the two preceding generations and can go generations prior as well. The client would also include the following generations as applicable.

Couple status is identified by connecting the two geometric shapes with a line moving slightly down and then across. This connection represents varying relationships, for example, marriage, if the connecting line is solid; separation, if the connecting line has one mark through it; and divorce, if there are two marks. Living together is indicated with dotted lines and in a "committed relationship" by a solid line with a dotted line above it (The Multicultural Family Institute, n.d.). Relationship status or patterns among the family system members are indicated by using a variety of lines. A straight line indicates a "normal," while double straight lines indicate a strong relationship. Jagged lines reflect conflict or hostility in the relationship, and dotted lines mean distance. A jagged line with an arrow indicates abuse in the relationship and the arrow denotes the individual being abused. Counselors often develop their own style or focus when completing these genograms with the client. For example, if substance abuse is a concern, the client may ask clients to indicate any observations they have regarding use within their system. The counselor and client may co-construct methods of indicating substance use and focus on any patterns that emerge. Religious and spiritual themes can be incorporated, or even color-coded, throughout genograms, providing insights into the impact of these themes on the client and the system (Hodge, 2013). The Transgenerational Trauma and Resilience Genogram (TTRG) was developed to assist counselors in assessing the impact of trauma on systems, identifying patterns, and understanding the transmission of trauma within systems and across generations (Goodman, 2013). Figure 12.2 provides some insight into how genograms may appear. When creating a genogram, each symbol represents something that is visually displayed. For example, in Figure 12.2, males are represented with a triangle, females are represented

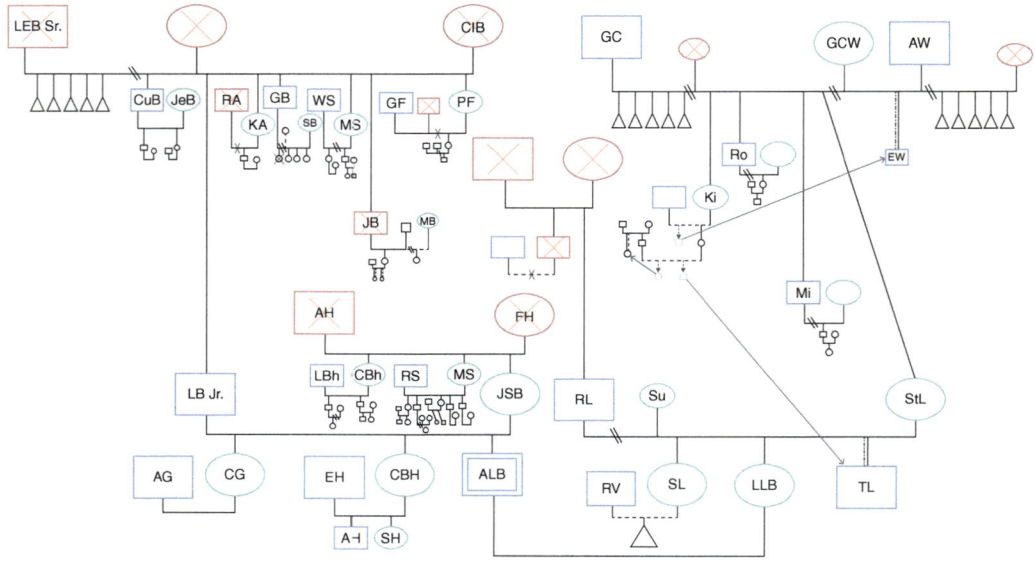

FIGURE 12.2. **Genogram.**

with a oval, births are represented with a direct solid line from the parent, x's are deaths, and broken relationships have a slash through the horizontal line between the people. You can use any symbols you want and get creative with your clients.

Incorporating a Developmental View of Narrative Strategies: Early Recollections

Alfred Adler believed that individuals develop life patterns or rules based on experiences from their earliest years. He theorized that a client's fundamental lifestyle beliefs could be ascertained by uncovering these rules about life, self, others, and the world. Further, because these are formed at an early age, understanding a person's very earliest, full memories or ER, in terms of feeling, cognitions, and activity, could inform the counselor in terms of second order change (Sweeney, 2019). In Adlerian therapy, ERs are generally gathered during the interview process, following a family constellation assessment (Sweeney, 2019). Assessing and identifying "Lifestyle" rule and maladaptive patterns help the clinician in forming a thorough case conceptualization and understanding the client's lifestyle convictions and patterns (Sperry & Sperry, 2020).

ERs are the first, complete memories that an individual has. Because the limbic system and hippocampus fully develop around 6 years or older (Van der Kolk, 2014), these memories generally occur after 6 years of age. Based on his observations of human behavior, Adler posited that the general timeframe in which an individual's lifestyle rules are developed is between 6 and 8. In addition, these events are remembered selectively because they have "significance to the individual in understanding, managing, and controlling life experiences" (Sweeney, 2019, p. 244). ERs must be complete stories with a beginning, middle, and end. To uncover these memories, counselors will ask the client to think back to a time when they were very young, as young as they can fully remember, where they can so vividly recall an event that took place that could be described as happening in the here and now. "What is your earliest recollection?" may be a good way to initiate the conversation. ERs that are quickly recalled may have the most impact on the client's current adaptive or maladaptive patterns. The counselor can guide the client(s) through a process of recalling these events, in first person if possible, and ensuring that there is mutual understanding using reflection statements and summarization. The client is the owner of their ERs; the counselor can listen, reflect, and help with interpretation, but we do not get in the client's way.

Interpretations of ERs are also co-constructed. The counselor may work with the client to determine if the recollections are active or passive; if the client is observer or participant; what movement, or pattern (if any), there is within the ERs; if the individual is alone or withdrawn; and relationship status to others (Sweeney, 2019). The counselors will also elicit feelings surrounding these ERs, as well as any cognitions the client remembers. Asking the client to give the ER a title or caption often provides insight into the client's pattern. Counselors will try to obtain three or more of these memories and look for patterns and themes that impact current client functioning.

Information from genograms and ERs is easily incorporated into the ICC and other models of case conceptualization. Genograms provide insight into family dynamics, rules, and expectations. They are easily adapted to focus on specific constructs such as religion or spirituality. ERs are used to identify underlying patterns in terms of lifestyle rules, behaviors, and interactions with others. These rules include movement that contributes directly to the ICC's pattern, as often clients' patterns are developed at an early age. These ERs can also be used for implementing a Developmental Counseling and Therapy–based interview intervention that is beyond the scope of this chapter. However, resources regarding this intervention are provided in *Adlerian Counseling and Psychotherapy: A Practitioner's Wellness Approach* (Sweeney, 2019).

INTERNATIONAL CLASSIFICATION OF FUNCTIONING, DISABILITY, AND HEALTH

Health has been defined in the WHO Constitution as "a state of complete physical, mental, and social well-being and not merely the absence of disease or infirmity" (WHO, n.d., para. 1). The *ICF* provides a scientific, operational basis for describing, understanding, and studying health and health-related states, outcomes, and determinants. In the *ICF*, the term *functioning* refers to all body functions, activities, and participation, whereas *disability* is an umbrella term for impairments, activity limitations, and participation restrictions. The *ICF* also lists environmental factors that interact with all these components. The *ICF* provides this model (Figure 12.3), which organizes information in two parts. Part I deals with functioning and disability, whereas part II covers contextual factors. Each part has two components:

1. Functioning and Disability:
   a. Body Functions and Body Structures
   b. Activities and Participation

2. Contextual Factors:
   a. Environmental Factors
   b. Personal Factors

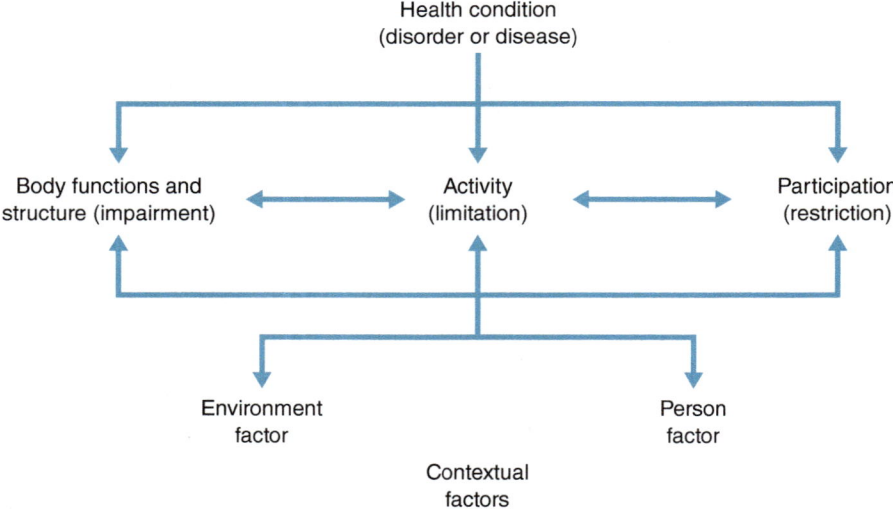

FIGURE 12.3. The *ICF* Model: Interaction between *ICF* components.
ICF, International Classification of Functioning, Disability, and Health.
Source: Chan, F., Yaghmaian, R., Chen, X., Wu, J.-R., Lee, B., Iwanaga, K., & Tao, J. (2020). The World Health Organization *International Classification of Functioning, Disability, and Health* as a framework for rehabilitation assessment. In D. R. Strauser, T. N. Tansey, & C. Fong (Eds.), *Assessment in rehabilitation and mental health counseling* (pp. 15–36). Springer Publishing Company.

The *ICF* conceptualizes a person's level of functioning as a dynamic interaction between their health conditions, environmental factors, and personal factors. It is a biopsychosocial model of disability, based on an integration of the social and medical models of disability. As illustrated in Figure 12.3, disability is multidimensional and interactive. All components of disability are important and any one may interact with another. Environmental factors must be taken into consideration as they affect everything and may need to be changed.

International Classification of Functioning, Disability, and Health Components

BODY FUNCTIONS AND STRUCTURES

The *ICF* model highlights two principal categories of body components: body functions and body structures. Body functions encompass the physical and psychologic functions of various body systems. This category includes mental functions, sensory functions and pain, voice and speech functions, and functions of the cardiovascular, hematologic, immunologic, and respiratory systems. It also covers functions related to the digestive, metabolic, and endocrine systems; genitourinary and reproductive functions; neuromusculoskeletal and movement-related functions; and functions of the skin and related structures.

In parallel to body functions, body structures are associated with anatomical parts of the body such as organs, limbs, and their components. These structures relate directly to their respective body functions. For instance, mental function (a body function) is connected to structures of the nervous system (a body structure). Specific segments of body structures contain structures of the nervous system; the eye, ear, and associated structures; structures involved in voice and speech; and structures of the cardiovascular, immunologic, and respiratory systems.

ACTIVITIES AND PARTICIPATION

Within the *ICF* model, the concepts of activities and participation play a crucial role in understanding how variations in bodily functions and structures translate into differences in individual and societal capacity and performance. Activities refer to the basic tasks performed by an individual, whereas participation represents involvement in community-level life activities. The *ICF* model identifies nine domains that encompass activities and participation: learning and applying knowledge; general tasks and demands; communication; movement; self-care; domestic life; interpersonal interactions; major life areas; and community, social, and civic life.

Participation can be understood as an individual's involvement in various life situations and roles, such as interpersonal relationships, academic pursuits, and employment. Furthermore, participation in life situations is influenced by the interactions between a person and their environment. These person-environment interactions significantly impact an individual's ability to engage in various life situations, highlighting the intricate and interconnected nature of activities and participation within the *ICF* model.

ENVIRONMENTAL FACTORS

Environmental aspects are the physical, social, and attitudinal environment in which people live and conduct their lives. These are either barriers to or facilitators of the person's functioning. Specific environmental factors include products and technology, which refer to both natural and man-made goods, systems, equipment, and technology present in an individual's immediate environment. Support and relationships involve the people or animals offering practical or emotional support, care, protection, assistance, and interpersonal connections in various settings of daily life. Attitudes embody the observable outcomes of customs, practices, ideologies, values, norms, factual beliefs, and religious beliefs held by people external to the individual described.

Progress Monitoring Tools and Routine Outcome Monitoring

Writing treatment plans and case reports can be a lengthy process, but it is important to remember that treatment plans and case reports are not stagnant. They will continually need to be changed and updated over time, as do the assessment tools that we utilize. We can use the assessment process to measure change over time and assist in updating reports, treatment plans, and even case conceptualizations. The updating of treatment plans and reports assists counselors in staying on track and with sharing information, particularly with integrated care teams. Further, clients may report and track progress that is being made during the course of treatment. Progress monitoring tools assist us with these tasks. *Progress monitoring tools* are forms of clinical assessments that can be used in mental health counseling to assess clients' progress in the treatment process and estimate the effectiveness of therapy. They are commonly brief, self-report questionnaires that can be administered in many settings (Lambert, 2010). School counselors and teachers often use progress monitoring tools to assess students' academic performance, quantify a student's rate of improvement or responsiveness to instruction or intervention, and assess social and emotional learning. Self-monitoring of progress enhances a client's ability to quantify changes and can lead to more self-reflection and self-insight. Additionally, progress monitoring has been shown to outperform models that do not engage in progress monitoring, resulting in decreased costs and a lower chance of patient decline while in treatment (Lewis et al., 2019).

Several progress monitoring tools are available for mental health counseling, and many double as clinical assessments. Some specific progress monitoring tools include the Beck Depression Inventory, Second Edition (BDI-II; Beck et al., 1996), the Beck Anxiety Inventory (BAI; Beck et al., 1988), and the Beck Hopelessness Scale (BHS; Beck et al., 1974). Specific progress monitoring tools can be used to assess response, which is the initial improvement in symptoms after treatment; remission, which is the absence of symptoms after treatment; relapse, which is the return of symptoms after a period of remission; and recovery, which refers to the restoration of functioning and quality of life after treatment. It is critical to note that progress monitoring tools in counseling should not be used as a singular basis for clinical decision-making. They should be used in conjunction with other assessment methods.

Routine outcome monitoring (ROM) refers to the regular use of standardized outcomes assessment, including progress monitoring tools, to assess treatment effectiveness and client progress throughout the therapeutic process. Within the beginning stages of therapy, the counselor and client work to establish a baseline for symptoms related to the presenting problem. Throughout the process, reassessment can occur at regular, intentional intervals so that both counselor and client can determine the effectiveness of treatment and clients are given the opportunity for an even more active role in the direction of their treatment. This information may be particularly salient for clients who experience chronic conditions, such as schizophrenia, or for those who are not progressing in treatment.

Rating scales, such as the Outcomes Rating Scale (ORS; Miller et al., 2003) and Clinical Outcomes Routine Evaluation-10 (CORE-10; Barkham et al., 2013) are available for counselors to use. The CORE-10 (Barkham et al., 2013) was designed to measure psychologic distress. The instrument is intended for use at the beginning of the session and is retrospective of the client's experience of symptoms over the past week. This assessment uses a 5-point scale to measure subjective well-being, anxiety, depression, physical problems, trauma, general functioning, close relationships (functioning), social relationships (functioning), risk to self, and risk to others. Ten items measure these domains, and clients respond in terms of 0 (not at all) to 4 (most of the time). The CORE-10 is scored by summing the responses to all items, with a possible range of 0 to 40. Higher scores indicate high levels of distress, with a cut off score of 11 for mild psychological distress (Barkham et al., 2013). As noted in the name, the counselors may use this instrument for ROM. Evidence of reliability includes a coefficient alpha of .90 and evidence of validity is provided through strong correlations with related instruments. The CORE-10 manual, along with helpful tips and the instrument itself, is available at www.core.uk.net/media/2311/perinatal-roms-manual-a4-final-print-december-2019.pdf.

ROM is used to assess common factors in the therapeutic process, such as therapeutic relationship and working alliance. In this way, counselors gain insight into the strength of the therapeutic alliance while also engaging in another common factor, collecting client feedback. Counselors can determine the client's perceptions regarding the strength of the relationship using assessments such as the Session Rating Scale (SRS; Duncan et al., 2003) and the Working Alliance Inventory (WAI-SR; Munder et al., 2010). The SRS is a four-item self-report measure of the client's perception of the relationship, goals and topics, approach or method, and overall response to the session, directly following a counseling session. Clients respond to these items by making a hash mark on a 10-cm line for which marks on the left represent more difficulty and marks on the right indicate fewer issues. Reliability is reported as high, with a coefficient alpha of .88, and evidence of good concurrent validity was reported when measuring the alliance (Duncan et al., 2003). Because of the issues with clients consistently reporting alliance on the upper side of this measure, counselors are encouraged to follow-up on any overall assessment score of 36 or any item score less than 9. In addition to this version, the SRS and the ORS were adapted for children. These measures, the Child Session Rating Scale (CSRS) and the Child Outcomes Rating Scale (CORS), are available for use in a variety of settings, including clinical mental health centers and school settings. In the CORS, the adapted version of the ORS, a frowny face appears on the left side of the scale and a smiley face on the right side. The child is prompted to make a mark on the scale, closest to how they are doing at that time, in response to questions such as, "How am I doing at school?", "How are things in my family?", and "How is everything going?" (Duncan et al., 2003). Similarly, the CSRS has the same images. The counselor prompts the child to respond in terms of the time they spent together that day, using the scale with opposing faces. The child can rate what happened in the session, how well the counselor listened, how important the session topics were, and the overall session direction (Duncan et al., 2003).

There is initial evidence that ROM impacts treatment in terms of improving dropout rates and symptom reduction (De Jong et al., 2021; Ogles et al., 2022). Additionally, a series of meta-analysis focused on evidence-based therapy relationships indicated that collecting client feedback is one of the elements that contributes to effective therapy (Norcross & Wampold, 2011). However, drawbacks are identified as well, including the difficulty in implementing this in a routine way, clients' increased awareness of symptoms, and reliability of the instruments themselves. Inclusion of multiple, different methods for ROM is encouraged. Ogles et al. advocate for the inclusion of semistructured, narrative interviews as a method of broadening data collection, noting that qualitative assessments may provide a more complex insight into the client's change process (2022).

CHECKING IN WITH JOHN

John has a previous diagnosis of PTSD and depression. He reports suffering from mental health issues following his military deployments and subsequent retirement. He is seeking treatment to reduce these symptoms and fully engage in his familial relationships.

1. What assessments might the counselor use to confirm these diagnoses and establish a baseline of symptoms for treatment?

2. What type (s) of progress monitoring tools might be most appropriate when working with John?

3. When/how often could these tools be used?

4. How can the counselor effectively integrate the outcomes of these assessments into treatment planning?

5. What is the ultimate goal of routine outcome monitoring for this client?

END-OF-CHAPTER RESOURCES

DISCUSSION QUESTIONS

1. How does assessment systemically impact the counseling process?

2. What is the role of assessment in case conceptualization and treatment planning? How do assessment results impact the development and ongoing evaluation of case conceptualizations and treatment plans?

3. How do ROM assessments contribute to the efficacy of counseling interventions, and in what ways can counselors influence the insights gained from these assessments to enhance the quality of client care and promote positive therapeutic outcomes?

4. How does common factors theory, specifically the working alliance and real relationship, impact how a counselor discusses assessment and assessment results with the client?

CLASS ACTIVITIES

1. Reflect on the case of Arturo. The counselor has worked with him to determine a diagnosis of Persistent Depressive Disorder and the counselor and client have agreed to an evidence-based treatment plan that includes methods for reconnecting with his religious group and spiritual self. In groups of three or more, discuss what types of assessments a counselor would consider using with Arturo. Which assessment would be part of ROM? At what intervals should the counselor use these? Identify the associated potential benefits and drawbacks.

2. Compare and contrast the various case conceptualization models. What are the strengths and weaknesses of each? Which model are you most likely to employ? What model are you least likely to use and why?

3. Identify resources that give more insight into the model you are most likely to use. Create a presentation of the tenets and principles of this model. Identify how and why assessments are used through the case conceptualization process.

4. In dyads, use the genogram provided in this chapter to role-play a client and counselor. The counselor will work with the client to discuss the assessment, make connections, and draw treatment-related conclusions. Respond to "how would you as a counselor integrate this assessment in your therapeutic work?"

PERSPECTIVE FROM THE FIELD

Chapter 12 covers the integration and use of assessment data in the counseling process. This podcast interview provides valuable insight from Dr. Jon Sperry, coauthor of *Case Conceptualization: Mastering This Competency With Ease and Confidence*. Dr. Sperry discusses the ICC model of case conceptualization, including tips and tools for effective data integration. He gives unique insights into thorough diagnostic formulations, including understanding clients' individual pattern of responding to others. Dr. Sperry talks about the importance of spiri-
tuality and religion as part of cultural formulation and the qualitative assessment data that can result from understanding the clients' ERs. Dr. Sperry is a core faculty member in the clinical mental health counseling program at Lynn University. Dr. Sperry's area of expertise is competency-based instruction and outcomes-focused evaluation. He engages in teaching, research, writing, and conference presentations on case conceptualization in counseling practice. Dr. Sperry is also very active in the research and theory of individual psychology; he has spent the last 12 years researching, publishing, and presenting about this counseling approach. He was president of the North American Society of Adlerian Psychology (NASAP) from 2017 to 2018 and is currently the coeditor in chief of the *Journal of Individual Psychology* (*JIP*). In 2018, he was appointed as a board member of the International Committee for Adlerian Summer Schools and Institutes (ICASSI), which focuses on individual psychology counseling techniques and is hosted in a new country each year. Dr. Sperry has coauthored four books, including *Cognitive Behavior Therapy of the* DSM-5 *Personality Disorders* and *Psychopathology and Psychotherapy: DSM-5 Diagnosis, Case Conceptualization, and Treatment*.

Access podcasts via the QR code or http://connect.springerpub.com/content/book/978-0-8261-8913-4/chapter/ch00.

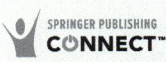 A robust set of instructor resources designed to supplement this text is located at http://connect.springerpub.com/content/book/978-0-8261-8913-4. Qualifying instructors may request access by emailing textbook@springerpub.com.

REFERENCES

American Psychiatric Association. (2022). *Diagnostic and statistical manual of mental disorders* (5th ed., text rev.). https://doi.org/10.1176/appi.books.9780890425787

Barkham, M., Bewick, B., Mullin, T., Gilbody, S., Connell, J., Cahill, J., Mellor-Clark, J., Richards, D., Unsworth, G., & Evans, C. (2013). The CORE-10: A short measure of psychological distress for routine use in the psychological therapies. *Counselling and Psychotherapy Research, 13*(1), 3–13. https://doi.org/10.1080/14733145.2012.729069

Beck, A. T., Epstein, N., Brown, G., & Steer, R. (1988). An inventory for measuring clinical anxiety: Psychometric properties. *Journal of Consultation in Clinical Psychology, 56*(6), 893–897. https://doi.org/10.1037//0022-006x.56.6.893

Beck, A. T., Steer, R. A., & Brown, G. K. (1996). *Beck Depression Inventory (BDI-II): Manual and questionnaire*. The Psychological Corporation.

Beck, A. T., Weissman, A., Lester, D., & Trexler, L. (1974). The measurement of pessimism: The hopelessness scale. *Journal of Consulting and Clinical Psychology, 42*(6), 861–865. https://doi.org/10.1037/h0037562

Bronfenbrenner, U. (1979). *The ecology of human development: Experiments by nature and design*. Harvard University Press.

Council for Accreditation of Counseling and Related Educational Programs. (2023). *2024 CACREP standards*. https://www.cacrep.org/wp-content/uploads/2023/06/Combined-version-6.21.23.pdf

Darling, N. (2007). Ecological systems theory: The person in the center of the circles. *Research in Human Development, 4*(3–4), 203–217. https://doi.org/10.1080/15427600701663023

De Jong, K., Conjin, J. M., Gallagher, R. A. V., Reshetnikova, A. S., Heij, M., & Lutz, M. C. (2021). Using progress feedback to improve outcomes and reduce drop-out, treatment duration, and deterioration: A multilevel meta-analysis. *Clinical Psychology Review, 85*, 102002. https://doi.org/10.1016/j.cpr.2021.102002

Duncan, B., Miller, S., Sparks, J., Claud, D. A., Reynolds, L., Brown, J., & Johnson, L. D. (2003). The Session Rating Scale: Preliminary psychometric properties of a "working" alliance measure. *Journal of Brief Therapy, 3*, 3–12.

Fitzpatrick, S., & Rizvi, S. L. (2022). Dialectical behavior therapy: Assessment and case conceptualization. In A. Masuda & W. O'Donohue (Eds.), *Behavior therapy: First, second, and third waves* (pp. 173–193). Springer International Publishing.

Gill, C. S., Dailey, S. F., Karl, S., & Barrio Minton, C. (2024). *DSM-5-TR learning companion for counselors* (2nd ed.). Alexandria, VA: American Counseling Association.

Gill, C. S., Harper, M., & Dailey, S. (2019). Assessing the client's spiritual domain. In C. S. Cashwell & J. S. Young (Eds.), *Integrating religion and spirituality in counseling: A guide to competent practice* (3rd ed.). American Counseling Association.

Goodman, R. D. (2013). The transgenerational trauma and resilience genogram. *Counselling Psychology Quarterly, 26*(3–4), 386–405. https://doi.org/10.1080/09515070.2013.820172

Haynes, S. N., & O'Brien, W. H. (2000). Clinical case formulation. In S. N. Haynes & W. H. O'Brien (Eds.), *Principles and practice of behavioral assessment: Applied clinical psychology*. Springer. https://doi.org/10.1007/978-0-306-47469-9_13

Hodge, D. R. (2013). Assessing spirituality and religion in the context of counseling and psychotherapy. In K. I. Pargament (Ed.), *Handbook of psychology, religion, and spirituality: Vol. 2. An applied psychology of religion and spirituality* (pp. 92–123). American Psychiatric Association. https://doi.org/10.1037/14046-005

Howden, J. (1992). *Development and psychometric characteristics of the spiritual assessment scale* (Dissertation Services). Bell & Howell Company.

Lambert, M. J. (2010). *Prevention of treatment failure: The use of measuring, monitoring, and feedback in clinical practice*. American Psychological Association. http://dx.doi.org/10.1037/12141-000

Lewis, C. C., Boyd, M., Puspitasari, A., Navarro, E., Howard, J., Kassab, H., Hoffman, M., Scott, K., Lyon, A., Douglas, S., Simon, G., & Kroenke, K. (2019). Implementing measurement-based care in behavioral health: A review. *JAMA Psychiatry, 76*(3), 324–335. https://doi.org/10.1001/jamapsychiatry.2018.3329

Luedke, A. J., Peluso, P. R., Diaz, P., Freund, R., & Baker, A. (2017). Predicting dropout in counseling using affect coding of the therapeutic relationship: An empirical analysis. *Journal of Counseling & Development, 95*(2), 125–134. https://doi.org/10.1002/jcad.12125

Macneil, C. A., Hasty, M. K., Conus, P., & Berk, M. (2012). Is diagnosis enough to guide interventions in mental health? Using case formulation in clinical practice. *BMC Medicine, 10*, 1–3. https://doi.org/10.1186/1741-7015-10-111

McGoldrick, M., Gerson, R., & Petry, S. (2020). *Genograms: Assessment and intervention* (4th ed.). W. W. Norton.

Miller, S., Duncan, B., & Brown, J. (2003). The outcome rating scale: A preliminary study of the reliability, validity, and feasibility of a brief visual analog measure. *Journal of Brief Therapy, 2*, 91–100.

Munder, T., Wilmers, F., Leonhart, R., Linster, H. W., & Barth, J. (2010). Working Alliance Inventory-Short Revised (WAI-SR): Psychometric properties in outpatients and inpatients. *Clinical Psychology & Psychotherapy, 17*(3), 231–239. https://doi.org/10.1002/cpp.658

Nahum, D., Alfonso, C. A., & Sönmez, E. (2019). Common factors in psychotherapy. In A. Javed & K. Fountoulakis (Eds.), *Advances in psychiatry* (pp. 471–481). Springer. https://doi.org/10.1007/978-3-319-70554-5_29

Norcross, J. C., & Wampold, B. E. (2011). Evidence-based therapy relationships: Research conclusions and clinical practices. *Psychotherapy, 48*(1), 98–102. https://doi.org/10.1037/a0022161

Ogles, B. M., Goates-Jones, M. K., & Erekson, D. M. (2022). Treatment success or failure? Using a narrative interview to supplement ROM. *Journal of Clinical Psychology, 78*(10), 1986–2001. https://doi.org/10.1002/jclp.23345

Pargament, K. I., Feuille, M., & Burdzy, D. (2011). The brief RCOPE: Current psychometric status of a short measure of religious coping. *Religions, 2*(1), 51–76. https://doi.org/10.3390/rel2010051

Peluso, P. R., & Freund, R. R. (2018). Therapist and client emotional expression and psychotherapy outcomes: A meta-analysis. *Psychotherapy, 55*(4), 461–472. https://doi.org/10.1037/pst0000165

Ridley, C. R., Jeffrey, C. E., & Roberson, R. B. III (2017). Case mis-conceptualization in psychological treatment: An enduring clinical problem. *Journal of Clinical Psychology, 73*(4), 359–375. https://doi.org/10.1002/jclp.22354

Sperry, L. (2005). Case conceptualization: A strategy for incorporating individual, couple and family dynamics in the treatment process. *The American Journal of Family Therapy, 33*(5), 353–364. https://doi.org/10.1080/01926180500341598

Sperry, L. (2010). *Core competencies in counseling and psychotherapy: Becoming a highly competent and effective therapist*. Routledge.

Sperry, L., & Sperry, J. (2020). *Case conceptualization: Mastering this competency with ease and confidence* (2nd ed.). Routledge.

Stoupas, G., Binensztok, V., & Sperry, L. (2018). Understanding the spiritual domain through case conceptualization. In C. S. Gill & R. R. Freund (Eds.), *Spirituality and religion in counseling: Competency-based strategies for ethical practice* (pp. 64–82). Routledge.

Strauser, D. R., & Greco, C. E. (2020). Introduction to assessment in rehabilitation. In D. R. Strauser, T. N. Tansey, & C. Fong (Eds.), *Assessment in rehabilitation and mental health counseling* (pp. 3–14). Springer Publishing Company.

Sulmasy, D. P. (2002). A biopsychosocial-spiritual model for the care of patients at the end of life. *The Gerontologist, 42*(Suppl. 3), 24–33. https://doi.org/10.1093/geront/42.suppl_3.24

Sweeney, T. J. (2019). *Adlerian counseling and psychotherapy: A practitioner's wellness approach* (6th ed.). Routledge.

Testa, R. J., Habarth, J., Peta, J., Balsam, K., & Bockting, W. (2015). Development of the gender minority stress and resilience measure. *Psychology of Sexual Orientation and Gender Diversity, 2*(1), 65–77. https://doi.org/10.1037/sgd0000081

The Multicultural Family Institute. (n.d.). *Standard symbols for genograms*. https://stanfield.pbworks.com/f/explaining_genograms.pdf

Van der Kolk, B. (2014). *The body keeps the score: Brain, mind, and body in the healing of trauma*. Penguin Books.
Wampold, B. E. (2015). How important are the common factors in psychotherapy? An update. *World Psychiatry, 14*(3), 270–277. https://doi.org/10.1002/wps.20238
World Health Organization. (n.d.). *Constitution*. Revised September 15, 2005. https://www.who.int/about/governance/constitution
World Health Organization. (2001, May 22). *International classification of functioning, disability, and health (ICF)*. https://www.who.int/standards/classifications/international-classification-of-functioning-disability-and-health
Zea, M. C., Asner-Self, K. K., Birman, D., & Buki, L. P. (2003). The abbreviated multidimensional acculturation scale: Empirical validation with two Latino/Latina samples. *Cultural Diversity and Ethnic Minority Psychology, 9*(2), 107–126. https://doi.org/10.1037/1099-9809.9.2.107

13

Looking Ahead: Future Direction of Assessment and Testing in Counseling

CLARA BOSSIE AND CARMAN S. GILL

2024 CACREP STANDARD

3.E.5. application of technology related to counseling

In the early 2000s, fresh out of graduate school, my world of counseling was largely analog. Picture this: a young counselor, adept with pen and paper, navigating through mazes of fireproof filing cabinets. It was a time when the term electronic medical record (EMR) was beginning to ripple through our professional circles. I often joke about it being akin to the adage of walking a mile in the snow, but transitioning from paper to digital was a pivotal moment in my career. In my first counseling position, I was given a significant task: to review and choose an EMR system for our practice. This shift felt monumental. It wasn't just about replacing physical files with digital ones; it was about rethinking our entire approach to storing, encrypting, and sharing sensitive client data. This posed a daunting challenge for many of us, particularly those not well-versed in technology. There were legitimate fears about privacy breaches and uncertainties about what would constitute the new standard of care in this digital age. I remember the initial resistance, both within myself and among colleagues. The comfort of tangible, paper-based records was hard to let go of. Yet, as I delved deeper into the world of EMRs, I began to appreciate their potential. The shift wasn't just about efficiency; it was a gateway to more comprehensive, accessible, and secure client care. As I spearheaded the transition in our practice, the early years of the digital revolution in counseling were fraught with questions and learning curves. We moved from fireproof filing cabinets to firewalls and backup servers. I recall the countless hours spent training the team, troubleshooting issues, and reassuring concerned colleagues about the security and efficacy of our new system. Fast forward over a decade, and the landscape of digital tools in counseling has become more refined and expansive. EMRs have evolved into sophisticated platforms that store data; offer assessment, analysis tools, and therapeutic treatments; and integrate with telehealth services. This journey has reshaped my approach to counseling, making assessments more dynamic and client-centered. Reflecting on this transition, I realize how it mirrored the broader evolution within the counseling profession. The initial skepticism gradually gave way to acceptance, and then enthusiasm as the benefits of digital integration became undeniable. The journey has been transformative, from apprehensions about technology and privacy concerns to embracing digital solutions for better client care.

FROM PAPER TRAILS TO DIGITAL FOOTPRINTS

As we stand on the brink of a new era in the counseling field, it is important to recognize the dynamic and evolving nature of counseling assessments. Many of the novel assessment tools we see today are fundamental to understanding our clients and a reflection of the broader changes in technology, society, and our understanding of mental health. As discussed throughout the text, the current state of counseling assessments is rich with traditional techniques and emerging innovations. As counselors in training, you are entering a profession where the tools of our trade are rapidly adapting to the needs of a diverse, technologically advanced, and ethically complex society. This chapter aims to guide you through the anticipated developments in the realm of assessments, preparing you for today's realities and tomorrow's exciting possibilities. We will examine how future counselors can prepare for and adapt to these changes. The landscape of counseling assessments is not just changing but inviting us to grow, learn, and evolve. As we embark on this exploration, remember that the core of our profession remains unchanged: the commitment to understanding and aiding those who seek our help. The tools and methods may evolve, yet our mission remains steadfast. Welcome to a glimpse of the future of counseling in the ever-evolving world of counseling assessments.

TECHNOLOGICAL ADVANCEMENTS IN COUNSELING ASSESSMENTS

Platforms of Plenty

In counseling assessments, counselors are presented with various technology tools. These range from cloud-based solutions and web-based platforms to desktop and application-based software and mobile-optimized tools. Such diversity means these tools can be hosted on the internet, accessed through web browsers, or installed as applications on various devices, including personal computers and mobile phones. The new generation of counselors must be familiar with these varied platforms and understand their unique features and implications. Each platform carries risks and benefits, from data security concerns in cloud-based tools to the accessibility challenges of desktop software (see Table 13.1). Being informed about these differences is key to making judicious choices when selecting assessment tools.

When evaluating tools and their corresponding platforms, counselors must consider several questions: How does the platform ensure client data privacy and security? Is the tool easily accessible to clients of different demographics? Does the platform align with the counselor's methodological approach and the specific needs of their clients? Understanding these nuances will empower counselors to choose the most appropriate, effective, and ethical tools for their practice, ensuring that they meet the diverse needs of their clients in a rapidly evolving digital landscape.

Digitalization and Online Assessments

INNOVATION IN COUNSELING ASSESSMENT TOOLS

The digital revolution has transformed countless aspects of our lives, and counseling assessments are no exception. We have seen a surge in technology's role in mental health, leading to a significant shift toward digital and online assessment tools. EMR platforms like

TABLE 13.1 **PLATFORM PANORAMA: MAPPING COUNSELING ASSESSMENT TECHNOLOGIES**

Type of Tool	Description	Key Features	Considerations
Cloud-Based	Hosted on cloud servers, accessible over the internet	No local installation, accessible across devices	Data security, internet reliability, accessibility
Web-Based	Accessed directly through a web browser	Browser as the primary interface	Browser compatibility, data storage location
Application-Based	Requires downloading an app on a device	Available as mobile or desktop apps, may sync with cloud services	Device compatibility, app updates, user experience
Desktop-Based	Installed and run on a desktop or laptop computer	Works independently of the internet, data stored locally	Software updates, data backup, hardware requirements
Mobile-Based	Designed for smartphones and tablets	Tailored for mobile use, often with specific features and interfaces	Mobile accessibility, app usability, screen size
Hybrid Systems	Integrates multiple platforms, such as desktop applications syncing to cloud	Combines features of desktop and cloud-based systems	Integration efficiency, synchronization reliability

TherapyNotes, TheraPlatform, and SimplePractice offer integrated online assessment tools where counselors can administer and score assessments directly within the platform. These platforms offer remarkable benefits, including increased accessibility for clients in remote or underserved areas and greater flexibility in scheduling and format.

Digital assessments are administered through various devices, ensuring clients can access them most conveniently and comfortably. For instance, Quenza allows for the remote delivery of customizable assessments and supplemental activities that clients can complete on their smartphones or tablets. Pearson's Q-interactive system and Psychological Assessment Resources (PAR) also provide interactive tools and standardized tests, delivering dynamic, engaging, formal assessment experiences in clinical, educational, and rehabilitation settings. Platforms like OQ Measures enhance real-time data collection and routine outcome measuring, providing immediate insights into client responses during sessions.

Artificial Intelligence and Machine Learning

Before exploring the transformative impact of artificial intelligence (AI) and machine learning (ML) in counseling assessments, it is crucial to understand what these technologies are and how they function. At its core, AI refers to the simulation of human intelligence in machines that are programmed to think and learn. The term encompasses various technologies that enable machines to perceive, understand, act, and learn to perform human-like tasks. ML, a subset of AI, is the process through which computers use statistical techniques to "learn" from data. In ML, algorithms are used to analyze patterns in data, make predictions, or help make decisions based on new information. These algorithms improve automatically through experience, making ML particularly powerful in adapting to new data without being explicitly programmed to do so. In the context of counseling assessments, AI and ML work together to greatly enhance the tools and methods used. AI algorithms can process and analyze vast amounts of assessment data, identifying patterns and making predictions about a client's mental health. This analysis is not static; as new data become available, ML algorithms enable these systems to update their understanding, improving their accuracy and relevance.

AI and ML are set to revolutionize counseling assessments by offering more personalized and accurate insights into clients' mental health. AI algorithms can analyze vast amounts of assessment data to identify patterns and predict outcomes, offering a level of detail and precision previously unattainable. These technologies can also assist in identifying early signs of mental health issues, potentially leading to earlier intervention and better outcomes. Moreover, AI-driven assessments can continually learn and adapt based on new data, ensuring they remain relevant and accurate. For instance, Ellipsis Health leverages AI to analyze language, assess mental well-being, and provide immediate insights. In a similar vein, AI-powered chatbots like AI-Therapy and Woebot are making significant strides in mental health support. While Woebot, relying on conversational AI, has stirred some controversy for sidestepping traditional human interaction, it offers real-time assessments and guidance grounded in cognitive-behavioral therapy principles. Meanwhile, AI-Therapy's online CBT program customizes therapy modules based on AI-driven analysis of user responses, ensuring that therapeutic content is highly relevant and tailored to individual needs. This trend of AI-driven interaction, poised to grow with new tools, is instrumental in identifying mood patterns and providing therapeutic interventions. Many digital services, such as Ginger.io (now part of Headspace Health), employ evidence-based digital assessment measures to deliver immediate, widespread mental healthcare. Ginger.io, aspiring to serve as a comprehensive employee assistance program (EAP), melds AI with human expertise. This blend facilitates initial assessments and steers users toward appropriate resources or therapists. The AI component in Ginger.io critically evaluates user input to determine the necessary level of care, thus enabling referral between clients and mental health professionals. However, AI's innovative use in counseling brings significant ethical considerations. It is imperative to ensure that these advanced tools are beneficial and remain sensitive to client needs. Here, counselors must remain vigilant about the potential biases inherent in AI systems and ensure that these tools are used to augment, not replace, the human element in counseling. As these examples illustrate, AI in counseling assessments is not just about automation; it is about enhancing the understanding of mental health, increasing access to resources, and improving the efficacy of interventions.

Virtual Reality and Augmented Reality

Virtual reality (VR) and augmented reality (AR) are groundbreaking technologies reshaping the presentation of counseling assessments. Understanding their definitions and differences is key to appreciating their potential in mental healthcare. *Virtual reality (VR)* is a completely immersive digital environment that replaces the user's real-world environment. This is typically achieved through VR headsets or goggles. In counseling, VR can create controlled simulations and environments, enabling counselors to observe clients' reactions and behaviors in scenarios that are difficult or impossible to replicate in a traditional office setting. For instance, VR has been effectively used in exposure therapy for clients with specific phobias or PTSD, allowing them to confront and process traumatic memories or fears in a safe, controlled environment. In contrast, *augmented reality (AR)* overlays digital information onto the real world. Unlike VR, which creates a wholly artificial environment, AR enhances the real world with digital elements, such as images or information projected onto the user's field of vision. In counseling assessments, AR offers opportunities for interactive

TABLE 13.2 NEW TECHNOLOGY IN VIRTUAL AND AUGMENTED REALITY

Technology	Tool	Use	Description
VR	Bravemind	PTSD assessment and treatment	A VR exposure therapy tool specifically designed for PTSD assessment and treatment, allowing counselors to measure responses to trauma-related stimuli
VR	Limbix	Adolescent mental health assessment	Provides VR scenarios aimed at adolescents, facilitating the assessment of mental health issues like anxiety and depression in a relatable, immersive environment
AR	Augment Therapy	Pediatric behavioral and cognitive assessment	An AR platform for children that gamifies physical and mental health exercises, aiding in the assessment of cognitive and behavioral patterns in a playful, engaging manner
AR	Reflectly	Mood tracking and emotional assessment	An AI-driven journal app that uses AR to help users reflect on their day, provides insights into mood patterns and emotional well-being, and is useful for self-assessment

AI, artificial intelligence; AR, augmented reality; PTSD, posttraumatic stress disorder; VR, virtual reality.

and engaging experiences, which is particularly useful in pediatric and adolescent mental health. For example, AR games can assess children's cognitive functions and emotional states, making the assessment process less intimidating and more engaging.

These technologies are not just futuristic concepts but also practical tools that reshape how counselors understand and interact with their clients, where digital elements blend seamlessly with physical surroundings (see Table 13.2). As we look to the future, the possibilities are boundless. As these technologies evolve, we may see more sophisticated assessments incorporating biometric data through VR and AR, providing deeper insights into physiological responses during assessments. Integrating AI with these technologies can offer more personalized and adaptive assessment experiences. Staying informed and adept with these emerging technologies is crucial for counseling professionals. They present novel ways to assess clients, offering insights that might not be as readily accessible through traditional methods. However, ethical considerations, such as privacy and the digital divide, must also be at the forefront of their application to develop best practice policies.

ETHICS AND PRIVACY IN A DIGITAL AGE

Data Privacy and Security

In an era where digital and online assessments are becoming the norm, safeguarding client data has never been more crucial. Future counselors must be well-versed in the ethical handling of sensitive information. This includes understanding and complying with laws and regulations concerning data protection, such as the Health Insurance Portability and Accountability Act (HIPAA) in the United States, as well as being aware of international regulations like the General Data Protection Regulation (GDPR) in Europe, especially for global or online practices. Equally important for school counselors is familiarity with the Family Educational Rights and Privacy Act (FERPA). As noted in Chapter 2, FERPA is a federal law that protects the privacy of student education records. For school counselors, this means ensuring that any digital assessment platform complies with FERPA's requirements regarding handling, accessing, and sharing student educational records. FERPA's implications are particularly significant when sharing student information with third parties, requiring explicit parental consent in many cases, or ensuring that these third parties operate under the same privacy conditions as the school. Secure digital platforms must be used for administering assessments and storing results to prevent unauthorized access to client data. Counselors should proactively ensure that any assessment technology meets stringent security standards. Moreover, establishing well-defined policies concerning access to assessment data and its storage duration is essential. To this end, securing a business associate agreement (BAA) is an important aspect of data security. A BAA is a contract between a HIPAA-covered entity and a vendor who has access to protected health information (PHI). This agreement ensures the vendor appropriately safeguards PHI and adheres to specific requirements for handling and securing data. In digital counseling assessments, a BAA is crucial when using any third-party digital platforms or tools that may store or process client information. These agreements confirm that the technology providers are committed to maintaining HIPAA's privacy and security standards. Consulting with a developer or security specialist can be invaluable for counselors who may not be well-versed in technology. This consultation can ensure the selection of tools that adhere to industry standards and enhances understanding of their functionalities. Such knowledge is crucial for internal operations and confidently discussing privacy and security with clients.

Informed Consent in the Digital Age

The concept of informed consent must evolve alongside technological advancements in counseling assessments. Counselors may fully inform clients about what assessments entail, how their data will be used, and the measures in place to protect their privacy. This information is presented clearly and understandably, free from jargon so that clients can make informed decisions. Counselors should also be prepared to discuss digital assessments' potential risks and benefits with their clients (see Table 13.3). This includes addressing clients' concerns about digital data collection and storage and reassuring them about the steps taken to mitigate these risks.

The Role of Counselors in Upholding Ethical Standards

As technology becomes more integral to counseling assessments, counselors must stay informed about ethical issues and best practices in digital assessments. This includes ongoing education and training in data protection, cyber security, and the ethical use of AI and other emerging technologies. Counselors must also advocate for their clients, protecting their rights and privacy. This may involve partnerships with technology developers to improve assessment tools' security and ethical standards and lobbying for stronger regulations and protections at the industry or government level. The future will undoubtedly present new ethical challenges as the field of counseling assessments continues to evolve. Counselors must be prepared to navigate these complex situations with a strong ethical framework and some technology know-how. This involves adhering to professional codes of ethics and engaging in critical reflection and consultation with peers and supervisors when faced with difficult decisions.

TABLE 13.3 **BENEFITS AND RISKS OF DIGITALLY DELIVERED ASSESSMENTS**

Aspect	Benefits	Risks
Accessibility	• Increased access for clients in remote areas • Flexible scheduling	• Potential digital divide, limiting access for clients without reliable internet or technology
Convenience	• Can be completed from the comfort of home • Saves travel time	• Technical difficulties or interruptions during assessments
Privacy and Confidentiality	• Secure platforms offer strong data protection • Private participation	• Risk of data breaches or unauthorized access • Dependence on platform's security measures
Engagement	• Interactive and user-friendly tools • Can be more appealing, especially to younger clients	• Overreliance on technology can reduce human interaction • May not suit all client preferences
Real-Time Feedback	• Immediate results and analysis • Quicker intervention possible	• Automated feedback may lack personalization or miss nuances
Innovation	• Use of AI, VR, and AR for more comprehensive assessments	• New technologies may have unaddressed issues or be less tested in real-world settings
Cost	• Can be more cost-effective than traditional methods	• Initial setup costs for technology and training can be high
Adaptability	• Tools can be quickly updated or customized	• Requires ongoing learning and adaptation by both clients and counselors

AI, artificial intelligence; AR, augmented reality; VR, virtual reality.

COLLABORATIVE AND CLIENT-CENTERED APPROACHES

In addition to the innovations of technology, our ideas about assessment are also expanding. The future of counseling assessments lies in a more collaborative and client-centered approach. This paradigm shift recognizes clients as active participants in their assessment process rather than passive subjects. Involving clients directly in the assessment process can lead to greater ownership and engagement in treatment planning. Collaboration also allows assessments to be more tailored to individual needs and preferences, enhancing their relevance and effectiveness.

Collaboration in counseling assessments extends beyond the counselor-client dynamic and increasingly involves interdisciplinary teamwork. Today, technology plays a pivotal role in this collaborative process, offering seamless ways to share assessment data effectively among different healthcare providers. Future counselors are expected to work closely with a diverse range of professionals, including psychologists, psychiatrists, social workers, educators, and holistic health practitioners. This allows for a more well-rounded understanding of clients, considering various aspects of their lives and well-being. This collaborative approach to assessment and treatment is often called integrated care, where assessments inform a comprehensive plan involving various professionals as needed (see Table 13.4).

Multidisciplinary communication is facilitated by digital tools such as electronic healthcare records (EHR) systems like Epic or Cerner, which allow for the secure sharing of client

TABLE 13.4 **INTEGRATED CARE TEAMS**

Healthcare Professional	Role in Integrated Care	Data Sharing Relevance
Clinical Psychologists	Mental health diagnosis and therapy	Share insights on mental health diagnoses and treatment plans
Psychiatrists	Medication management, psychiatric evaluations	Coordinate on medication effects and psychiatric conditions
Social Workers	Client advocacy, resource coordination	Share socioeconomic factors impacting mental health
School Counselors	Academic and emotional support for students	Collaborate on student assessments and support plans
Educators	Academic development and support	Insights on academic performance, learning challenges, and social interactions in educational settings
Occupational Therapists	Enhance client's daily living and working skills	Share assessments related to client's daily functioning
Physical Therapists	Improve physical wellness and mobility	Exchange information on physical health and its impact
Nutritionists/ Dietitians	Dietary planning and education	Discuss nutritional impacts on mental health
Holistic Health Practitioners	Alternative therapies (e.g., acupuncture, yoga)	Share insights on complementary treatments and responses
General Practitioners	Overall healthcare and monitoring	Coordinate on physical health issues affecting mental well-being
Nurses	Patient care and education	Share observations from clinical settings and patient responses

information across different medical practices. Additionally, behavioral health and wellness platforms like Healthie or SimplePractice provide integrated care teams with tools for scheduling, telehealth, and documentation, ensuring that each team member is informed and in sync regarding client care. Secure messaging apps like TigerConnect or Siilo enable real-time communication between team members, allowing for prompt consultation and decision-making. This integrated care approach, where assessments inform a comprehensive treatment plan, is greatly enhanced by such digital solutions. They facilitate a holistic understanding of clients by considering various aspects of their lives and well-being, and ensure that all professionals involved in their care can collaborate effectively, even when working from different practices.

EVIDENCE-BASED PRACTICES AND RESEARCH

The Role of Research in Shaping Future Assessments and Adapting to Emerging Needs

The development and refinement of counseling assessments are deeply rooted in ongoing research. Future trends in counseling assessments will likely be driven by evidence-based practices, with a strong emphasis on empirical research to validate the effectiveness of new tools and techniques. There will be more focus on validating assessment tools for various cultural applications and translations. Further, counseling assessments must evolve in response to emerging trends and needs in mental health. To this end, we are already seeing the need to develop and refine assessments to address issues such as digital addiction, pandemic-related stress, and other emerging challenges. Keeping assessments relevant and effective in the face of changing mental health landscapes is crucial for the future of the counseling profession.

INNOVATION IN COUNSELING RESEARCH ASSESSMENT TOOLS

The evolution of research assessment tools in counseling has also brought sophisticated software for qualitative data analysis to the forefront, such as NVivo. NVivo is a powerful tool widely used in counseling research to analyze complex qualitative data, like interview transcripts, open-ended survey responses, and social media content. This software helps identify themes, patterns, and narratives, providing depth and nuance to counseling research findings. Its advanced data coding and query features allow counselors and researchers to dive deep into the qualitative aspects of client experiences and therapeutic outcomes. Moreover, platforms like Qualtrics and SurveyMonkey have become indispensable for quantitative data collection and analysis in counseling research. Qualtrics offers robust survey creation and data analysis capabilities, ideal for conducting sophisticated research. Its flexibility allows for creating detailed surveys that capture various psychologic data. With its user-friendly interface, SurveyMonkey is frequently used for initial screenings and data gathering in various counseling contexts.

Together, these tools represent a significant leap forward in counseling research. They enable the collection, analysis, and interpreting of quantitative and qualitative data, providing comprehensive insights. This integration of diverse methodologies enriches the research landscape and supports evidence-based practices in counseling, guiding the development of more effective assessment techniques and therapeutic interventions.

COUNSELOR EDUCATION IN THE ERA OF EVOLVING ASSESSMENTS

As the counseling field advances into a future enriched with technological developments and evolving societal needs, the preparation of counselors in training is becoming increasingly vital. The crux of this preparation is mastering software applications and embedding these digital competencies seamlessly into counseling practice. These technological advancements have significantly influenced counselor education and the assessment of counseling student competencies. In response to the COVID-19 pandemic and this new era, accrediting bodies like the Council for Accreditation of Counseling and Related Educational Programs (CACREP) have developed specific terminology and standards for digitally delivered counselor education, reflecting technology integration in training with platforms such as Canva, Zoom, and various other tools (CACREP, n.d.). Counselors will find themselves navigating a field where digital tools, ranging from data analysis platforms like NVivo and SPSS for research to VR environments for experiential learning, become integral to their toolkits. For instance, VR tools such as Bravemind, developed at the University of Southern California Institute for Creative Technologies, are used in training programs to simulate exposure therapy sessions, offering students a realistic practice environment. Similarly, e-learning platforms and online practicums are becoming commonplace, allowing for a blend of theoretical learning with practical, real-world scenarios. This technological integration extends to the methods used to assess counseling students. Digital assessments, online simulations, and interactive case studies are increasingly employed to evaluate student competencies, ensuring a comprehensive and modern approach to counselor education. Training programs thus emphasize a mix of simulation-based learning, extensive practicums, and exposure to varied assessment scenarios.

Developing a discerning approach to these new tools is crucial. Future counselors must critically evaluate new digital tools for their reliability, validity, and adherence to ethical standards. This critical analytical skill is essential to ensure that their chosen tools are apt for the diverse needs and contexts they will encounter in their professional practice. As technology reshapes our ideas of counselor education and assessment, future counselors must be theoretically knowledgeable and practically adept in utilizing these diverse and evolving tools. The goal is to ensure that as the methods and tools evolve, counselors are well-prepared to provide effective, ethical, and client-centered care in an increasingly digital world.

EMBRACING THE FUTURE OF COUNSELING ASSESSMENTS

In a field that's continually reshaped by new research and technologies, the learning journey for a counselor never truly ends. This ongoing journey is marked by a commitment to professional development, a pursuit that keeps counselors aligned with the latest advancements in their field. This alignment is about immersing oneself in an ongoing educational process that spans a counselor's career. Equally important is networking and collaboration, as the collective wisdom of a professional community offers unparalleled opportunities for learning and growth. Engaging actively with peers, sharing experiences, and collaborating on various initiatives opens doors to new perspectives and deepens a counselor's understanding of evolving assessment methodologies. Staying connected with academic and clinical research forms another cornerstone of a counselor's continuous education. Counselors ensure that the latest insights and evidence always inform their practice by engaging with current research findings, contributing to scholarly discussions, and participating in research initiatives. Adaptability and flexibility in this ever-changing field become beneficial and essential traits. The ability to integrate new information and adapt assessment methods accordingly ensures that a counselor's practice remains relevant, effective, and responsive to the shifting needs of their clients. Lastly, the ethical dimension of counseling assessments is an area that requires continuous attention and learning. As new tools and methods emerge, so do their ethical considerations and implications. Engaging in continuous ethical education is imperative to navigate these complexities responsibly, ensuring the highest standards of client care are upheld.

As we draw this exploration to a close, it becomes evident that counseling assessments are poised on the cusp of significant transformation. This journey through the emerging trends and innovations in assessments has illuminated the path ahead and underscored our profession's enduring core: the commitment to understanding, supporting, and aiding those who seek our help. Integrating advanced technologies, from AI-driven tools to immersive VR environments, signals a future where assessments are more nuanced, precise, and accessible. Yet, as we embrace these technological strides, the essence of counseling, human connection, and understanding remains paramount. It is this balance between technological advancement and human empathy that will define the future effectiveness of counseling assessments.

CHECKING IN WITH SARAH

Sarah has been working with her counselor and registered dietitian weekly for the past 8 months. Additionally, she meets with her psychiatrist for medication maintenance every other month. Sarah has accomplished many of her treatment goals, as evidenced by her active participation and feedback from her multidisciplinary team, which includes her family, counselor, dietitian, psychiatrist, general practitioner, school counselor, and cheer coach. Further, she shows an increase in skills, self-care, and mood via a self-reported weekly diary card accessed through a mobile application. Sarah is ready and excited to plan for a transition to college. She will remain in the state to attend a university a few hours from her home. Fortunately, Sarah's counselor's practice offers digital delivery, allowing Sarah to maintain continuity of care through virtual sessions. This delivery change prompted Sarah's counselor to provide her with the Software Services and Telehealth Consent form. In preparation for the transition, Sarah's counselor uses an online assessment platform to send Sarah an invitation to retake several of the supplementary diagnostic assessments that she took at the start of her treatment. This allows the counselor to monitor progress and set new goals. Sarah's counselor will prompt the assessment platform to send routine outcome measures (ROMs) every month during Sarah's first semester away. To help Sarah take over the management of her own treatment schedule and billing account, the counselor provides her with a portal invitation for her practice software system. Sarah can request and change appointments, manage her billing account, and log in to her virtual sessions here. Sarah's parents will also have access to the account. The first telehealth session encountered initial challenges, with Sarah logging in from her car en route to a café where she intended to have her session. The counselor asked Sarah to find a parking spot and then rejoin the session. During that visit, most of the time was spent orienting Sarah to telehealth etiquette and the boundaries of digital services. To help Sarah cope ahead, they identified the best time of day for a standing session, potential private locations, and paralleling the in-person environments when in the digital environment. As she adapted, Sarah successfully utilized telehealth for her weekly counseling sessions, bi-monthly dietetic appointments, and quarterly medication management reviews. To keep abreast of progress, Sarah receives an email prompt periodically to complete ROMs. The measures are scored by the system and distributed to her multidisciplinary treatment team. Looking towards the future, Sarah's counselor plans to introduce AR sessions, utilizing an Apple headset, as a new dimension to telehealth counseling. Sarah will be one of her first clients to join sessions using this new digital platform.

1. Sarah's counselor felt that telehealth was an effective option for Sarah as she transitioned to college. Would you continue digitally delivered treatment or refer Sarah to a provider near her university? Why?

2. The counselor provided Sarah with the Software Services and Telehealth Consent Form. What type of information must be included in this form? What additional information might a counselor want to include that outlines telehealth and online etiquette?

3. Suppose the ROMs begin to show a slight decline in wellness toward the end of the semester. As a telehealth provider, how might you navigate this with Sarah?

4. Sarah can benefit from creating a digital toolkit so that, while at college, she has go-to skills immediately available on her device. What mobile applications are beneficial for clients to consider when building a digital toolkit?

END-OF-CHAPTER RESOURCES

DISCUSSION QUESTIONS

1. How do you think the integration of AI and ML in counseling assessments will change the traditional approaches to diagnosing and understanding mental health conditions? Discuss potential benefits and challenges.

2. With the rise of digital and online assessments, what ethical dilemmas do you foresee for future counselors? How should they navigate issues related to data privacy, security, and the digital divide?

3. VR and AR are becoming more prevalent in counseling assessments. Discuss how these technologies can enhance the assessment process and what limitations they might have, especially in understanding complex human behaviors.

4. Considering the rapid advancement in assessment technologies, how should counselor education programs adapt to prepare future counselors? Discuss the importance of practical training with digital tools versus traditional methods.

5. How can counselors effectively use digital tools to collaborate with other healthcare professionals in the context of integrated care? Discuss the importance of interdisciplinary communication and data sharing in providing comprehensive client care.

CLASS ACTIVITIES

1. **Digital Assessment Tool Evaluation:** Consider digital assessment tools (e.g., PsychSurveys). Work in pairs to research one tool, focusing on how it works, its applications in counseling, its advantages and limitations, and any ethical considerations. Prepare a brief presentation to share findings with the class, including a possible demonstration (e.g., a walkthrough of the tool's interface or features). Following the presentations, facilitate a discussion about the future of digital tools in counseling, encouraging others to consider how these tools might evolve and the skills they will need to utilize them effectively.

2. **Creation of a Client Bill of Rights and Informed Consent for Digital Tools and Assessments:** Working in groups of three or four, draft a "Client Bill of Rights" for digital counseling services. This document should outline clients' rights regarding digital tools, data privacy, confidentiality, and access to their information. The Bill of Rights should address:

    - the right to be informed about the nature and purpose of digital assessment tools
    - the right to confidentiality and how data are protected
    - the right to access or refuse the use of digital services
    - the right to be informed about data breaches or security issues

In the same groups, create an informed consent form that counselors will provide to clients before using digital tools and assessments. The form should cover:

- detailed information about the digital tools and services being used (e.g., types of digital assessments, teletherapy platforms)
- the potential risks and benefits of using these digital tools
- data storage, security measures, and the handling of digital records
- the client's right to withdraw consent at any time

Reflection on Ethical Implications: As a group, write a brief reflection on the ethical implications of using digital tools in counseling, discussing the importance of the Client Bill of Rights and informed consent in upholding ethical standards.

Using the case example given, demonstrate how you would present the Client Bill of Rights and the informed consent form to the client, tailoring the approach to the specific needs and context of the scenario.

3. **VR Simulation Exercise:** Divide into small groups. Each group will be given a VR headset and access to a VR counseling simulation (e.g., a VR exposure therapy session for phobias). Take turns experiencing the VR environment and then role-play as both the counselor and client in a simulated session. After the exercise, each group discusses their experience, focusing on VR's benefits, challenges, and potential applications in counseling. Finally, in class, discuss and share insights and reflections from the group discussions.

 ## PERSPECTIVE FROM THE FIELD

In this concluding chapter on the future of counseling assessment, we delve into the transformative role of technology in reshaping counseling and assessment practices. We present the insights of Clara Bossie, a licensed marriage and family therapist, and Aldo Gonzalez, a software architect, whose unique partnership and expertise bridge the gap between the realms of mental health and technological innovation. Clara and Aldo offer a forward-looking perspective on the integration of technology in counseling assessment. This dialogue anticipates future trends and encourages emerging counselors to consider how digital advancements can be harnessed to foster more effective, accessible, and compassionate therapeutic interventions. Clara is the owner of Wisely Wellness, a counseling, clinical supervision, and consulting firm. She brings almost two decades of experience in clinical care and the innovative use of digital tools to enhance client care and program development. Joining the discussion is Aldo, a technology expert with a 25-year background in building software solutions. He is the president of Total Tech Consulting and the Chief Technology Officer at Client Support Software. Additionally, Clara and Aldo are both Mindful Self-Compassion teachers, with Aldo particularly passionate about bringing soft skills into the tech world.

Access podcasts via the QR code or http://connect.springerpub.com/content/book/978-0-8261-8913-4/chapter/ch00.

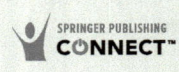

A robust set of instructor resources designed to supplement this text is located at http://connect.springerpub.com/content/book/978-0-8261-8913-4. Qualifying instructors may request access by emailing textbook@springerpub.com.

REFERENCES

Council for Accreditation of Counseling and Related Educational Programs. (n.d.). *Digital delivery of programs statement*. https://www.cacrep.org/for-programs/digital-delivery/#digital-delivery-of-programs-statement

Council for Accreditation of Counseling and Related Educational Programs. (2023). *2024 CACREP standards*. https://www.cacrep.org/wp-content/uploads/2023/06/Combined-version-6.21.23.pdf

14

Resources for Assessment in Counseling

CARMAN S. GILL, KELLY EMELIANCHIK-KEY, AND AYSE TORRES

DIAGNOSTIC INTERVIEW

In this video, the counselor works with Elphie, the client, to conduct a thorough diagnostic interview. He introduces the assessment and the purpose of the assessment, determines the client's presenting problem, and completes a series of questions toward understanding mental health symptoms. The counselor utilizes an encouragement-based approach to gathering the information necessary to begin a comprehensive and accurate case conceptualization. Both individuals are student volunteers, and this scenario is fictitious (i.e., meant for training purposes only). *Access the video via the QR code or* http://connect.springerpub.com/content/book/978-0-8261-8913-4/chapter/ch00.

CASE CONCEPTUALIZATION: MEGHAN

Presenting Problem and Context: Meghan is a 16-year-old White high school student referred to counseling after an accident that was suspected to be a suicidal gesture. She is a competitive gymnast, and her most recent accident has injured her to where she can no longer train or compete. She was referred to therapy partly to gather information on her mental wellbeing to clarify insurance-related concerns surrounding the accident. She was also restricted from competing until her team receives confirmation from her therapist that she is mentally well enough to do so. She presents in therapy with agitated, defensive mood and congruent affect. She communicates aggressively and abrasively and displays likely depressive symptoms and suicidal ideation, as evidenced by past incidents involving bodily harm and statements like "dying would have solved my problems." Her presentation was precipitated by the accident, and Meghan otherwise denies the need for counseling, stating that she is simply engaging to get the "professional opinion" that will clear her to compete in gymnastics again. Additionally, Meghan has been babysitting the children of her middle-aged gymnastics coach, Sy, and recently Sy's ex-wife informed Meghan that they wish for her to stay away from the children, as the children are becoming too attached to Meghan, which may have precipitated Meghan's depression and likely suicidality. Meghan also reports a romantic and sexual relationship with Sy, which has caused confusion and distress in Meghan's life. Meghan is guarded and defensive in therapy. Her movement is toward and then away from others, initially seeking attention to remain safe and then moving away in fear of rejection. Thus, her relationships to others are intensely unstable, aligning with the borderline personality style and a depressive disorder and possible eating disorder.

Mental Status Exam: Meghan dresses appropriately with clean clothes and good hygiene and appears to be oriented x4. Her mood ranges from depressed to euphoric, to angry and guarded. She appears to have an above-average IQ, as evidenced by her ability to articulate thoughts and her reports of performing at a high level academically. Meghan appears to have a functioning short-term and long-term memory, and her difficulty recalling information appears at times to be voluntary and at times due to trauma and mood symptoms, complicating self-reporting. She demonstrates poor insight, as evidenced by her limited awareness of the nature of her relationship with her gymnastics coach, her and her teammates' relationships with food, and her parents' divorce. Meghan's judgment is poor, as evidenced by her engagement with her gymnastics coach and her involvement in multiple accidents and high-risk behaviors including getting out of a car in the rain and breaking a picture frame in the therapist's office. Meghan's parents wonder if she has engaged in self-injurious behavior and suicidal ideation, though she has not explicitly reported suicidal ideation, plan, or intent.

Developmental History and Dynamics: Little is known about Meghan's family history outside of relational conflict and divorce between her parents. She reports being an only child and was put into competitive gymnastics at a young age, which became the focus point of her household. This placed Meghan in a position to be scrutinized and held to a high standard from early childhood, contributing to her sense of responsibility regarding her parents' divorce and father's later relational issues. She expressed the love she knows her father has for her yet does not view him as truly supportive or present in her life.

Meghan recalls one of her early recollections (ERs) during her first year of gymnastics when she failed to execute a move at practice and was reprimanded by her coach. She states that she remembers clearly thinking that she would prove that she could complete the move perfectly, but her timing was just off. Her coach raised his voice at her, stating "anyone could have done better." Meghan reports feelings of betrayal, as she trusted her coach, and was angry with herself for not getting his approval. From this experience, she began developing the core belief that her performance in gymnastics dictated the acceptance she earned from loved ones, and she began equating her value with her athletic performance. This belief continues to be prominent today, as she believes she must perform at a high level to be loved and deemed worthy. Her pattern is rooted in the movement toward others for love and acceptance, then away for fear of disappointment and rejection. Meghan's ER also shows her ability to self-reflect but also her tendency toward self-blame and anger. Meghan's parents' eventual divorce perpetuated Meghan's belief of her inferiority and lack of value, and further complicated her feeling secure and safe in relationships and her own identity.

Social History and Cultural Dynamics: Meghan is a teenager in an upper middle-class, White, single-parent household. She is presumably heterosexual and cisgender and reports a limited social life due to the time commitment of competitive gymnastics. She reports that her most significant relationship is with her middle-aged gymnastics coach Sy, with whom she is currently romantically and sexually involved. This exacerbated Meghan's social difficulties, as her teammates have grown jealous and resentful of her for her close relationship with Sy. She reports having no time to socialize outside of her school, gymnastics, and babysitting responsibilities. However, she was recently informed she would no longer be babysitting, reducing her socialization with Sy's family. Meghan's immediate family culture is unknown, and her involvement in gymnastics appears to be the most operative factor in her cultural identity, as it has influenced her self-image, eating habits, and interpersonal relationships.

Health History and Health Behaviors: Meghan's current health considerations are her potentially disordered eating habits and her physical injuries sustained in her most recent accident. She is physically active and engages in a rigorous training regimen for gymnastics.

She reports pressure on her to have a thin physique, which could influence unsafe eating habits and future health complications. She reports no alcohol or illicit substance use, and no preexisting health conditions or genetic predispositions for illness. She reports no current or past prescription medications.

Client Resources: Meghan appears to have a lack of adaptive support. Her primary relationships include her mother, Sy, and her gymnastics teammates, though none appear sufficiently supportive of her mental wellness. She appears to be in the precontemplation stage of change, as evidenced by her limited insight into the severity of her accidents and possible desire for self-harming. She does not seem to comprehend the need for treatment and has developed a skewed perception of adult support due to her parents' divorce and her relationship with Sy. She has displayed an increased capacity for self-disclosure in therapy. However, she will need to continue increasing her ability to utilize her therapist as a resource for guidance and support. She demonstrates strengths including consistency, intelligence, and self-discipline, and she can incorporate these skills into therapy to assist her in achieving the goals outlined in her treatment plan.

Diagnostic Formulation: Meghan meets seven of the nine diagnostic criteria for Borderline Personality Disorder. She demonstrated frantic efforts to avoid abandonment in her first session with the therapist, questioning his investment in her and his intentions (1). She demonstrates a pattern of unstable interpersonal relationships, and both idealizes and devalues herself and others, particularly Sy and her parents (2). Her involvement in gymnastics has exacerbated her identity disturbance and self-image and her performance in school (3). Her destructive behaviors, such as breaking the picture frame, and her relationship with Sy reflect self-damaging impulsivity (4). She has been involved in two accidents that are assumed to be suicidal gestures (5). Meghan has displayed mood inconsistencies and unpredictability with her mood, ranging from euphoric to angry or depressed with congruent affect (6). Similarly, Meghan has displayed inappropriate, intense anger with Sy and her therapist, reflecting her inability to control her anger and her temper (8).

Diagnostic and Statistical Manual of Mental Disorders **(5th ed., Text Revision;** *DSM-5-TR*) **Diagnosis:** F60.3 Borderline Personality Disorder
   More information is needed to determine whether a diagnosis of Depressive Disorder is warranted and to differentiate between suicidal behavior and nonsuicidal self-injury (NSSI). Thorough assessment is needed in terms of ruling out an Anorexia Nervosa diagnosis.

Clinical Formulation: Meghan's agitated, defensive mood and depressive symptoms (*presentation*) seem to be her reaction to her most recent accident and the wife of her gymnastics coach discouraging her from coming to their house (*precipitant*). Meghan seeks attention and validation from others while also clashing with others by sizing them up and anticipating harm (*maladaptive pattern*). Meghan's presenting problems are understandable when viewed from the perspective of her lifestyle. Her style of relating to others relates directly to the conditional support received from her parents and childhood coach, as it compels her to seek acceptance and love in any way available. She reports a self-view of superiority, though this is likely an attempt at masking her low self-worth and self-image. Meghan's self-view is presumably that she is only as valuable as her achievements and measurable performance within her role obligations. This self-view is challenged by her romantic and sexual involvement with her current coach, who is admired and whose attention is sought after by her peers. Meghan views others as demanding and unsupportive, and she views the world as a judgmental, conditional place in which she must accomplish things athletically and academically to earn value and acceptance. Her life strategy appears to be centered in aiming for perfection, and she believes that by striving for accolades and meeting the demands and needs of others, she will avoid rejection and abandonment (*predisposition*). Furthermore, her strategy of appeasing others and degrading herself when she falls short of perfection is perpetuated by her lack of emotion regulation skills and the excessively high-intensity and high-pressure environment of competitive gymnastics (*perpetuants*).

Cultural Formulation: Meghan identifies as White and a competitive gymnast (*cultural identity*). She reports no difficulties with her racial identity, though her identification as a highly accomplished gymnast is operative in her presentation. Her self-image, eating habits, mood symptoms, and maladaptive interpersonal relationships are impacted by the enmeshed nature of her personality, resulting from her involvement in the sport (*culture-acculturation*). Meghan believes that her current presentation is a product of the turmoil in her parents' marriage and the pressure she feels from family and her gymnastics coach (*cultural explanation*). Meghan's personality dynamics are more operative than her culture, as her borderline personality style manifests as inappropriate anger, mood swings, inconsistent self-image, presumed self-harm, and fear of abandonment. However, the implications of Meghan's cultural identity as a competitive gymnast must be considered in her treatment, as they are clinically relevant and directly amplify symptoms and borderline personality traits (*culture vs. personality*).

Treatment Formulation and Plan: The treatment pattern is to establish movement toward others to relate to them in an adaptive, emotionally safe manner with less projection of harm and abandonment. Treatment will also work to reduce depressive symptoms and implications of her borderline personality style (*treatment pattern*). First order goals will be to reduce Meghan's depressive symptoms and suicidal behaviors, and address/reduce her angry outbursts. Second order goals will be to reduce Meghan's maladaptive pattern of ambivalent movement and projection in relationships and perfectionistic ideals and behaviors. The therapist will increase Meghan's capacity for adaptive interpersonal interactions and address her dependency and need for acceptance, validation, and attention. The therapist will attempt to reduce high-risk behaviors for meeting needs and identify consequences associated with sizing up others and behaving out of fear of abandonment. In pursuing third order goals, Meghan will develop the ability to self-regulate negative emotions in the moment and utilize adaptive coping strategies to avoid angry outbursts and self-harm. She will identify red flag behaviors and cognitions and manage depressive symptoms without the direct guidance of the therapist. She will be self-directed in reality testing and monitoring cognitive distortions to improve interpersonal effectiveness (*treatment goals*). The focus will be to increase Meghan's awareness of her aggressive, fearful thoughts and behaviors, and the consequences associated, as well as her capacity for emotion regulation and interpersonal effectiveness (*treatment focus*). The therapist will work to improve Meghan's ability to correlate perfectionism and unreasonably high expectations of gymnastics, and her emotional wellness and behaviors in other areas of life. Additionally, the treatment strategy will include increasing Meghan's capacity for self-acceptance and improve her self-image to reduce engagement in high-risk behaviors including sex and self-harm (*treatment strategy*). The therapist will utilize motivational interviewing to encourage Meghan to identify problematic elements with sleeping with a married middle-aged man and facilitate dialogue about adaptive relationships, boundaries, sexual abuse, and her relationship with food. Similarly, Motivational Interviewing will focus on encouraging Meghan to discuss the negative implications of being immersed in competitive gymnastics. The therapist will educate Meghan on skills including reality testing and cognitive distortions (overgeneralization, catastrophic thinking, projection) to increase awareness of her own maladaptive pattern and interpersonal ineffectiveness. The therapist will use the solution-focused "exception period" and encourage Meghan to identify a time in her life when she was better able to manage impulsivity and when she was not compelled to self-harm. The concept of "deviation amplification" will be used to reintroduce skills and strategies that increase contentment and fulfillment in her life outside of gymnastics. The therapist will encourage Meghan to meet with a psychiatrist for medication consultation. Lastly, the therapist will introduce dialectical behavior therapy (DBT), focusing on mindfulness skills including meditation, breathing, counting, tapping exercises, and the use of mantras to regulate and reduce anger and aggression in emotionally tense moments (*treatment interventions*).

Because of Meghan's borderline personality style, the therapist anticipates that Meghan could terminate treatment due to a lack of trust that the therapist cares for her, or due to a perceived attack or fear of abandonment. This underscores the importance of the therapist fostering a safe, secure therapeutic environment and alliance. It is possible that Meghan's coach may pressure her to terminate treatment, due to his ability to manipulate and control her and her demanding gymnastics training schedule. Meghan is a presumably moderate to high risk for NSSI and/or suicidal behavior, and therefore further acts of self-harm could interrupt treatment. The therapist will need to regularly assess Meghan's suicidal ideation. If the therapist provides Meghan with an assessment permitting her to return to her normal life, it is possible Meghan could terminate treatment (*treatment obstacles*). The therapist will need to provide treatment in a competent and sensitive way, considering her cultural identity as a competitive gymnast. The therapist will need to place attention on compassionate, nonjudgmental, validating, and accepting communication and treatment. Moreover, the therapist will need to consider the implications of Meghan's identity as a child of divorced parents to concentrate on consistency and dependability to strengthen the therapeutic alliance (*treatment-cultural*). Meghan's prognosis is fair if she demonstrates willingness to comply with treatment and share honestly with the therapist about her history of depressive symptoms and suicidality. Her borderline personality style prevents her prognosis from being good, but if she is able to increase awareness and utilizes adaptive skills to regulate emotion and distress, her prognosis will be improved (*treatment-prognosis*).

CASE CONCEPTUALIZATION ELEMENTS WORKSHEET: MEGHAN

Presentation	Meghan presents with an agitated, defensive mood and congruent affect. She appears controlling with aggressive, abrasive, demanding speech. Meghan demonstrates paranoia at times regarding a report written about her and her therapist's communication with her mother and demonstrates the skill deficit of emotion regulation (sadness, anger). Meghan displays possible depression and suicidal ideation, as evidenced by passive behaviors and remarks related to suicide (deliberately hurting herself, stating "dying would have solved my problems" then quickly denying she meant anything by it).
Precipitant	Meghan was involved in an accident in which she collided with a moving car in traffic. It is presumed that this was a suicidal gesture or passive suicidal behavior, and it was the catalyst for Meghan's referral to treatment. Meghan immediately states her intentions for therapy, claiming she is strictly there for a "professional opinion" to be cleared to return to compete in gymnastics. Her recent accident was precipitated by her gymnastics coach's wife discouraging her from coming to their house because the children were becoming too attached to Meghan.

(continued)

CASE CONCEPTUALIZATION ELEMENTS WORKSHEET: MEGHAN (*continued*)

Maladaptive Pattern	Meghan demonstrates an ambivalent pattern: She moves toward others to get attention and feel worthwhile but pays a high price and becomes compromised (perfectionism in gymnastics, sex with her middle-aged coach, causing physical harm to herself). She moves against others by sizing them up but expecting them to harm her (taunting therapist using his books and his daughter, sarcastically mocking his education and competency, then accuses therapist of not caring about her).
Predisposition	**Biological:** No significant biological factors are mentioned, though client is possibly engaging in disordered eating. Meghan's neck and arms are currently injured from her recent accident. **Psychological (personality style, coping capacity)** *Personality style*: borderline personality style *Skill deficits*: emotion management and regulation, distress tolerance, assertive communication, impulse control **Self–Other Schemas** *Self-view*: Meghan appears to speak and think more highly of herself than the other girls on her gymnastics team, though this is likely an attempt at masking her low self-worth. Her presumed inferiority is evidenced by her high level of involvement in the perfectionistic culture of competitive gymnastics. Her self-view is challenged by her romantic and sexual involvement with her coach, who is admired and whose attention is sought after by her peers. *Worldview*: Meghan views the world as a place that demands achievement from her, and she must succeed to earn acceptance and love from others. She views the world as judgmental, inconsistent, and overwhelming. **Life strategy:** Meghan's life strategy is to aim for perfection. She attempts to please those around her, particularly her parents and her coach, by striving for athletic accolades and providing sex to avoid rejection and reprimanding. **Social:** Meghan appears to have limited to no social life outside of gymnastics. Between attending school and practice, she sounded surprised when the therapist asked her "how's life?" because gymnastics appears to be most or all of her life. **Strengths/Resiliencies:** Meghan has demonstrated the capacity for commitment and dedication, courageous self-disclosure, intelligence, and some awareness.
Perpetuants	Meghan's maladaptive pattern is maintained by her lack of emotion regulation skills, lack of insight into her own depressive symptoms, and the excessively high-intensity and high-pressure environment of competitive gymnastics.
Cultural Identity	No significant cultural elements are mentioned. Meghan is presumably middle-class to upper-middle-class and White. She belongs to the highly competitive, idealistic culture of competitive gymnastics. This element of her identity is clinically relevant and exacerbates symptoms. She is presumably cisgender and female, neither of which are operative in her current presentation.
Acculturation	Meghan has a high level of acculturation related to certain elements of her cultural identity (race, gender) but is experiencing high acculturative stress regarding her involvement in the gymnastics culture.
Cultural Explanation	Meghan believes that her current presentation is a product of the turmoil in her parents' marriage, as well as the pressure she feels from family and her gymnastics coach.
Culture vs. Personality	Meghan's personality dynamics are more operative than her culture, as her borderline personality style manifests as inappropriate anger, mood swings, inconsistent self-image, presumed self-harm, and fear of abandonment.

(*continued*)

CASE CONCEPTUALIZATION ELEMENTS WORKSHEET: MEGHAN (*continued*)

Treatment Pattern	The treatment pattern is to establish movement toward others to relate to them in an adaptive, emotionally safe manner with less projection of harm and abandonment. Treatment will also work to reduce depressive symptoms and implications of her borderline personality style.
Treatment Goals	**First order:** reduce depressive symptoms and suicidal behaviors. Address and reduce angry outbursts. **Second order:** reduce maladaptive pattern of abrasiveness and projection in relationships. Reduce perfectionistic ideals and behaviors and increase adaptive interpersonal interactions. Address dependency and need for acceptance, validation, and attention and reduce high-risk behaviors for meeting needs. Identify consequences associated with sizing up others and behaving out of fear of abandonment. **Third order:** Meghan will have the ability to self-regulate negative emotions in the moment and utilize adaptive coping strategies to avoid angry outbursts and self-harm. She will identify red flag behaviors and cognitions and manage depressive symptoms without direct guidance of the therapist. She will be self-directed in reality testing and monitoring cognitive distortions to improve interpersonal effectiveness.
Treatment Focus	The focus is to increase Meghan's awareness of her aggressive, fearful thoughts and behaviors and the consequences associated. It also involves increasing her capacity for emotion regulation and interpersonal effectiveness.
Treatment Strategy	The strategy is to improve Meghan's ability to correlate perfectionism and unreasonably high expectations of gymnastics, and her emotional wellness and behaviors in other areas of life. Another goal is to increase Meghan's capacity for self-acceptance and improve her self-image to reduce engagement in high-risk behaviors including sex and self-harm.
Treatment Interventions	Use Motivational Interviewing to encourage Meghan to identify problematic elements with sleeping with a married middle-aged man and facilitate dialogue about adaptive relationships, boundaries, sexual abuse, and her relationship with food. Use Motivational Interviewing to encourage Meghan to discuss the negative implications of being immersed in competitive gymnastics. Educate Meghan on skills including reality testing and cognitive distortions (overgeneralization, catastrophic thinking, projection) to increase awareness of her own maladaptive pattern and interpersonal ineffectiveness. Use solution-focused "exception period" and encourage Meghan to identify a time in her life when she was better able to manage impulsivity and when she was not compelled to self-harm. Use "deviation amplification" to reintroduce skills and strategies that increase contentment and fulfillment in her life outside of gymnastics. Encourage Meghan to meet with a psychiatrist for medication consultation. Teach Meghan dialectical behavior therapy (DBT) skills, particularly mindfulness skills including meditation, breathing, counting, and tapping exercises, and the use of mantras to regulate and reduce anger and aggression in emotionally tense moments.
Treatment Obstacles	Because of Meghan's borderline personality style, Meghan may terminate treatment due to a lack of trust that the therapist cares for her, or due to a perceived attack or fear of abandonment. This emphasizes the importance of the therapist fostering a safe, secure therapeutic environment and alliance. It is possible that Meghan's relationship with her coach could pressure her to terminate treatment, due to his ability to manipulate and control her and her demanding gymnastics training schedule. Meghan is a presumably moderate to high suicide risk, and therefore further acts of self-harm could interrupt treatment. The therapist will need to regularly assess Meghan's suicidal ideation. If the therapist provides Meghan with an assessment permitting her to return to her normal life, it is possible Meghan could terminate treatment.

(*continued*)

CASE CONCEPTUALIZATION ELEMENTS WORKSHEET: MEGHAN (*continued*)

Treatment Cultural	The therapist must provide treatment in a competent and sensitive way, considering her cultural identity as a competitive gymnast. The therapist will need to place attention on compassionate, nonjudgmental, validating, and accepting communication and treatment.
Treatment Prognosis	Meghan's prognosis is fair if she demonstrates willingness to comply with treatment and share honestly with the therapist about her history of depressive symptoms and suicidality. Her borderline personality style prevents her prognosis from being good, but if she is able to increase awareness and utilizes adaptive skills to regulate emotion and distress, her prognosis is improved.

PERCENTILE CONVERSIONS WITH Z-SCORES

Standard Scores and Percentiles

Z-score	Percentile	Z-score	Percentile	Z-score	Percentile	Z-score	Percentile
−3.5	00.02	−1.00	15.87	0.00	50.00	1.1	86.43
−3.0	00.13	−0.95	17.11	0.05	51.99	1.2	88.49
−2.9	00.19	−0.90	18.41	0.10	53.98	1.3	90.32
−2.8	00.26	−0.85	19.77	0.15	55.96	1.4	91.92
−2.7	00.35	−0.80	21.19	0.20	57.93	1.5	93.32
−2.6	00.47	−0.75	22.66	0.25	59.87	1.6	94.52
−2.5	00.62	−0.70	24.20	0.30	61.79	1.7	95.54
−2.4	00.82	−0.65	25.78	0.35	63.68	1.8	96.41
−2.3	01.07	−0.60	27.43	0.40	65.54	1.9	97.13
−2.2	01.39	−0.55	29.12	0.45	67.36	2.0	97.72
−2.1	01.79	−0.50	30.85	0.50	69.15	2.1	98.21
−2.0	02.28	−0.45	32.64	0.55	70.88	2.2	98.61
−1.9	02.87	−0.40	34.46	0.60	72.57	2.3	98.93
−1.8	03.59	−0.35	36.32	0.65	74.22	2.4	99.18
−1.7	04.46	−0.30	38.21	0.70	75.80	2.5	99.38
−1.6	05.48	−0.25	40.13	0.75	77.34	2.6	99.53
−1.5	06.68	−0.20	42.07	0.80	78.81	2.7	99.65
−1.4	08.08	−0.15	44.04	0.85	80.23	2.8	99.74
−1.3	09.68	−0.10	46.02	0.90	81.59	2.9	99.81
−1.2	11.51	−0.05	48.01	0.95	82.89	3.0	99.87
−1.1	13.57	−0.00	50.00	1.00	84.13	3.5	99.98

A caution regarding percentile from Z-score conversion tables is that using rounded Z-scores can lead to inaccurate conclusions. Rounding Z-scores incorrectly can result in imprecise percentiles and probabilities, which may affect the accuracy of statistical analysis and comparisons. It is commonly recommended to use unrounded Z-scores for maximum precision and avoid potential statistical calculation inaccuracies. Additionally, when interpreting Z-scores and percentiles, it is important to note that if the percentile is below 50, the corresponding Z-score will be negative, as all Z-scores to the left of the mean are negative.

A more precise percentile is calculated using the formula from a Z-score: $p = \Pr(Z < z^*)$.

- p is the percentile (as a probability). The resulting probability represents the percentile. Percentile tells you the proportion of values in the distribution that fall below the given z^* score.

- Pr is probability. This calculates the probability that a randomly selected Z value is less than the specific z^* value.

- Z is the standard random variable. This is a normal distribution (mean of 0 and a standard deviation of 1). The random variable Z follows this distribution.

- z^* is a specific Z-score value. This standardized score informs you how many standard deviations away from the mean a data point is. It is calculated using $(X - \mu) / \sigma$, where X is the raw score, μ is the population mean, and σ is the population standard deviation.

To use this formula:

1. Calculate or obtain the Z-score (z^*) for your data point (as mentioned in Chapter 6).

2. Use a standard normal distribution table or statistical software to find the probability that Z is less than z^*.

3. The resulting probability is the percentile.
   For example, if $z^* = 1.5$ and you find that $\Pr(Z < 1.5) = 0.9332$, this means a Z-score of 1.5 corresponds to the 93.32nd percentile.
   This method provides a precise way to calculate percentiles.

CLASS ACTIVITIES

1. Consider the case of Elphie. What additional assessments might assist the counselor and the client toward fully understanding her treatment needs?

2. For the case of Meghan, the therapist is considering engaging this character/client in a genogram for assessment and intervention. What would this look like? How would you proceed and what information would you hope to gain?

3. Meghan's case conceptualization indicates that a thorough assessment is needed to differentiate between suicidal behavior and NSSI. How would you as the therapist proceed?

4. Golda has a court-mandated session with you after she was found guilty of breaking and entering, as well as stealing food. The Bear family reported her to the police after finding her in their youngest child's bed, fast asleep. Golda has a history of breaking into homes but states that she doesn't remember engaging in the activity. She reports frequent gaps in her memory, a desire to run away from home, and a history of abuse by her stepmother. She is an only child whose father was killed shortly after he remarried.

What specific assessment(s) could impact this character's story and influence the counseling sessions, moving Golda in a positive manner and direction? How could a therapist intervene, using assessment, to fully understand and care for her? What are the ethical implications of using assessment with a court-mandated client?

ADDITIONAL RESOURCES

American Counseling Association. (n.d.). *The American Counseling Association (ACA) position statement on high stakes testing.* https://aarc-counseling.org/wp-content/uploads/2020/04/American-Counseling-Association-ACA-Position-Statement-on-High-Stakes-Testing.pdf

American Psychiatric Association. (2024). DSM-5-TR *online assessment measures.* https://www.psychiatry.org/psychiatrists/practice/dsm/educational-resources/assessment-measures

American Psychological Association. (2020). *Assessment tools (caregivers).* https://www.apa.org/pi/about/publications/caregivers/practice-settings/assessment/tools

American Psychological Association & APA Task Force on Psychological Assessment and Evaluation Guidelines. (2020). *APA guidelines for psychological assessment and evaluation.* https://www.apa.org/about/policy/guidelines-psychological-assessment-evaluation.pdf

Association for Assessment and Research in Counseling. (n.d.). *AARC's free assessment database.* https://docs.google.com/spreadsheets/d/1ooqa37vxHhjklN6qpRAMKc5kj6f2j5jivcqOv8sxloo/edit#gid=0

Association for Assessment and Research in Counseling. (2021). *AARC diversity inclusion and social justice committee resources list.* https://aarc-counseling.org/wp-content/uploads/2021/10/AARC-Diversity-Inclusion-and-Social-Justice-Resource-List-May-2021.pdf

Banks-VanAllen, C. (2023, May). Conceptualizing diagnosis through a social justice lens. *Counseling Today.* https://www.counseling.org/publications/counseling-today-magazine/article-archive/article/legacy/conceptualizing-diagnosis-through-a-social-justice-lens

Bennett, C., Blount, A., Gerlach, J., Chroede, K., Ausloos, C. D., Bloom, Z., Goodrich, K. M., Hollenbaugh, K. M., & Taylor, J. (2021). *Standards of care for assessment in group work.* https://aarc-counseling.org/wp-content/uploads/2021/09/Standards-for-Assessment-in-Group-Work-March-2021.pdf

Bray, B. (2021, September). Assessment, diagnosis, and treatment planning: A map for the journey ahead. *Counseling Today.* https://www.counseling.org/publications/counseling-today-magazine/article-archive/article/legacy/assessment-diagnosis-and-treatment-planning-a-map-for-the-journey-ahead

Gleeson, S. (2022, October). 'Not a monster': Destigmatizing borderline personality disorder. *Counseling Today.* https://www.counseling.org/publications/counseling-today-magazine/article-archive/article/legacy/not-a-monster-destigmatizing-borderline-personality-disorder

National Board of Forensic Evaluators. (2024, January 1). *Can licensed mental health counselors administer and interpret psychological tests?* https://www.nbfe.net/resources/Documents/Can%20Counselors%20Test.pdf

Rhodes, L. R. (2023, September). Taking a culturally responsive approach to suicide assessment. *Counseling Today.* https://www.counseling.org/publications/counseling-today-magazine/article-archive/article/legacy/taking-a-culturally-responsive-approach-to-suicide-assessment

Sperry, J., & Sperry, L. (2020, December). Case conceptualization: Key to highly effective counseling. *Counseling Today.* https://www.counseling.org/publications/counseling-today-magazine/article-archive/article/legacy/case-conceptualization-key-to-highly-effective-counseling

Index

AARC. *See* Association for Assessment and Research in Counseling
abilities, assessment of, 173–174, 177–179
abuse, 265–267
   of adults with disabilities, 266–267
   of child, 251, 266
   of older adults, 266–267
ACA. *See* American Counseling Association
Academic Optimism of School Surveys, 189
ACCESS for ELLs assessments, 184
accessibility, of tests, 45
accessibility bias, 46
acculturation, 51, 53–54
acculturative stress, 54
ACE. *See* Adverse Childhood Experiences questionnaire
achievement, assessments of, 183–184
achievement tests, 174
ACT. *See* American College Testing
actuarial risk assessment instruments (ARAIs), 264
addiction, 267
ADHD Rating Scale-5, 236
Adler, Alfred, 287
Adlerian therapists, 105
Adlerian therapy, 278, 282, 287
ADOS-2. *See* Autism Diagnostic Observation Schedule
Advanced Warning of RElapse (AWARE) questionnaire 3.0, 269
Adverse Childhood Experiences (ACE) questionnaire, 250, 251
AERA. *See* American Educational Research Association
age-equivalent norms, 139
ageism, 58
aging populations, 53, 57–58
AI-Therapy, 300
Alcohol, Smoking, and Substance Involvement Screening Test (ASSIST), 268
Alcohol Use Disorders Identification Test-C (AUDIT-C), 268
American College Testing (ACT), 185
American Counseling Association (ACA), 8, 12, 21, 24, 100
   Code of Ethics, 25, 26, 28, 29, 30, 31, 58, 79, 247–248
   Values and Statements, 42
American Educational Research Association (AERA), 3, 44
   Standards for Educational and Psychological Testing, 3, 8, 28, 151, 160
American Institutes for Research Conditions for Learning Survey, 189
American Mental Health Counselors Association (AMHCA), 58
American Psychiatric Association Practical Guidelines, 257
American Psychological Association (APA), 27, 79, 229
   Guidelines for Test User Qualifications, 27
American School Counselor Association (ASCA), 12, 49, 58
   Define, Manage, Deliver, and Assess, 188
   Ethical Standards for School Counselors, 13
   National Model, 188
American Society of Addiction Medicine (ASAM), 267
AMHCA. *See* American Mental Health Counselors Association
ancillary tests, in interviews, 77
anxiety, phobias, and fear, assessment of, 229–232
anxiety disorder assessments, 232
APA. *See* American Psychological Association
application-based tools, 299
aptitude, assessments of, 184–185
aptitude tests, 173–174, 183, 196
   assessments of, 184–185
ARAIs. *See* actuarial risk assessment instruments
arrangement projective techniques, 224
art-based assessment methods, 92
artificial intelligence and machine learning and, 299–300
artistic individuals, 201
ASAM. *See* American Society of Addiction Medicine
ASCA. *See* American School Counselor Association
ASD. *See* autism spectrum disorder
ASK. *See* Attitudes, Skills, and Knowledge
assessment. *See also individual entries*
   administering, 29
   cases studies and, 14–16
   conceptualizing and diagnosing clients for, 6–7

321

assessment (*continued*)
  in counseling, guidance for, 8–13
  as counselor, 5–6
  definition and meaning of, 3–4
  information, formats to access, 125–126
  intentionality in, 277–278
  issues in, 22–24
  laws and education in, 33–35
  legal issues in, 31–33
  multicultural-and diversity issues in, 29
  norm-, criterion-, and self-referenced, 5
  progress evaluation for, 7–8
  quantitative and qualitative, 4–5
  scoring and interpretation of, 29–30
  screening and, 6
  treatment plan and goal setting for, 7
assessment methods
  direct and indirect techniques of, 69–74
  formal and informal, 83
  formats of, 86–92
  initial interviews and, 74–77
  interview guidelines and, 77–83
  standardized and nonstandardized, 84–86
ASSIST. *See* Alcohol, Smoking, and Substance Involvement Screening Test
Association for Assessment and Research in Counseling (AARC), 8, 12
  Scientist Practitioner Model, 13
  Standards for Multicultural Assessment, 13
Association of Assessment in Research and Counseling, 27
association projective techniques, 224
Attitudes, Skills, and Knowledge (ASK) approach, 189–190
AUDIT-C. *See* Alcohol Use Disorders Identification Test-C
auditory processing, 178
augmented reality, 300–301
Augment Therapy, 301
authentic assessments, 129
Autism Diagnostic Observation Schedule (ADOS-2), 237
autism spectrum disorder (ASD), 235–236
autobiographical methods, of data assessment, 92
autonomy, 25
AWARE. *See* Advanced Warning of RElapse questionnaire 3.0

BAA. *See* business associate agreement
BAI. *See* Beck Anxiety Inventory
Bar-On Emotional Quotient Inventory: Youth Version (Bar-OnEQ-i:YV), 186
Bar-OnEQ-i:YV. *See* Bar-On Emotional Quotient Inventory: Youth Version
BASC-3PRS. *See* Behavior Assessment System for Children
BDD-SS. *See* Body Dysmorphic Disorder Symptom Scale
BDI and BDI-II. *See* Beck Depression Inventory

Beck Anxiety Inventory (BAI), 232, 290
Beck Depression Inventory (BDI), 4, 26, 229
  Second Edition (BDI-II), 290
Beck Hopelessness Scale, 290
behavioral interviews, 73–74
Behavior Assessment System for Children (BASC-3PRS), 186
Behavior Intervention Monitoring Assessment System (BIMAS-2), 186
bell curve, 135
BFI. *See* Big Five Inventory
bias
  minimization of, 48–49
  of tests, 45
Big Five Inventory (BFI), 197
BIMAS-2. *See* Behavior Intervention Monitoring Assessment System
Binet, Alfred, 21, 174
Binet-Simon Intelligence Scale, 174
biofeedback, 88
biological measures, 88
biopsychosocial assessments, 6
biopsychosocial-spiritual (BPSS) model, 75–76, 249, 283
  components of, 75
Bipolar Spectrum Diagnostic Scale (BSDS), 231
Blueprint (software), 107
Body Dysmorphic Disorder Symptom Scale (BDD-SS), 235
body mapping, 92
body size, 52, 57
box plot, 135
BPSS. *See* biopsychosocial-spiritual model
Bracken School Readiness Assessment (BSRA-4), 184
Bravemind, 301, 305
Brief Symptom Inventory (BSI), 238
BSDS. *See* Bipolar Spectrum Diagnostic Scale
BSI. *See* Brief Symptom Inventory
BSRA-4. *See* Bracken School Readiness Assessment
burnout, 252
business associate agreement (BAA), 302

CACREP. *See* Council for Accreditation of Counseling and Related Educational Programs
CAGE questionnaire, 267–269
CAGE-AID questionnaire, 269
California Psychological Inventory (CPI), 220
CAPS-5. *See* Clinician-Administered PTSD scale for *DSM-5*
career assessments, 195–197
  cultural considerations in, 198–199
  in online platforms, 197–198
  tools of, 200–208
  for veterans, 209–211
  for youth with disabilities, and transition, 208–209

career thoughts inventory (CTI), 211
carryover effects, 152, 156
CARS-2. *See* Childhood Autism Rating Scale
case conceptualization, 6–7, 282–283
    components of, 284–285
    functions of, 284
    worksheet of, 315–318
CASEL. *See* Collaborative for Academic, Social, and Emotional Learning
Cattell, James, 20
Cattell, Raymond, 177
Cattell-Horn-Carroll (CHC) theory, of cognitive abilities, 177–179
CBCL. *See* Child Behavior Checklist
CBT. *See* cognitive behavioral therapy
CDRS. *See* Children's Depression Rating Scale
Center for Epidemiologic Studies Depression Scale (CES-D) and Scale for Children (CES-DC), 230
Cerner, 303
CES-DC. *See* Center for Epidemiologic Studies Depression Scale (CES-D) and Scale for Children
CFA. *See* confirmatory factor analysis
CFI. *See* cultural formulation interview
ChEAT. *See* Child Eating Attitudes Test
checklists, 87
    in interviews, 77
child abuse, 266
Child Behavior Checklist (CBCL), 238
Child Eating Attitudes Test (ChEAT), 234
Childhood Autism Rating Scale (CARS-2), 237
Child Outcomes Rating Scale (CORS), 291
Children's Depression Rating Scale (CDRS), 230
Child Session Rating Scale (CSRS), 291
choice arrangement technique, 227
CI. *See* confidence intervals
classic test theory (CTT), 151, 152, 167
clinical approach, 264
clinical assessments
    of anxiety, phobias, and fear, 229–232
    common, 238–239
    in counseling, 217–228
    of depression and bipolar disorder, 228–229, 230–231
    of eating disorders, 232–234
    formats of, 217–218
    of neurodevelopmental disorders, 235–237
    of obsessive-compulsive and related disorders, 234–235
    personality assessments and, 219–223
    of psychotic disorders and related disorders, 238
    subjective and unstructured personality assessments and, 223–228
    and use, in settings, 218–219
Clinical Outcomes Routine Evaluation-10 (CORE-10), 290–291

Clinician-Administered PTSD Scale for *DSM-5* (CAPS-5), 251
cloud-based tools, 299
code of ethics, 24
coefficient alpha, 157–158
coefficient of determination (R^2), 143
CogAT test, 184, 190
cognitive behavioral therapy (CBT), 104, 105
collaborative and client-centered approaches, 303–304
Collaborative for Academic, Social, and Emotional Learning (CASEL), 186, 189
collateral information, 7
collateral information gathering, in interviews, 77
college entrance exam scores, 138
Columbia-Suicide Severity Rating Scale (C-SSRS), 4, 257
Commission on Rehabilitation Counselor Certification (CRCC), 13, 58
communication, integrated approach to, 278–279
    assessment findings and, 279–280
    assessment report writing and, 280–281
    case conceptualization and, 282–283
    International Classification of Functioning, Disability, and Health and, 288–291
    treatment planning and, 281–282
compassion fatigue, 252
completion projective techniques, 224
computer-based scoring, 129
conceptual equivalence, 23
Concise Manual for the Professional Quality of Life Scale, 253
concurrent validity, 162
confidence interval (CI), 154
confidentiality, 31–32
confirmability, 164
confirmatory factor analysis (CFA), 161–162
Conners' Rating Scales (CRS), 236
construction projective techniques, 224
construct irrelevance, 160
construct-irrelevant variance, 43, 47
constructs, 3, 4, 150
construct underrepresentation, 45, 47, 160
construct validity, 161–162
content bias, 46
content-oriented assessment, 165
content sampling error, 153
content validity, 160–161, 165
continuous variables, 123–124
conventional individuals, 202
convergent validity, 161
correlation, 140
correlation coefficient, 140
CORS. *See* Child Outcomes Rating Scale
Council for Accreditation of Counseling and Related Educational Programs (CACREP), 3, 8, 305
Counselor Burnout Inventory, 162
counselor education, 305–306

counselors, as agents of change, 51–58
Counselors Preparation Comprehensive Examination (CPCE), 127
CPCE. *See* Counselors Preparation Comprehensive Examination
CPI. *See* California Psychological Inventory
CRCC. *See* Commission on Rehabilitation Counselor Certification
credibility, 164
crisis, 248
criterion-referenced assessments, 5
criterion-referenced tests, 130
criterion-related validity, 162–163
Cronbach's alpha. *See* coefficient alpha
CRS. *See* Conners' Rating Scales
crystallized intelligence, 177
CSRS. *See* Child Session Rating Scale
C-SSRS. *See* Columbia-Suicide Severity Rating Scale
CTI. *See* career thoughts inventory
CTT. *See* classic test theory
cultural and contextual tailoring, in interviews, 77
cultural formulation interview (CFI), 113
cultural humility and multicultural competence, 41–43
culturally responsive assessment, recommendations for, 51–53
cultural sensitivity, 110
  of tests, 45
culture and diversity considerations, 41
  counselors as agents of change and, 51–58
  culturally responsive assessment and, 58–59
  fairness in testing and, 43–49
  high-stakes testing and, 49–50
  multicultural competence and cultural humility in assessment counseling and, 41–43
culture-relevant assessment tools, 113
curves, 135–136
cyclical model, of assessment process, 277, 278

Darwin, Charles, 20
DASS. *See* Depression Anxiety and Stress Scales
data, analyzing, 81
data distribution, 135–136
DBC. *See* Developmental Behavior Checklist
DBT. *See* dialectical behavior therapy
DBT Chain Analysis, 74
decay, 87
Delaware Social-Emotional Competency Scale (DSECS–S), 187
delayed alternate-form reliability, 155–156
Deliberate Self-Harm Inventory, 261
dependability, in qualitative assessment, 164
depression and bipolar disorder, assessment of, 228–229, 230–231
Depression Anxiety and Stress Scales (DASS), 239
descriptive statistics, 123
desktop-based tools, 299
DESSA. *See* Devereaux Student Strengths Assessment

Developmental Behavior Checklist (DBC), 237
developmental norms, 139–140
Devereaux Student Strengths Assessment (DESSA), 187
deviation IQ scores, 138
diagnosis, 7
Diagnostic and Statistical Manual of Mental Disorders (DSM)
  diagnostic assessment, 106
  history and philosophy of, 98–101
diagnostic assessment
  conducting, 103–112
  endorsement of, 116
  history of, 97–101
  individualizing care and understanding varying abilities and, 114–116
  as multifaceted, 101–103
  protective, risk factors, and warning signs in, 112–113
  theoretical perspectives of, 105
diagnostic interview, 311
dialectical behavior therapy (DBT), 104, 105
diary card, 73
Dialectical Behavior Therapy Case Conceptualization, 283
diary card tool, 73
DIF. *See* differential item functioning
differential item functioning (DIF), 46
differential test functioning (DTF), 47
digital footprints, 298
digitalization and online assessments and, 298–299
digitally delivered assessments, benefits and risks of, 303
Direct and Indirect Self-Harm Inventory, 261
direct assessments, 69–70
direct observations, 91
disaster, 248
DISC. *See* discrimination and stigma scale
discrete quantitative variables, 123
discriminant validity, 161
discrimination and stigma scale (DISC), 113
discrimination index measures, 167
distal stressors, 55
diversity and disability, in assessment, 23–24
document analysis, 88
documentation and outcome reporting, 81–82
drawing/expression techniques, 225
drift, 87
DSECS–S. *See* Delaware Social-Emotional Competency Scale
DSM. See *Diagnostic and Statistical Manual of Mental Disorders*
DSM-5-TR diagnostic assessment, 106, 228, 232, 234, 259, 267, 284
  Diagnostic and Statistical Manual Cross-Cutting Symptom Measures (DSM-XC), 106–107
  supplemental diagnostic tools and, 107–112
DTF. *See* differential test functioning

early recollections, 284, 287–288
EAT-26. *See* Eating Attitudes Test
Eating Attitudes Test (EAT-26), 233
Eating Disorder Examination (EDE-Q), 233
Eating Disorder Inventory (EDI-3), 233
eating disorders, assessment of, 232–234
Ecological Systems Theory, 283
EDE-Q. *See* Eating Disorder Examination
EDI-3. *See* Eating Disorder Inventory
ED School Climate Surveys, 189
EFA. *See* exploratory factor analysis
EHR. *See* electronic healthcare records
EIS. *See* ethnic identity scale
elderly adults. *See* older adults
electronic healthcare records (EHR), 303–304
Ellipsis Health, 300
Emotional Intelligence (EQ), 186–187
enterprising individuals, 201
Epic, 303
EQ. *See* Emotional Intelligence
equity, 46
error source, 152–153
Esquirol, Jean-Étienne Dominique, 20
ESSA. *See* Every Student Succeeds Act
ethics and law, 24–25
    assessment administration and, 29
    assessment scoring and interpretation and, 29–30
    client rights and, 26
    competence and, 26–27
    decisions and codes and, 25–26
    forensic evaluation and, 31
    informed consent and privacy and, 27–28
    instrument selection and, 28–29
    mental health disorder diagnosis and, 28
    multicultural and diversity issues in assessment and, 29
    stigmatization and client rights and, 28
    test security and integrity and, 30
ethics and privacy, in digital age
    counselors' role in ethical standards and, 302
    data privacy and security and, 301–302
    informed consent and, 302
ethnic identity scale (EIS), 113
event sampling, 89
Every Student Succeeds Act (ESSA), 49
evidence-based practices and research, 304–305
examiner's language bias, 47
experiential and expressive approaches, in interviewing, 77
experimental validity. *See* treatment validity
exploratory factor analysis (EFA), 161–162

face validity, 161
FACT. *See* Fair Access to Testing
factor analysis, 161
Fair Access to Testing (FACT), 12
fairness, in testing, 43–44
    in constructs measured, 47–48

    as deficit of instrument, measurement, and cultural bias, 46–47
    evaluation of, 45
    promotion of, 48–49
    in treatment during the process, 44–46
    in validity of interpretations, 48
Family CAGE-AID questionnaire, 269
Family Educational Rights and Privacy Act (FERPA), 32–33, 301–302
FASM. *See* Functional Assessment of Self-Mutilation
feedback and appeals, of tests, 45
FERPA. *See* Family Educational Rights and Privacy Act
fidelity, 26
Five Factor Wellness Evaluation of Lifestyle, 4
Five Factor Wellness Inventory, 22
Five Ps, 283
five-step model (Strauser and Greco), 277
fluid intelligence, 177
forensic evaluation, 31
forensic rehabilitation, 207
formal and standardized techniques, 4
formal assessments, 83, 163
formal observations, 89
Frames of Mind (Gardner), 179
frequency polygons, 132, 133
Functional Assessment of Self-Mutilation (FASM), 261

"g" factor, 175–176
GAD-7. *See* Generalized Anxiety Disorder 7
GAF. *See* Global Assessment of Functioning scale
Galton, Francis, 20, 174
Gardner, Howard, 179–180
GDPR. *See* General Data Protection Regulation
GDS. *See* Geriatric Depression Scale
gender bias, 56
Gender Dysphoria, 100
gender identity, 52, 55–56
Gender Minority Stress and Resilience Measure, 52, 56, 285
General Data Protection Regulation (GDPR), 301
Generalized Anxiety Disorder 7 (GAD-7), 231
generosity error, 87
genograms, 284, 285–287
Geriatric Depression Scale (GDS), 230
Ginger.io, 300
Global Assessment of Functioning (GAF) scale, 114
goal setting, 7
Goddard, Henry, 21, 23
grade-equivalent norms, 139–140
Graduate Record Examination (GRE), 22, 127, 130, 153, 185–186
graphic assessment methods, 92
GRE. *See* Graduate Record Examination
group assessments, 85
group intelligence testing, 21

halo effect, 87
HAM-D. *See* Hamilton Depression Rating Scale
Hamilton Depression Rating Scale (HAM-D), 231
hand scoring, 129
harm, 253–265
   nonsuicidal self-injury (NSSI), 259–262
   to others, risk of, 262–265
   suicide, 253–258
HCR-20. *See* Historical Clinical Risk Management-20
Healthie, 304
Health Insurance Portability and Accountability Act (HIPAA), 32, 280, 301
Helms Individual Differences (HID) fairness model, 44
heteronormativity, 55
hierarchical model of intelligence, 177, 178
hierarchical regression, 144
high-stakes testing, 49–50
   pros and cons of, 50
HIPAA. *See* Health Insurance Portability and Accountability Act
HIRE model, 260
histograms, 132, 133
Historical Clinical Risk Management-20 (HCR-20), 265
historical perspectives, 19–22
Holland Codes. *See* RIASEC model
House-Tree-Person, 227
humanistic therapists, 105
hybrid systems-based tools, 299

IAM. *See* Integrated Acculturation Model
IAMFC. *See* International Association of Marriage and Family Counselors
ICD. See *International Classification of Diseases*
ICF. *See International Classification of Functioning, Disability, and Health*
ICP. *See* Inventory of Common Problems
IDEA. *See* Individuals with Disabilities Education Act
indirect assessments, 70
indirect observations, 91
individual assessments, 85
Individuals with Disabilities Education Act (IDEA), 208
Indivisible Self, The: An Evidence-Based Model of Wellness (ISWEL), 22
inductive reasoning, 176
inequitable social consequences, 47
informal and nonstandardized techniques, 4
informal assessments, 83, 163
informal observations, 89
informed consent, 27, 79, 127, 302
initial intake assessment, 77–83
   clinical intake interviews and, 78–80
   diagnostic interviews and, 76–77
   initial contact and, 78
   interviewing children and, 82–83
   synthesis and, 81–82

innovation, in counseling assessment tools, 298–299, 305
instruments, 4
insufficient standardization practices, 47
Integrated Acculturation Model (IAM), 54
integrated care teams, 304
Integrative Case Conceptualization, 283–285
   early recollections and, 287–288
   genograms and, 285–287
intelligence quotient, 174
intelligence tests, 174
   cultural and ethical considerations in administration of, 182–183
   definitions and theories of, 175
   measures of, 180–183
interdisciplinary communication and continuation of care, 101–102
interest inventories, 196, 200
interindividual scoring, 130
internal consistency reliability, 156–158
International Association of Marriage and Family Counselors (IAMFC), 58
International Classification of Diseases (ICD), 99, 104
International Classification of Functioning, Disability, and Health (ICF), 283, 288–289
   components of, 289–290
   progress monitoring tools and routine outcome monitoring and, 290–291
International Society for Traumatic Stress Studies (ISTSS), 250
Interpersonal-Psychological Theory of Suicide (IPTS), 259
interquartile range, 134
interrater reliability, 158–159
inter-scorer differences. *See* content sampling error
interval recordings, 71
   common approaches to, 72
intervals, 132
interval scales, 131
interviewing strategies, 77
intraindividual scoring, 130
Inventory of Common Problems (ICP), 239
Inventory of Statements About Self-Injury (ISAS), 261
investigative individuals, 201
Iowa Assessments, 184, 185, 190
IPTS. *See* Interpersonal-Psychological Theory of Suicide
IQ. *See* intelligence tests
IRT. *See* item response theory
ISAS. *See* Inventory of Statements About Self-Injury
ISTSS. *See* International Society for Traumatic Stress Studies
ISWEL. *See* Indivisible Self, The: An Evidence-Based Model of Wellness
item analysis, 166
item bias, 46
item difficulty, 166–167

item discrimination, 166
item response theory (IRT), 167
item sampling error. *See* content sampling error
iterative process, in interviews, 77

JCTP. *See* Joint Committee on Testing Practices
Joint Committee on Testing Practices (JCTP), 12
justice, 25

Kaufman Test of Educational Achievement (KTEA-3), 183–184
Kinetic-House-Tree-Person, 227–228
KTEA-3. *See* Kaufman Test of Educational Achievement
Kuder–Richardson method, 158

language, in counseling, 51, 54–55
latent constructs, 161
law and ethics, 24–31
leadership style scale, 203
learning environment scale, 203
Level of Service Inventory-Revised (LSI-R), 265
Life Events Checklist for *DSM-5*, 250–251
Likert scales, 87, 141, 200
Limbix, 301
line of best fit, 143
local independence, 167
long-term storage and retrieval, 178
LSI-R. *See* Level of Service Inventory-Revised

machine learning, 299–300
mandated testing, 49
MAP. *See* Measures of Academic Progress Standardized Assessments
Mayer–Salovey–Caruso Emotional Intelligence Test (MSCEIT), 187
MBTI®. *See* Myers-Briggs Type Indicator®
MCI. *See* My Class Inventory
MCMI-IV. *See* Millon Clinical Multiaxial Inventory
MDQ. *See* Mood Disorder Questionnaire
mean, 133–134
measure, 4
measurement bias, 46
measurement errors, 151–152
measurement invariance, 161
Measures of Academic Progress Standardized Assessments (MAP), 183
measures of central tendency, 133–134
measures of variability, 134–136
  data distribution and curves and, 135–136
median, 134
MEIM. *See* multigroup ethnic identity measure
memory, 176
mental abilities, primary, 176
Mental Measurement Yearbook (MMY), 125
mental status exam (MSE), 79–80
  domains of, 80
Millon Clinical Multiaxial Inventory (MCMI-IV), 221

Minnesota Multiphasic Personality Inventory (MMPI), 22
Minnesota Multiphasic Personality Inventory-3 (MMPI-3), 219, 221
minority stress
  meaning and significance of, 55
  Meyer's theory of, 55, 56
MMPI. *See* Minnesota Multiphasic Personality Inventory
MMPI-3. *See* Minnesota Multiphasic Personality Inventory-3
MMY. *See* Mental Measurement Yearbook
mobile-based tools, 299
mode, 134
momentary time sampling (MTS), 72
Mood Disorder Questionnaire (MDQ), 230
MSCEIT. *See* Mayer–Salovey–Caruso Emotional Intelligence Test
MSE. *See* mental status exam
MTS. *See* momentary time sampling
multicultural competence and cultural humility, 41–43
multidisciplinary approach, in interviews, 77
multifactor theory, 176
multigroup ethnic identity measure (MEIM), 113
multiple intelligences, 179–180
multiple regression, 143
My Class Inventory (MCI), 187
Myers-Briggs Type Indicator® (MBTI®), 221, 223

narrative approach, to interviewing, 77
narrative recordings, 70–71
National Board for Certified Counselors (NBCC), 12, 79
National Center on Safe Supportive Learning Environments (NCSSLE), 189
National Counseling Examination (NCE), 127, 130
National Institute for Children's Health Quality (NICHQ) Vanderbilt Assessment Scales, 141
National Vocational Guidance Association (NVGA), 21
NBCC. *See* National Board for Certified Counselors
NCE. *See* normal curve equivalent scores
NCLB Act. *See* No Child Left Behind Act
NCSSLE. *See* National Center on Safe Supportive Learning Environments
NEO Personality Inventory (NEO-PI), 22
  Revised NEO Personality Inventory-3 (NEO-PI-3), 223
NEO-PI. *See* NEO Personality Inventory
neurodevelopmental disorders, assessment of, 235–237
neurofeedback, 88
NICHQ Vanderbilt Assessment Scales. *See* National Institute for Children's Health Quality (NICHQ) Vanderbilt Assessment Scales

No Child Left Behind (NCLB) Act, 49
nominal scales, 130–131
nonmaleficence, 25
nonstandardized assessments, 84–86
nonsuicidal self-injury (NSSI), 259
　Assessment Tool (NSSI-AT), 261
　formal assessments of, 260–261
　informal assessments of, 259–260
　initial and ongoing assessment of, 259
　integrated approaches of, 262
　inventories of, 261
nontraditional methods, 92
nonverbal assessments, 85
normal curve equivalent (NCE) scores, 138
normal distribution, 135
norm groups, 5
norming sample, 139
norm-referenced tests, 5, 130
NSSI. *See* nonsuicidal self-injury
numerical ability, 176
numerical scales, 87
NVGA. *See* National Vocational Guidance Association
NVivo, 305

objective assessments, 86
observation bias, 90
observations, 88–90
　challenges with, 90–91
　direct and indirect, 91
　in interviews, 77
observed scores, 151–152
obsessive-compulsive and related disorders, assessment of, 234–235
Obsessive-Compulsive Inventory-Revised (OCI-R), 235
Occupational Information Network (O*NET), 199
　Interest Profiler, 197, 205–206
OCI-R. *See* Obsessive-Compulsive Inventory-Revised
older and disabled adults, abuse of, 266–267
omega coefficient, 162
O*NET. *See* Occupational Information Network
ongoing evaluation, of tests, 45
online assessments, 298–299
online career assessments, 197
　strengths of, 197–198
　weaknesses of, 198
OQ Measures, 299
ordinal scales, 131
Outcomes Rating Scale, 290

PAI. *See* Personality Assessment Inventory
PAR. *See* Psychological Assessment Resources
parallel/alternate form reliability, 155–156
PARDI. *See* Pica, ARFID, and Rumination Disorder Interview
Parsons, Frank, 21, 98

partial-interval recording, 72
Patient Health Questionnaire 9 (PHQ-9), 230
Peabody Picture Vocabulary Test (PPVT), 237
Pearson's correlation, 141
peer debriefing, 164
people with disabilities (PWDs), 52, 56–57
percentage, 136
percent agreement, 158, 159
percentile scores, 136–137, 318
Perceptual Reasoning Index, 181
perceptual speed, 176
performance assessments, 128
Personality Assessment Inventory (PAI), 220
personality assessments, 196–197, 219–223
personality tests, 219
PHI. *See* protected health information
phi coefficient, 142
PHQ-9. *See* Patient Health Questionnaire 9
Pica, ARFID, and Rumination Disorder Interview (PARDI), 234
PLACHECK. *See* planned activity check
planned activity check (PLACHECK), 72
plop phenomenon, 30
population variance, 134
posttraumatic growth, 253
posttraumatic stress (PTS), 248
posttraumatic stress disorder (PTSD), 248–249
Posttraumatic Stress Disorder Symptom Scale Interview, 101
PPVT. *See* Peabody Picture Vocabulary Test
practical-mechanical spatial ability, 177
predictive bias, 47
predictive validity, 163
prescreening phase, 78
privacy, 27–28
privileged communications, 32
processing speed, 179
Processing Speed Index, 181
Proem Behavioral Health (software), 107
professional associations, 126
Professional Quality of Life Scale (ProQOL), 252–253
Professional School Counselors (PSCs), 183, 187–188
progress monitoring tools, 290
PROIE methodology, 282
projective assessments, 88
projective tests, 223
　description of, 224–225
Prolonged Grief Disorder, 100
ProQOL. *See* Professional Quality of Life Scale
protected health information (PHI), 302
proximal stressors, 55
PSCs. *See* Professional School Counselors
psychiatry and counseling, comparison of, 98
psychoanalytic theory, 223
Psychological Assessment Resources (PAR), 299
Psychology Tools and Therapist Aid, 282
psychometrics, 4

psychometric properties, 4
psychotic disorders and related disorders, assessment of, 235, 238
PsychSurveys (software), 107
PTS. *See* posttraumatic stress
PTSD. *See* posttraumatic stress disorder
publisher catalogs and manuals, 125
publisher scoring, 129
PWDs. *See* people with disabilities

Q-interactive system, 299
q-sort tests, 87
qualitative assessments, 4, 164
   bias reduction in, 164–165
qualitative variables, 124
quality assessments, developing, 165–167
Qualtrics, 305
quantitative assessments, 4
quantitative reasoning, 177
quantitative variables, 123
questionnaires, in interviews, 77

Rafferty, Janet E., 226
RAND Education Assessment Finder, 186, 188–189
random error, 151, 152
range, 134
rank-ordered variables, 141
rank-order scales, 87
rating scales, 86–87
ratio scales, 131
raw scores, understanding, 131–132
   developmental norms and, 139–140
   measures of central tendency and, 133–134
   measures of variability and, 134–136
   score comparison and, 136–137
   standard scores and, 137–139
readiness, 183
   assessments of, 184
reading and writing ability, 178
realistic individuals, 201
Reflectly, 301
reflexivity, 164–165
regression, 143–144
Rehabilitation Act, 208
rehabilitation counseling, 218
   counselor educators and supervisors, 12
relationships, measuring, 140–145
   regression and, 143–144
reliability, 149, 150–154
   classic test theory and, 151
   combination with validity, 150
   error source and, 152–153
   estimation of, 154–159
   measurement error and, 151–152
   quality assessments and, 165–167
   standard error of measurement and, 153–154
   of tests, 45
   test validity and, 159–165

reliability coefficient, 155
research role, in future assessments and adapting to needs, 304–305
resource allocation and regulatory compliance, 103
Responsibilities of Users of Standardized Tests (RUST), 12, 28, 149
RIASEC model, 201–202, 205, 211
risk assessment, 262–263
   of harm, methods for, 264–265
   initial and ongoing assessment of, 263–264
   tools, significance of, 262–263
risk management and ongoing monitoring, 102–103
risk-taking scale, 203
ROM. *See* routine outcome monitoring
Rorschach, Hermann, 225
Rorschach Inkblot Test, 225–226
Rotter, Julian B., 226
Rotter Incomplete Sentences Blank, 226–227
routine outcome evaluation, 277
routine outcome monitoring (ROM), 290, 291
RUST. *See* Responsibilities of Users of Standardized Test

SAD PERSONS scale, 255–256
SAEBRS. *See* Social, Academic, and Emotional Behavior Risk Screener
SAFE-T. *See* Suicide Assessment Five-Step Evaluation and Triage
SAMHSA. *See* Substance Abuse and Mental Health Services Administration
sample variance, 134
sampling, 4
sandtray technique, 227
SASSI-4. *See* Substance Abuse Subtle Screening Inventory-4
SAT. *See* Scholastic Aptitude Test
Saving Inventory-Revised (SIR), 235
SCARED. *See* Screen for Child Anxiety Related Disorders
scatter plots, 141
Scholastic Aptitude Test (SAT), 21–22, 127, 130, 185, 190
school climate assessments, 187
school counselor model and assessment, 187–188
SCL-90-R. *See* Symptom Checklist-90-Revised
score comparison, 136–137
scoring, of assessments, 45, 128–131
   advantages and disadvantages of, 129
   interpretation of, 130
   measurement scales for, 130–131
Screener and Opioid Assessment for Patients with Pain (SOAPP)© Version, 268
Screen for Child Anxiety Related Disorders (SCARED), 232
screening inventories, 86
SDQ. *See* Strengths and Difficulties Questionnaire

SDS. *See* self-directed search
secondary traumatic stress, 252
SEE. *See* standard error of estimate
Séguin, Édouard, 20
Seguin Form Board Test, 20
self-concept, 219
self-directed search (SDS), 211
self-esteem, 219
 assessments, 220
Self-Harm Behavior Questionnaire (SHBQ), 261
Self-Harm Inventory (SHI), 261
Self-Injurious Thoughts and Behaviors Interview (SITBI), 261
Self-Injury Questionnaire (SIQ), 261
self-monitoring, 72–73
self-referenced tests, 5
self-reporting, 218
self-scoring, 129
SEM. *See* standard error of measurement
semantic differential scales, 87
semi-structured interviews, 75
Session Rating Scale (SRS), 291
sexual/affectional orientation, 52, 55
SHBQ. *See* Self-Harm Behavior Questionnaire
SHI. *See* Self-Harm Inventory
short-term memory, 178
SII. *See* Strong Interest Inventory
Siilo, 304
Simon, Theodore, 21, 174
Simon-Binet Scale. *See* Binet-Simon Intelligence Scale
simple linear regression, 143
SimplePractice, 299, 304
simultaneous alternate-form reliability, 155
SIQ. *See* Self-Injury Questionnaire
SIR. *See* Saving Inventory-Revised
SITBI. *See* Self-Injurious Thoughts and Behaviors Interview
situational evaluation, 207–208
Sixteen Personality Factor Questionnaire, 138, 220
skewed curve, 136
SMART framework, 282
SOAPP©. *See* Screener and Opioid Assessment for Patients with Pain Version
SOARS model, 260
Social, Academic, and Emotional Behavior Risk Screener (SAEBRS), 187
social/emotional domain assessments, 186–187
 examples of, 186–187
social desirability, 153
social desirability bias, 47
social individuals, 201
Social Phobia Inventory (SPIN), 232
Society for Sexual, Affectional, Intersex, and Gender Expansive Identities, 100
spatial visualization, 176
Spearman, Charles Edward, 175
Spearman's rank correlation coefficient, 141
Spearman-Brown Formula, 157
SPIN. *See* Social Phobia Inventory
SPJ. *See* structured and professional judgment
split-half reliability method, 156–157
SPS. *See* Suicide Probability Scale
SPSS, 305
SRS. *See* Session Rating Scale
STAI-CH. *See* State-Trait Anxiety Inventory (STAI) Inventory for Children
standard deviation, 134–135
standard error of estimate (SEE), 144
standard error of measurement (SEM), 153–154
standardized assessments, 84–86
standardized testing procedures, 42
standard scores, 137–139
Standards for Educational and Psychological Testing, 3, 8, 28, 151, 160
Stanford-Binet scale, 21, 174, 180–181
Stanford-Binet test, 176
stanines, 138
State-Trait Anxiety Inventory (STAI) Inventory for Children (STAI-CH), 232
Static-99, 265
Statistical Manual for the Use of Institutions for the Insane, 97–98
statistics, significance of, 123. *See also individual entries*
sten, 138
stereotypes, of tests, 45
Stern, William, 174
stigmatization and client rights, 28
Strengths and Difficulties Questionnaire (SDQ), 187
stress, 248
Strong Interest Inventory (SII), 21, 196, 200
 basic interest scales of, 202
 general occupational themes of, 200–202
 occupational scales of, 202–203
 personal style scales, 203–204
 tips for counselors and, 204–205
structured and professional judgment (SPJ), 264–265
Structured Clinical Interview for *DSM-5*, 238
structured interviews, 74–75
student voice, in assessment, 189–190
subjective and unstructured personality assessments, 223–228
subjective assessments, 86
Subjective Units of Distress (SUD) scale, 249
subjectivity, 90, 153
Substance Abuse and Mental Health Services Administration (SAMHSA), 257, 267
Substance Abuse Subtle Screening Inventory-4 (SASSI-4), 124, 269–270
substance use disorders, 267–270
SUD. *See* Subjective Units of Distress scale
suicidal behavior, 254
suicide, 253–258
 assessment resources of, 258
 formal inventories to assess, 256–258
 initial and ongoing assessment of, 254–256

Suicide Assessment Five-Step Evaluation and Triage (SAFE-T), 256, 257–258
suicide attempt, 254
Suicide Probability Scale (SPS), 256
supplemental diagnostic tools
　adaptability in, 108
　comprehensiveness in, 107
　in enhancing therapeutic alliance, 110–111
　ethics in, 111–112
　legalities in, 111
　multidisciplinary framework in, 108
　for risk identification, 108–109
SurveyMonkey, 305
Symptom Checklist-90-Revised (SCL-90-R), 238
systematic error, 152
systems therapy, 105

TAT. *See* Thematic Apperception Test
team orientation scale, 204
technological advancements
　artificial intelligence and machine learning and, 299–300
　digitalization and online assessments and, 298–299
　platforms of plenty and, 298
　virtual reality and augmented reality and, 300–301
technological integration, in interviews, 77
Tennessee Self Concept Scale (TSCS), 220
Terman, Lewis, 21, 175
test, significance of, 4
test administration, 127–128
test reliability evidence, 149
test-retest coefficient, 155
test-retest reliability, 155, 156
test selection, 123
　steps in, 124–126
Tests in Print (TIP), 125
test standardization, 42, 44
test-taker preparation, 45
test validity. *See* validity
test validity evidence, 149
test worthiness and assessment practice, 163–165
Thematic Apperception Test (TAT), 226, 227
TheraPlatform, 299
TherapyNotes, 299
Thorndike, Edward, 21, 22
three stratum theory, 177
Thurstone, Louis Leon, 177
TigerConnect, 304
time sampling, 89, 90
time sampling error, 152
TIP. *See* Tests in Print
transferability, in qualitative assessment, 164
Transferable Skills Analysis (TSA), 211
Transgenerational Trauma and Resilience Genogram (TTRG), 286
transparency, of tests, 45
transphobia, 56

transtheoretical model (TTM), 270
trauma, 247
　assessment, and initial risk, 249–253
　events, formal assessment of, 250–251
　symptom related assessments, primary and secondary, 251–253
　understanding and assessing, 248–253
traumatic events, 248
treatment plans, 7
　and case reports, significance of, 290
　diagnostic assessment in, 102
treatment validity, 163
Trevor Project, 100
true score, 151
truthful, in client relationships, 26
TSA. *See* Transferable Skills Analysis
T-scores, 138
TSCS. *See* Tennessee Self Concept Scale
TTM. *See* transtheoretical model
TTRG. *See* Transgenerational Trauma and Resilience Genogram

unidimensionality, 167
universal design bias, 46
University of Rhode Island Change Assessment Scale (URICA), 270
unstructured interviews, 75
URICA. *See* University of Rhoda Island Change Assessment Scale
U.S. Department of Veteran Affairs, 250, 252

validity, 149, 159–165
　combination with reliability, 150
　evidence, sources of, 160–163
　of tests, 45
　test worthiness and, 163–165
values assessments, 197
Vanderbilt ADHD Rating Scales, 236
variance, 134
verbal assessments, 85
verbal comprehension, 176
Verbal Comprehension Index, 181
verbal-educational ability, 177
Vernon, Philip E., 177, 178
Veterans Administration, 200
Veterans and Military Occupations Finder (VMOF), 211
Violence Risk Appraisal Guide-Revised (VRAG-R), 265
virtual reality, 300–301
visual processing, 178
visual-spatial reasoning, 176
VMOF. *See* Veterans and Military Occupations Finder
vocational evaluation, 206–207
vocational interests, 199
vocational rehabilitation, 206
VRAG-R. *See* Violence Risk Appraisal Guide-Revised
vulnerable adults, 266

WAIS. *See* Wechsler Adult Intelligence Scale
WAI-SR. *See* Working Alliance Inventory
web-based tools, 299
Wechsler, David, 21, 174, 181
Wechsler Adult Intelligence Scale (WAIS), 21, 130, 174, 181–182, 190
Wechsler Intelligence Scale for Children (WISC-V), 181
weight bias, 57
Western Psychological Services (WPS), 256
WHO-5 Well-Being Index, 238
WHODAS. *See* World Health Organization Disability Assessment Schedule 2.0
whole interval recording, 72
WIDA consortium, 184
WIOA. *See* Workforce Innovation and Opportunity Act
WISC-V. *See* Wechsler Intelligence Scale for Children
Woebot, 300
Woodcock–Johnson Tests of Achievement, 183
Woodcock–Johnson Tests of Cognitive Abilities, 182
Woodworth Personal Data Sheet, 22
Woodworth Psychoneurotic Inventory, 22

word fluency, 176
Workforce Innovation and Opportunity Act (WIOA), 208
Working Alliance Inventory (WAI-SR), 291
working memory, 176
Working Memory Index, 181
work style scale, 203
Work Values Inventory (WVI), 197
World Health Organization Disability Assessment Schedule (WHODAS) 2.0, 114–115
  applications of, 115
  for children (WHODAS-Child), 115
  psychometrics in, 116
WPS. *See* Western Psychological Services
Wundt, Wilhelm, 20
WVI. *See* Work Values Inventory

Yale-Brown Obsessive Compulsive Scale (Y-BOCS), 235
Y-BOCS. *See* Yale-Brown Obsessive Compulsive Scale
YMRS. *See* Young Mania Rating Scale
Young Mania Rating Scale (YMRS), 231

Z-scores, 138, 318